THE MIND IN CONTEXT

The Mind in Context

Edited by

BATJA MESQUITA
LISA FELDMAN BARRETT
ELIOT R. SMITH

THE GUILFORD PRESS
New York London

A Division of Guilford Publications, Inc.
72 Spring Street, New York, NY 10012
www.guilford.com

Printed in the United States of America

This book is printed on acid-free paper.

Last digit is print number: 9 8 7 6 5 4 3 2 1

Library of Congress Cataloging-in-Publication Data

The mind in context / edited by Batja Mesquita, Lisa Feldman Barrett, Eliot R. Smith.
p. cm.
Includes bibliographic references and index.
ISBN 978-1-60623-553-9 (hbk.)
1. Context effects (Psychology) I. Mesquita, Batja. II. Barrett, Lisa Feldman. III. Smith, Eliot R.
BF315.2.M56 2010
153.7—dc22

2009039737

About the Editors

Batja Mesquita, PhD, is Professor of the Psychology of Emotion and Motivation at the Center for Cultural and Social Psychology at the University of Leuven in Belgium. Most of her research focuses on the constitutional role of cultural contexts in emotion. Dr. Mesquita has published widely on topics related to cultural differences in emotions and on acculturation and emotion. She has served as Associate Editor of *Cognition and Emotion* and *Emotion Review* and is currently on the editorial boards of *Emotion, Personality and Social Psychology Bulletin*, and *Social and Personality Psychology Compass.* Dr. Mesquita is a Fellow of the Royal Netherlands Academy of Arts and Sciences, the Association for Psychological Science, the Society for Personality and Social Psychology, the American Psychological Association, and the Society of Experimental Social Psychology.

Lisa Feldman Barrett, PhD, is Professor of Psychology and Director of the Interdisciplinary Affective Science Laboratory at Boston College, with appointments at Harvard Medical School and Massachusetts General Hospital. Her research focuses on the nature of emotion from social-psychological, psychophysiological, cognitive science, and neuroscience perspectives, and takes inspiration from anthropology, philosophy, and linguistics. Dr. Barrett is the recipient of numerous awards, most recently a National Institutes of Health's Pioneer Award and a National Institute of Mental Health's Independent Scientist Research Award. She is Co-Editor-in-Chief of *Emotion Review* and sits on the editorial boards of other top-tier journals in the field. Dr. Barrett has published over 100 papers and chapters and is coeditor (with Peter Salovey) of *The Wisdom in Feeling: Psychological Processes in Emotional Intelligence* and (with Paula Niedenthal and Piotr Winkielman) *Emotion and Consciousness.*

She is a Fellow of the American Association for the Advancement of Science, the Association for Psychological Science, the American Psychological Association, the Society of Experimental Social Psychology, and the Society for Personality and Social Psychology.

Eliot R. Smith, PhD, is Classes of the War Years Chancellor's Professor of Psychological and Brain Sciences at Indiana University. His research interests include the role of emotion in prejudice and intergroup behavior, as well as socially situated cognition. Dr. Smith's research has been recognized by the 2004 Thomas M. Ostrom Award for lifetime contributions to social cognition from Indiana University, as well as the 2005 Theoretical Innovation Prize from the Society for Personality and Social Psychology. He has served as Editor of *Personality and Social Psychology Review* and as Associate Editor of the *Journal of Personality and Social Psychology: Attitudes and Social Cognition*. Dr. Smith is coeditor (with Gün R. Semin) of *Embodied Grounding* and (with Diane M. Mackie) of *From Prejudice to Intergroup Emotions*. He is a Fellow of the Association for Psychological Science, the Society for Personality and Social Psychology, the American Psychological Association, and the Society of Experimental Social Psychology.

Contributors

Glenn Adams, PhD, Department of Psychology, University of Kansas, Lawrence, Kansas

Mahzarin R. Banaji, PhD, Department of Psychology, Harvard University, Cambridge, Massachusetts

Lisa Feldman Barrett, PhD, Department of Psychology, Boston College, Boston, Massachusetts

Lawrence W. Barsalou, PhD, Department of Psychology, Emory University, Atlanta, Georgia

Mark E. Bouton, PhD, Department of Psychology, University of Vermont, Burlington, Vermont

Elizabeth C. Collins, PhD, Center for Social Research and Intervention, Higher Institute of Labor Science and Enterprise, Lisbon University Institute, Lisbon, Portugal

Yarrow Dunham, EdD, Department of Human and Community Development, University of California Merced, Merced, California

Lawrence V. Harper, PhD, Department of Human and Community Development, University of California Davis, Davis, California

Wendy Hasenkamp, PhD, Department of Mental Health, Atlanta Veterans Affairs Medical Center, Atlanta, Georgia

Toshie Imada, PhD, Institute of Child Development, University of Minnesota, Twin Cities, Minneapolis, Minnesota

Tuğçe Kurtiş, MA, Department of Psychology, University of Kansas, Lawrence, Kansas

Shinobu Kitayama, PhD, Department of Psychology, University of Michigan, Ann Arbor, Michigan

Janetta Lun, PhD, Department of Psychology, University of Virginia, Charlottesville, Virginia

Kerry L. Marsh, PhD, Department of Psychology, University of Connecticut, Storrs, Connecticut

Batja Mesquita, PhD, Department of Psychology, University of Leuven, Leuven, Belgium

Walter Mischel, PhD, Department of Psychology, Columbia University, New York, New York

Nia L. Phillips, MA, Department of Psychology, University of Kansas, Lawrence, Kansas

Kate M. Pickett, MA, Department of Psychology, University of Kansas, Lawrence, Kansas

Deborah A. Prentice, PhD, Department of Psychology, Princeton University, Princeton, New Jersey

Michael J. Richardson, PhD, Department of Psychology, University of Cincinnati, Cincinnati, Ohio, and Department of Psychology, Colby College, Waterville, Maine

Phia S. Salter, MA, Department of Psychology, University of Kansas, Lawrence, Kansas

R. C. Schmidt, PhD, Department of Psychology, College of the Holy Cross, Worcester, Massachusetts

Norbert Schwarz, DrPhil, Institute for Social Research, University of Michigan, Ann Arbor, Michigan

Yuichi Shoda, PhD, Department of Psychology, University of Washington, Seattle, Washington

Stacey Sinclair, PhD, Department of Psychology, Princeton University, Princeton, New Jersey

Eliot R. Smith, PhD, Department of Psychology, Indiana University, Bloomington, Indiana

Olaf Sporns, PhD, Department of Psychological and Brain Sciences, Indiana University, Bloomington, Indiana

Thomas E. Trail, MA, Department of Psychology, Princeton University, Princeton, New Jersey

Sari M. van Anders, PhD, Program in Neuroscience and Departments of Psychology and Women's Studies, University of Michigan, Ann Arbor, Michigan

Christine D. Wilson, MA, Department of Psychology, Emory University, Atlanta, Georgia

Contents

III. THE PERSON

IV. BEHAVIOR

1

The Context Principle

LISA FELDMAN BARRETT
BATJA MESQUITA
ELIOT R. SMITH

Scientific disciplines categorize. They divide their universe of interest into groupings or "kinds," name them, then set about the business of understanding those kinds in a scientifically valid way. This categorization process functions like a sculptor's chisel, dividing up the world into figure and ground, leading scientists to attend to certain features and to ignore others. One consequence of scientific categorization is that we sometimes essentialize our subject matter, then search for evidence of those essences, without considering how context might influence or contribute to its very nature. William James observed this a century ago, when he wrote, "Whenever we have made a word ... to denote a certain group of phenomena, we are prone to suppose a substantive entity existing beyond the phenomena, of which the word shall be the name" (1890, p. 195). James knew that words do not just name a category. They encourage a very basic form of essentialism that, Paul Bloom (2004) argues, is already present in how people often think about the events and objects in their everyday lives. A word can function like an "essence placeholder," encouraging psychological essentialism: A word can convince the perceiver that there is some deep reality to the category in the material world (Barsalou, Wilson, & Hasenkamp, Chapter 16, this volume; Medin & Ortony, 1989), even in young infants (e.g., Dewar & Xu, 2009; Xu, Cote, & Baker, 2005). The main consequence of essentializing is that people ignore the influence of context.

THE ESSENTIALISM ERROR: AN EXAMPLE FROM MOLECULAR GENETICS

A particularly salient example of this essentialism error comes from the study of genetics (also see Harper, Chapter 2, this volume). When molecular biologists first began to study the units of inheritance, inspired by Mendel, they searched for and found *genes*—bits of deoxyribonucleic acid (DNA) that make the proteins needed to constitute the human body. Yet only a small proportion of human DNA (estimated between 2 and 5%) was *genes*; the rest of the stuff (that does not directly produce proteins) was labeled "junk," on the assumption that it was largely irrelevant to the biological understanding of life. As it turns out, however, "junk DNA" has some rather important functions, including regulation of *gene expression* (i.e., turning on and off protein production) in a contextually sensitive fashion (for a generally accessible review, see Gibbs, 2003). Scientists have discovered that much of what makes us human, and what makes one person different from another, lurks in this junk. In fact, even with the completely sequenced human genome, it is not possible simply to produce a human being from scratch because a human is not computed from genes alone. It is not really possible to answer a question like "Which genotype causes depression?" without specifying the environments in which a person developed and in which depression occurred.

Even when scientists do consider the environment, the concept of a "gene" can mistakenly lead to the assumption that there is only a single environment in question. To some extent, this misses the important transactional process by which an organism determines which elements of the external world make up the functional environment at any one point in time. As a consequence, there are a variety of potential environments in any physical surrounding, with a creature's current state making certain environments more likely or impactful than other potential environments at the same moment in time. These observations mean that even a static model of *gene–environment interaction* (where the genes determine an organism's capacity or tendency that is released by the environment) is still too essentialist (for a discussion, see Lewontin, 2000).

These sorts of observations have produced nothing short of a revolution in molecular genetics. Scientists now know that genes, in and of themselves, do not provide a sufficient recipe for life. The unit of selection is not the gene, but the individual, who, for the purposes of molecular genetics, can be thought of as a bundle of genes that are turned on and off by the rest of our DNA, which is regulated by the epigenetic context. The building blocks of evolution are a set of context-dependent processes, not a set of unitized elements.

THE ESSENTIALISM ERROR IN PSYCHOLOGY

The essentialism error—with its disregard of context—is particularly notable in the Western psychological tradition. Western models of the mind chunk and name phenomena with nouns (which encourage essentialism) as opposed to words that refer to processes (e.g., verbs; see Barsalou et al., Chapter 16, this volume). The process of categorizing and naming in much of psychology seems to have produced a deep commitment to the view that behaviors and mental states, and even people themselves, are determined by deep and unchanging internal forces. The goal (at least in Western psychology) is often to identify mental states, behaviors, and traits as natural entities that "cut nature at its joints," often without considering the influence from the environment. Even behaviorists like John Watson were psychological essentialists. John Watson observed and wrote about tremendous variability in emotional behaviors with the same name (e.g., *fear*), yet he assumed that a Platonic behavioral pattern must exist for each emotion even though he could not see it—very ironic for a behaviorist.

Of course, psychologists cannot dispense with naming categories, and categories call for names. But a name does not necessarily point to an essence.

In psychology, there is a great risk of confusing words with the phenomena that are of real interest. The questions that psychologists ask and the interpretations we offer often reinforce our natural (Western) tendencies toward psychological essentialism and away from the importance of context. Take, for instance, research on what is referred to as *fear learning*. In much of this research, rats are placed in a 9" × 12" spare box with grating on the floor. An auditory tone is paired with electric shock (delivered through the floor), so that when the animal hears the tone alone, it freezes (i.e., does not move except for respiration; e.g., LeDoux, Cicchetti, Zagoraris, & Romanski, 1990). The amygdala is necessary to produce this freezing response, leading many scientists to argue that the amygdala is the brain locus of fear. But, as it turns out, rats do not always freeze when faced with a threat. When the context gives them the opportunity (e.g., in a multiarmed testing chamber), rats escape from threat (e.g., Vazdarjanova & McGaugh, 1998). At other times, rats kick up their bedding in the direction of the threat (called *defensive treading*; Reynolds & Berridge, 2002, 2003, 2008). Physiology follows the behavior, not the category of emotion. When rats are restrained during threat, their blood pressure goes up; when they are free to escape, their blood pressure goes down (Iwata & LeDoux, 1988). In using the word *fear* to refer to behaviors as varied as freezing, escape, and defensive treading, not to mention feelings of worry, dread, and viewing startled looking faces, scientists are lulled into thinking these behaviors all share a deep property, and they will spend years searching for it in vain.

This example often prompts researchers to ask what the amygdala's function is, if not to create fear. An answer can be found in other research findings. The uncertainty of shock predicts sympathetic nervous system responses (organized by the central nucleus of the amygdala) better than does the intensity of shock during classical conditioning (Arntz, Van Eck, & de Jong, 1992). The amygdala is reliably responsive to novel objects (e.g., Breiter et al., 1996; Schwartz, Wright, Shin, Kagan, & Rauch, 2003; Weierich, Wright, Negreira, Dickerson, & Barrett, in press; Wilson & Rolls, 1993; Wright, Wedig, Williams, Rauch, & Albert, 2006) and novel (neutral) faces across the lifespan (Wright at al., 2008). Amygdala activity is associated with orienting responses (e.g., Holland & Gallagher, 1999), and amygdala lesions disrupt normal responses to novelty in primates (e.g., Burns, Annett, Kelley, Everitt, & Robbins, 1996; Mason, Capitiano, Machado, Mendoza, & Amaral, 2006; Prather et al., 2001). When uncertainty increases, so too does the amygdala's response (Herry et al., 2007), yet the amygdala habituates quickly to fearful faces (Wright et al., 2003). The findings together suggest that the amygdala functions to help direct attention (Holland & Gallagher, 1999) toward sensory stimulation when the predictive value of that stimulation for well-being and survival is unknown or uncertain, or when the appropriate response to a stimulus is unclear. Some people might argue that uncertainty is an ingredient of fear, and this might be so, but it is surely not specific to or interchangeable with the category "fear." But more importantly, uncertainty is inherently a context-dependent phenomenon.

The pervasiveness of essentialism has shaped Western psychology to its very core. Models of the mind have become fragmented as psychologists have come to assume that emotion, memory, the self, attitudes, personality traits, and so on, are different entities with distinct organizing principles and causes (Bruner, 1990). Furthermore, relationships between these entities are referred to as *interactions*. Cognition and emotion, for example, are said to influence one another, as if they are independent and separable mental phenomena.

Psychological essentialism has also led researchers to ignore variation and to treat it as psychological noise. In many cases, variation in psychological states or behaviors referred to by the same name is considered to be error (i.e., the measured variance that is not of interest). Moreover, studies are designed to control the context either experimentally or statistically minimize variability. By focusing on a mental state or behavior in isolation, it is easy to miss its embeddedness in a larger system that gives it its nature. It is easy to miss the forest for the trees.

FROM ESSENTIALISM TO CONTEXT

Amid this essentialism has lurked the idea that psychological states, traits, and behaviors are not entities but events constructed out of a more basic set of processes (Gendron & Barrett, 2009). And processes, unlike entities, are shaped by context. Mental events and human behaviors can be thought of as states that emerge from moment-by-moment interaction with the environment rather than proceeding in autonomous, invariant, context-free fashion from preformed dispositions or causes. Inherently, a mind exists in context. We call this the *context principle.*

Context, of course, can refer to many things. One process within the brain or body can serve as a context for another process (e.g., Sporns, Chapter 3, this volume). One psychological process can serve as the context for another psychological process or its product (e.g., Dunham & Banaji, Chapter 10; Schwarz, Chapter 6, this volume). The immediate physical surroundings or the social context (i.e., other people) can serve as the context (e.g., Bouton, Chapter 12; Dunham & Banaji, Chapter 10; Harper, Chapter 2; Mesquita, Chapter 5; Mischel & Shoda, Chapter 8; Prentice & Trail, Chapter 13; Richardson, Marsh, & Schmidt, Chapter 15; Sinclair & Lun, Chapter 11; Smith & Collins, Chapter 7; van Anders, Chapter 4, this volume). Phase of life or sociocultural environment can serve as a context (e.g., Adams, Salter, Pickett, Kurtiş, & Phillips, Chapter 14; Kitayama & Imada, Chapter 9, this volume). Even time can serve as a context (e.g., Bouton, Chapter 12, this volume). The basic idea is that the observables of psychology—thoughts, feelings, actions—are not driven by single causes but are the emergent results of multiple transactive processes.

History of the Context Principle in Psychology or "the Mind in Context"

The context principle has a long history in psychology. It can be observed in Wundt's attempt to understand psychological events as psychic compounds that are embedded and influenced by the social surroundings (Wundt, 1894/1998). Wundt advocated an early form of *emergentism*, where thoughts, emotions, actions, and so forth, are not static things or entities but are instead "psychical compounds" or composites that constitute "psychical elements" (that are simple and irreducible in a psychological sense) (Gendron & Barrett, 2009). He wrote about psychological phenomena as acts or processes rather than as static entities or objects with constant properties (see also Mesquita, Chapter 5, this volume). Furthermore, Wundt explicitly wrote about the social and cultural context as a necessary contribution to each individual person's mental life (what Wundt called *Volkerpsychologie*, which means social or cultural psychology but was mistranslated by Edward Titchener as "folk psychology"; for a discussion, see Danziger, 1983). According to psychological historian Kurt Danziger's description of Wundt's *Volkerpsychologie*,

> Psychological laws were not abstract principles, conceived on the model of classic mechanisms, that could be applied analogously on the individual and on the social level. Rather, they were developmental principles that expressed the kinds of changes that mental contents underwent in interaction with a medium (Wundt, 1886b). That medium was environmental and social as well as physiological. (Danziger, 1983, p. 307)[1]

The context principle can also be found in John Dewey's (1896) discussion of the reflex arc. Dewey denied that sensations were the stimuli, that responses were the effects, and that both were separable bits and pieces, like parts of a machine. Rather, both were like ingredients in a recipe, coordinated over a series of iterations to produce some mental event serving some kind of function. In Dewey's view, a response provides the context for the next round of sensation, and the "stimulus" itself emerges out of this coordination (see also Richarson et al., Chapter 15, this volume). This idea of context ran counter to that of the standard stimulus–cognition—response logic offered contemporaneously by Baldwin (1891) and rediscovered during the cognitive revolution in psychology. Ignoring the arc, in Dewey's words, erroneously leads psychologists to search for the explanation of behavior "in either an external pressure of 'environment,' or else in an unaccountable spontaneous variation from within the 'soul' or the 'organism' " (1896, p. 360). It leads psychologists toward a false kind of dualism that mistakenly essentializes either the stimulus or the person.

The context principle is most clearly embodied in the basic assumptions of social psychology, which developed in the early part of the 20th century as the scientific discipline devoted to the study of situational influences on the mind and behavior. The context principle is clearly embodied in Kurt Lewin's (1935) heuristic equation $B = f(P, E)$, where a behavior at a given point in time is a function of the person and his or her momentary context. Although earlier formulations of Lewin's equation took a more essentialist stance on context, examining the *influence* of the situation on mental events and behaviors, Lewin's later views were more nuanced, treating the person and the situation as transactional factors that realize behavior. From this perspective, mental events and behaviors are performances of context (Markus, 2008; Steele, 1997). Persons and situations are not separable sources of variation that interact and influence each other. They help to constitute each other. Similar considerations led Walter Mischel to study personality as a set of context-contingent regularities, highlighting that behavior is not the expression of some sort of essential "trait," but rather materializes in a transactional, context-specific manner (Mischel, 1968; Mischel & Shoda, Chapter 8, this volume).

In the mid-20th century, Egon Brunswik (1955a, 1955b) emphasized that the science of psychology should pay as much attention to the properties of the environment as it does to the organism itself. He emphasized the idea of *object sampling*, meaning that in experiments, various aspects of psychological environment should be explicitly sampled from the larger physical environment, just as subjects are sampled from a larger population of individuals. In Brunswik's view, elements of the environment were not essentialized but were themselves contextually determined. Like Dewey's discussion of the reflex arc, Brunswik's lens model specified a transactional (or what we might now call *recursive*) relation between the organism and its immediate environment, so that the outcome of one psychological state (be it a perception or a behavior) is the prior condition that set the stage for the next. Like Dewey, Brunswik criticized the artificiality inherent in the classic stimulus–organism–response (S-O-R) experiment. Person and context mutually constitute each other rather than interacting in a strict, independent fashion. Beginning in the mid-1960s, this view was developed considerably by Mischel, who demonstrated (as noted above) that even a personality cannot be understood without reference to the context (see Mischel & Shoda, 1995, and Chapter 8, this volume).

During the cognitive revolution, Jerome Bruner (1988, 1990) proposed that the study of cognition should focus on a contextualized understanding of the human mind. Bruner argued that psychology's task was to "discover and to describe formally the meanings that human beings created our of their encounters with the world, and then to propose hypotheses about what meaning-making processes were implicated" (1990, p. 2). Bruner's main argument was that human psychology is about meaning, which by definition "itself is a culturally mediated phenomenon that depends upon the prior existence of a shared symbol system" (p. 69). Thus, according to Bruner, context shapes the human mind. "It does so by imposing the patterns inherent in the culture's symbolic systems—its language and discourse modes, the forms of logical and narrative explication, and the patterns of mutually dependent communal life" (p. 4). Bruner's ideas form the foundation of cultural psychology, whose basic thesis is that many, though not all, of our mental models are cultural and shared in nature (Markus & Kitayama, 2003; Nisbett, 2003; Shore, 1996; Shweder, 1991b). This is not to say that culture determines thought in a homogenized fashion. Rather, the artifacts of culture—the ways that relationships are organized and structured—afford certain ways of thinking and feeling (Markus, Mullally, & Kitayama, 1997).

Implications of the Context Principle

The context principle helps scientists understand that the very definition of something as basic to psychology as "behavior" is contextually determined. Social psychologists who study person perception distinguish between *behaviors* (intentional, bounded events) and *actions* (descriptions of physical movements) (e.g., Vallacher & Wegner, 1987).[2] These meaning-filled events are neither observer-independent nor context-independent. Social psychology has accumulated a large and nuanced body of research on how people come to see the physical movements of others as meaningful "behaviors" by inferring the causes for those movements (usually by imputing an intention to the actor; for a review, see Gilbert, 1998). People and animals are constantly moving and doing things—that is, they are constantly engaging in a flow of "movements." A perceiver automatically and effortlessly partitions continuous movements into recognizable, meaningful, discrete acts using category knowledge about people and animals (Vallacher & Wegner, 1987). As we discussed earlier, a rat that kicks up bedding at a threatening creature is said to be defensive treading or in a state of fear. Similarly, standing still in response to a sudden tone that predicts an electric shock can be called freezing or fear. It can also be called an alert, behavioral stance that allows an organism to martial all its attentional and sensory resources to quickly learn more about a stimulus when its predictive value is uncertain (cf. Barrett, Lindquist, Bliss-Moreau, et al., 2007).

Moreover, cultural settings have a role in translating an action into a behavior. The "mutually interacting intentional states of the participants" constitute the meaning of behavior (Bruner, 1990, p. 19). These intentional states have been shown to vary across contexts of meaning. For instance, in highly interdependent cultures and relationships, withdrawal from the relationship may be recognized as an expression of anger; this is less so in environments in which active engagement is less the norm (Mesquita, 1993). In Japanese kindergartens, teachers do not interfere in fights among the children because they believe that this behavior is conducive to the development of sympathy and perspective taking. In contrast, American teachers interpret this lack of intervention as neglectful. Similarly, in a North American context, voluntary actions are interpreted as "choices" originating from individual preferences and goals, but in an Indian context, they are understood as responses to social roles and the expectations of others (Savani, Markus, Naidu, & Kumar, 2009). These examples demonstrate that similar actions derive their meaning from the specific cultural framework in which they are produced and understood.

Even the "situation" is not elemental and is itself contextual, in part being determined by the person (who acts as a form of context). Physical surroundings exist separately from observers, but "situations" do not. A creature's ecological niche includes only those aspects of the physical surroundings that are relevant to its actions and activities. The same can be said about "situations." To borrow an example of the ecological niche from the evolutionary biologist Richard Lewontin (2000), two species of bird (phoebes and thrushes) live in exactly the same territory within the northeastern United States that includes both grasses and rocks, but whereas a phoebe's niche includes grass to build nests, a thrush requires rocks to crack open seeds. Rocks are physically present for a phoebe but go unnoticed; the same is true for grass and thrushes. For humans, the psychological situation includes only those aspects of the physical surroundings (or the nominal situation; Shoda, Mischel, & Wright, 1994) that are relevant to the goals of the perceiver, so that within the exact same physical surrounding there exist different "situations" for different people (or for a single individual at different points in time). This is the basic idea embodied in appraisal models of emotion. It is also consistent with the idea that the mind determines the "active ingredients," or psychological features, of the situation (Shoda et al., 1994; Wright & Mischel, 1988). There are features of the immediate physical surroundings that have significant meaning for some individuals (but not others) and that define their psychological niche. From this standpoint, a situation is not a description of the physical properties of the environment, but it can be characterized as containing just those aspects that are relevant to the thoughts, feelings, and behaviors of that particular person at that particular point in time. In effect, the mind determines the nature of the situation, so that a "situation" does not exist separately from the person. A personality might be thought of as the mind creating a psychological niche with some consistency (for a similar view, see Mischel, 2004).

Similarly, cultural environments exist by virtue of the people who constitute them. These individual perceptions create central cultural goals, or *models*. For example, not only are self-esteem-enhancing instances more readily recognized in American than in Japanese contexts, but they are also created more often. People praise each other more in American than in Japanese contexts, and all kinds of awards and trophies are created in American contexts (D'Andrade, 1984; Mesquita & Markus, 2004). On the other hand, self-criticism is ritualized and instantiated in Japanese contexts, where schoolchildren reflect on their mistakes of the day, and where criticisms are a prevalent part of daily conversations (Heine, Lehman, Markus, & Kitayama, 1999; Lewis, 1995). Similarly, in cultural contexts emphasizing harmony, relationships and interactions are often scripted according to detailed rules of politeness and social roles (Briggs, 1970; Cohen, 1999). These situations are extensions of the culturally shaped mind, and in turn shape it. No clear boundaries indicate where the mind stops and the cultural ecology of situations starts. Mind and culture mutually constitute each other (Shweder, 1991a).

Recent Developments of the Context Principle

The context principle is key to a powerful new intellectual movement that has emerged across many areas of psychology and cognitive science, termed *situated cognition* (Smith & Semin, 2004). This perspective critiques the older idea that behavior is explained by abstract inner information processing or computation, replacing it with a focus on the detailed, moment-by-moment interaction between an organism and its environment as the locus of explanation. For example, instead of postulating that humans and other animals construct detailed inner representations of the world around them to which they refer in making judgments or planning behavior, the situated cognition perspective holds that organisms rely on immediate perception of their surroundings to guide thought and action. Some situated cognition theorists have gone so far as to deny any role to inner representations (at least as conventionally conceptualized) in behavior. Like any broad intellectual movement, the situated cognition approach has had some clear victories but also faces intellectual challenges (see Smith & Collins, Chapter 7, this volume). The approach is one important reflection of the new emphasis on the role of context—the situation, the immediate environment—in the generation of behavior.

The context principle is also easy to identify in Larry Barsalou's highly contextualized view of the conceptual system (for reviews, see Barsalou, 2008, 2009; Barsalou et al., Chapter 16, this volume). Rather than viewing concepts as fixed, highly abstract entities, Barsalou's view is that conceptual knowledge is strongly situated (involving scenes, events, objects, actions, and mental states that go along with category exemplars). For example, people do not have one concept for the category named *anger*. They have a collection of concepts that can be associatively recombined in any number of diverse and flexible ways. For example, you have a concept of anger when another driver cuts you off in traffic, and you yell and wave your fist; when a disobedient child breaks a rule and you calmly reexplain; when you hear the voice of a disliked politician and you turn off the radio; when a colleague insults you, and you sit very still and perhaps even smile; when you tease a friend instead of criticize; when you stub your toe and kick the kitchen table; and so on. Consistent with the view of situated cognition, the conceptual knowledge that is called forth in a given instance is tailored to the immediate situation, is acquired from prior experience, and may be supported by language.

Other Examples of the Mind in Context

In addition to the chapters in this volume, there are many empirical examples of the context principle at every level of scientific inquiry in psychology. For example, evidence has existed since the 1920s that emotion perception is influenced by contextual factors (for a review of these early papers, see Hunt, 1941). Knowledge of the social situation (Carroll & Russell, 1996; Sherman, 1927; Trope, 1986; Trope & Cohen, 1989), body postures (Aviezer et al., 2008; Meeren, van Heijnsbergen, & de Gelder, 2005), voices (de Gelder, Böcker, Tuomainen, Hensen, & Vroomen, 1999; de Gelder & Vroomen, 2000), scenes (Righart & de Gelder, 2008), or other emotional faces (Masuda et al., 2008; Russell & Fehr, 1987) all influence which emotion is seen in the structural configuration of another person's facial muscles (for a review, see de Gelder et al., 2006). Consider the fact, for example, that 60–75% of the time, people see facial depictions of fear as "angry" when they are paired with contextual information typically associated with anger (Carroll & Russell, 1996; for more examples, see Fernandez-Dohls, Carrera, Barchard, & Gacitua, 2008). Recent evidence indicates that perceivers routinely encode the context during emotion perception (Barrett & Kensinger, in press). People remembered the context better when asked to perceive emotion (either fear or disgust) in the face than when asked to make an affective judgment (either to approach or to avoid) about the face. The need to categorize the facial expression as an emotion required that perceivers use all information available to them—both the information contained within the structural configuration of facial muscles and that in the broader context.

Furthermore, emotion words provide a context for perceiving emotion in another person (for a review, see Barrett, Lindquist, & Gendron, 2007). When the influence of words is minimized, both children (Russell & Widen, 2002) and adults (Lindquist, Barrett, Bliss-Moreau, & Russell, 2006) have difficulty with the seemingly trivial task of using structural similarities in facial expressions alone to judge whether or not they match in emotional content (we say trivial because the face sets used have statistical regularities built in). It is striking that 58% of the time, people have difficulty saying that two expressions of anger depict the same emotion, if they are neither provided any emotion words nor asked to generate them during the task (Lindquist et al., 2006). More recently, it has been shown that perceivers can detect small changes in the structural information that is available to distinguish one facial configuration from another, but they do not know which are psychologically meaningful in the absence of emotion words. When viewing morphs of chimpanzee expressions (structurally analogous to human emotion expressions), both experts and novices can detect perceptual distinctions all the way along the continuum, but without the influence of words, they do not prioritize specific distinctions as psychologically meaningful (Fugate, Gouzoules, & Barrett, 2009).

Emotion perception is not the only psychological process that is contextualized. The context principle is easily observed in other aspects of vision. Internal states influence visual perception. For example, when shown an ambiguous figure (e.g., a bistable image that could be seen either as a B or the number 13, or a horse-seal figure), people see whichever image is more pleasant for them (Balcetis & Dunning, 2006). A person's momentary affective state can also serve as a context to influence perception (for a review, see Barrett & Bar, 2009). Neutral faces are prioritized in consciousness when they invoke an affective state by being previously paired with negative gossip (Anderson, Bliss-Moreau, & Barrett, 2009). When a person is in a negative mood or in pain, hills appear to be steeper and distances seem longer than they really are (Stefanucci, Proffitt, Clore, & Parekh, 2008; Witt et al., 2008). Even physical exertion can make a hill seem steeper (Bhalla & Proffitt, 1999) or a distance seem longer (Proffitt, Stefanucci, Banton, & Epstein, 2003). When a person is standing on a high balcony, the perceived distance to the ground is correlated with a fear of falling (Teachman, Stefanucci, Clerkin, Cody, & Proffitt, 2008). Momentary behaviors also influence visual perception. For example, people using a tool to reach targets that are just beyond arm's reach see target objects as closer than when they intend to reach without the tool (Witt, Proffitt, & Epstein, 2005).

Currently active goals influence not only how people interpret a sensory array but also how they interpret and sample the sensory world in the first place (even when there is no overt shift of attention). For example, when viewing a hybrid face consisting of both high-frequency spatial information (depicting a happy woman) and low-frequency information (depicting a neutral-faced man), people sampled information differently depending on which sort of categorization task they were asked to perform. People asked to categorize the face as happy versus angry sampled high-frequency information and saw a happy woman. People asked to categorize the face as expressive versus unexpressive sampled low-frequency information and saw an expressionless man (Schyns & Oliva, 1999). Goal-based sensory sampling can be observed even at the level of neurons in primary visual cortex (or V1). Perceivers who are asked to focus on and remember the color or orientation of a stimulus show different feature-specific activation patterns in V1, indicating that goal-based sensory sampling occurs at very early stages of visual processing (Serences, Ester, Vogel, & Awh, 2009; for another example of how goals influence feedforward color processing, see Zhang & Luck, 2009). In fact, within about 100 ms after stimulus onset, subcortical brain structures receive highly processed sensory input from the cortex; as a result, even the brainstem, midbrain, and thalamus cannot be considered solely bottom-up structures that respond merely to sensory information from the world (for a review on the implications for vision, see Barrett & Bar, 2009).

The physical environment also influences normal object perception (for a review, see Bar, 2004; Oliva & Torralba, 2007). For example, embedding blurred images of objects (e.g., an image of a toaster or a computer) in a congruent context (e.g., in a kitchen or an office, respectively) helps perceivers to see an object more easily than when they are placed in an incongruent context (e.g., a toaster in an office). Objects placed in an incongruent context are misrecognized as something that belongs to the context (Palmer, 1975). These effects occur not only because visual information in the context constrains what we expect to see and where we look (Chun, 2000) but also because the brain makes a prediction about what visual sensations refer to or stand for in the world based on past experience and future behavior (Bar, 2007).

Even neurons are subject to the context principle (see Sporns, Chapter 3, this volume). The information signaled by a neuron depends on the features of the external context. For example, a recent study with rats demonstrates a functional remapping of cells in the nucleus accumbens (part of the ventral striatum)—sometimes they code for reward and other times for threat, depending on the degree of negativity in the context (Reynolds & Berridge, 2008). The information signaled by a neuron also depends in part on the assembly of neurons that serve as the context in which it is firing. For example, a recent study in ferrets showed that individual neurons respond to different type of sensory cues when participating in different neural assemblies, even in primary sensory areas in which receptive fields for neurons are supposed to be well defined (as in V1; Basole, White, & Fitzpatrick, 2003). Other evidence indicates that motivational context influences the functional connectivity between brain areas. For example, neural responding is more tightly coupled in areas of early vision cortex (V1 through V4) when viewing affective objects that are outside the focus of attention but have previously been paired with shock (and are more affectively significant) than when viewing objects that are neutral (Damaraju, Huang, Barrett, & Pessoa, 2009). Amygdala responses to emotional faces are influenced both by interpretive context (Kim et al., 2004) and by the amount of circulating stress hormone (Kukolja et al., 2008).

Nor is the context principle uniquely human (see Bouton, Chapter 12, this volume). As described earlier, rats do many things in "fear" (i.e., in the presence a threat). Other times they freeze. At still other times they escape. Sometimes they kick up their bedding in the direction of a threat (defensive treading).

The Context Principle Outside of Psychology

Although certain traditions within psychology have been concerned with the influence of context since its inception as a scientific discipline, the context principle is not specific to psychology. Biology, chemistry, and physics have all discovered the context principle. In biology, the importance of epigenetic factors in gene expression is only one example of the context principle. In chemistry, the context principle can be seen in the reactivity of *functional groups* (organic molecules or compounds). As molecular complexity increases, the context-dependent behavior scales accordingly, or maybe even in an exponential fashion. In physics, the paradigmatic example might be the theory of relativity. For many centuries, physicists struggled to comprehend time and space as absolute and unchanging entities—that is, until Einstein changed the terms of the questions entirely with his theory of relativity. Time and space are not rigidly independent categories; they are different ways of experiencing the same phenomenon, depending on the context.

THE PRESENT VOLUME

In psychology, if our field's task is mapping the various manifestations of the context principle, then the results might be similarly revolutionary. In this volume, we provide the interested reader with selected examples of how the external context (in the form of the physical, social, and cultural environments) configures with the internal context of the organism to produce the varied phenomena that make up the human mind (memories, emotions, behaviors, etc.). *The Mind in Context* contains 15 concise, forward-looking chapters that illustrate with empirical examples how the psychological phenomena of interest (from genes to personhood) emerge from the interaction between mind and context, while emphasizing future conceptual and empirical directions. We also include a final chapter (Barsalou et al., Chapter 16, this volume) that integrates the chapters into an analysis of why the error of essentialism occurs and how better to represent and discuss the context principle. By looking across various research programs, and traversing levels of analysis, we hope to illustrate that the "context principle" is finally picking up some speed as a major theoretical force in psychology.

If the context principle is correct, then, as Dewey observed over a century ago, psychologists must abandon the linear logic of an experiment as a metaphor for how the mind works. In the classic experiment, we present a participant (be it a human or some nonhuman animal) with some sensory stimulation (what we call a *stimulus*); then we measure some response. Correspondingly, psychological models of the mind (and brain) almost always follow a similar ordering (stimulus → organism → response). Neurons are presumed generally to lie quiet until stimulated by a source from the external world. Scientists talk about "independent variables" because we assume that they exist separate from the participant. But outside the lab, the brain (not an experimenter) selects what is a stimulus and what is not, in part by predicting what will be important in the future. Said another way, the current state of the human brain makes some sensory stimulation into "information" and relegates the rest to the psychologically impotent "physical surroundings." In this way, sensory stimulation from the world only modulates preexisting neuronal activity but does not cause it outright (Llinas, Ribary, Contreras, & Pedroarena, 1998), and the human brain contributes to every mental moment whether or not we experience a sense of agency (and usually we do not). This means that the simple linear models of psychological phenomena that psychologists often construct will never really offer true explanations of psychological events. As demonstrated in this volume's chapters, the context principle offers a more promising approach to understanding the mind.

ACKNOWLEDGMENTS

Preparation of this chapter was supported by a National Institutes of Health Director's Pioneer Award (No. DP1OD003312), a National Institute of Mental Health's Independent Scientist Research Award (No. K02 MH001981), grants from the National Institute of Aging (No. AG030311) and the National Science Foundation (Nos. BCS 0721260 and BCS 0527440), and a contract with the Army Research Institute (No. W91WAW), as well as by a James McKeen Cattell Award and a Sabbatical Fellowship from the American Philosophical Society to Lisa Feldman Barrett; and by a grant from the National Science Foundation (No. BCS 0527249) to Eliot R. Smith.

NOTES

1. As this aspect of Wundt's work largely remains untranslated into English, it is necessary to rely on secondary sources.
2. Ironically enough, other social psychologists use these words exactly the other way around (Bruner, 1990; Markus & Kitayama, 2003). Regardless of what one calls what, the point is that there are physical movements out of which the brain creates (not detects) psychologically meaningful events.

REFERENCES

Anderson, E., Bliss-Moreau, E., & Barrett, L. F. (2009). *The visual impact of gossip*. Manuscript under review.

Arntz, A., Van Eck, M., & de Jong, P. J. (1992). Unpredictable sudden increases in intensity of pain and acquired fear. *Journal of Psychophysiology, 6*, 54–64.

Aviezer, H., Hassin, R. R., Ryan, J., Grady, C., Susskind, J., Anderson, A., et al. (2008). Angry, disgusted, or afraid?: Studies on the malleability of emotion perception. *Psychological Science, 19*, 724–732.

Balcetis, E., & Dunning, D. (2006). See what you want to see: Motivational influences on visual perception. *Journal of Personality and Social Psychology, 91*, 612–625.

Baldwin, J. M. (1891). *Handbook of psychology: Feeling and will*. New York: Holt.

Bar, M. (2004). Visual objects in context. *Nature Reviews Neuroscience, 5*, 617–629.

Bar, M. (2007). The proactive brain: Using analogies and associations to generate predictions. *Trends in Cognitive Sciences, 11*, 280–289.

Barrett, L. F., & Bar, M. (2009). See it with feeling: Affective predictions in the human brain. *Philosophical Transactions of the Royal Society of London B, 364*, 1325–1334.

Barrett, L. F., Lindquist, K., Bliss-Moreau, E., Duncan, S., Gendron, M., Mize, J., et al. (2007). Of mice and men: Natural kinds of emotion in the mammalian brain? *Perspectives on Psychological Science, 2*, 297–312.

Barrett, L. F., Lindquist, K., & Gendron, M. (2007). Language as a context for emotion perception. *Trends in Cognitive Sciences, 11*, 327–332.

Barrett, L. F., & Kensinger, E. A. (2009). *Context is routinely encoded during emotion perception*. Manuscript under review.

Barsalou, L. W. (2009). Simulation, situated conceptualization, and prediction. *Philosophical Transactions of the Royal Society of London B, 364*, 1281–1289.

Barsalou, L. W. (2008). Grounded cognition. *Annual Review of Psychology, 59*, 617–645.

Basole, A., White, L. E., & Fitzpatrick, D. (2003). Mapping multiple features in the population response of visual cortex. *Nature, 423*, 986–990.

Bhalla, M., & Proffitt, D. R. (1999). Visual–motor recalibration in geographical slant perception. *Journal of Experimental Psychology: Human Perception and Performance, 25*(4), 1076–1096.

Bloom, P. (2004). *Descartes' baby: How the science of child development explains what makes us human.* New York: Basic Books.

Breiter, H. C., Etcoff, N. L., Whalen, P. J., Kennedy, W. A., Rauch, S. L., Buckner, R. L., et al. (1996). Response and habituation of the human amygdala during visual processing of facial expressions. *Neuron, 17,* 875–877.

Briggs, J. L. (1970). *Never in anger: Portrait of an Eskimo family.* Cambridge, MA: Harvard University Press.

Bruner, J. (1988). *Actual minds, possible worlds.* Cambridge, MA: Harvard University Press.

Bruner, J. (1990). *Acts of meaning.* Cambridge, MA: Harvard University Press.

Brunswik, E. (1955a). In defense of probabilistic functionalism: A reply. *Psychological Review, 62,* 236–242.

Brunswik, E. (1955b). Representative design and probabilistic theory in a functional psychology. *Psychological Review, 62,* 193–217.

Burns, L. H., Annett, L., Kelley, A. E., Everitt, B. J., & Robbins, T. W. (1996) Effects of lesions to amygdala, ventral subiculum, medial prefrontal cortex, and nucleus accumbens on the reaction to novelty: Implication for limbic–striatal interactions. *Behavioral Neuroscience, 110,* 60–73.

Carroll, J. M., & Russell, J. A. (1996). Do facial expressions signal specific emotions?: Judging emotion from the face in context. *Journal of Personality and Social Psychology, 70,* 205–218.

Chun, M. M. (2000). Contextual cuing of visual attention. *Trends in Cognitive Sciences, 4,* 170–178.

Cohen, D. (1999). "When you call me that, smile!": How norms for politeness, interaction styles, and aggression work together in Southern culture. *Social Psychology Quarterly, 62*(3), 257–275.

Damaraju, E., Huang, Y.-M., Barrett, L. F., & Pessoa, L. (2009). Affective learning enhances activity and functional connectivity in early visual cortex. *Neuropsychologia, 47,* 2480–2487.

D'Andrade, R. G. (1984). Culture meaning systems. In R. A. Shweder & R. A. Levine (Eds.), *Culture theory: Essays on mind, self, and emotion* (pp. 88–119). Cambridge, UK: Cambridge University Press.

Danziger, K. (1983). Origins and basic principles of Wundt's *Volkerpsychologie. British Journal of Social Psychology, 22,* 303–313.

de Gelder, B., & Vroomen, J. (2000). The perception of emotions by ear and by eye. *Cognition and Emotion, 14,* 289–311.

de Gelder, B., Böcker, K. B., Tuomainen, J., Hensen, M., & Vroomen, J. (1999). The combined perception of emotion from voice and face: Early interaction revealed by human electric brain responses. *Neuroscience Letters, 260*(2), 133–136.

de Gelder, B., Meeren, H. K. M., Righart, R., van den Stock, J., van de Riet, W. A. C., & Tamietto, M. (2006). Beyond the face: Exploring rapid influences of context on face processing. *Progress in Brain Research, 55,* 37–48.

Dewar, K., & Xu, F. (2009). Do early nouns refer to kinds or distinct shapes?: Evidence from 10-month-old infants. *Psychological Science, 20,* 252–257.

Dewey, J. (1896). The reflex arc concept in psychology. *Psychological Review, 3*, 357–370.

Fernandez-Dohls, J.-M., Carrera, P., Barchard, K. A., & Gacitua, M. (2008). False recognition of facial expressions of emotion: Cause and implications. *Emotion, 8*, 530–539.

Fugate, J. M. B., Gouzoules, H., & Barrett, L. F. (2009). *Reading chimpanzee faces: A test of the structural and conceptual hypotheses*. Manuscript under review.

Gendron, M., & Barrett, L. F. (2009). Reconstructing the past: A century of ideas about emotion in psychology. *Emotion Review, 1*, 1–24.

Gibbs, W. W. (2003). The unseen genome: Gems among the junk. *Scientific American, 289*, 47–53.

Gilbert, D. T. (1998). Ordinary personology. In D. T. Gilbert, S. T. Fiske, & G. Lindzey (Eds.), *The handbook of social psychology* (4th ed., Vol. 1, pp. 89–150). New York: McGraw-Hill.

Heine, S. J., Lehman, D. R., Markus, H. R., & Kitayama, S. (1999). Is there a universal need for positive self-regard? *Psychological Review, 106*(4), 766–794.

Herry, C., Bach, D. R., Esposito, F., Di Salle, F., Perrig, W. J., Scheffler, K., et al. (2007). Processing of temporal unpredictability in human and animal amygdala. *Journal of Neuroscience, 27*, 5958–5966.

Holland, P. C., & Gallagher, M (1999). Amygdala circuitry in attentional and representational processes. *Trends in Cognitive Sciences, 3*, 65–73.

Hunt, W. A. (1941). Recent developments in the field of emotion. *Psychological Bulletin, 38*, 249–276.

Iwata, J., & LeDoux, J. E. (1988). Dissociation of associative and nonassociative concomitants of classical fear conditioning in the freely behaving rat. *Behavioral Neuroscience, 102*, 66–76.

Kim, H., Somerville, L. H., Johnstone, T., Polis, S., Alexander, A. L., Shin, L. M., et al. (2004). Contextual modulation of amygdala responsivity to surprise faces. *Journal of Cognitive Neuroscience, 16*, 1730–1745.

Kukolja, J., Schalpfer, T. E., Keysers, C., Klingmuller, D., Maier, W., Fink, G. R., et al. (2008). Modeling a negative response bias in the human amygdala by noradrenergic–glucocorticoid interactions. *Journal of Neuroscience, 28*, 12868–12876.

LeDoux, J. E., Cicchetti, P., Zagoraris, A., & Romanski, L. M. (1990). The lateral amygdaloid nucleus: Sensory interface of the amygdala in fear conditioning. *Journal of Neuroscience, 10*, 1062–1069.

Lewin, K. (1935). *A dynamic theory of personality*. New York: McGraw-Hill.

Lewis, C. C. (1995). *Educating hearts and minds*. New York: Cambridge University Press.

Lewontin, R. (2000). *The triple helix: Gene, organism, and environment*. Cambridge, MA: Harvard University Press.

Lindquist, K., Barrett, L. F., Bliss-Moreau, E., & Russell, J. A. (2006). Language and the perception of emotion. *Emotion, 6*, 125–138.

Llinas, R., Ribary, U., Contreras, D., & Pedroarena, C. (1998). The neuronal basis for consciousness. *Philosophical Transactions of the Royal Society of the London B*, *353*, 1841–1849.

Markus, H. R. (2008). Pride, prejudice, and ambivalence: Toward a unified theory of race and ethnicity. *American Psychologist*, *63*, 651–760.

Markus, H. R., & Kitayama, S. (2003). Models of agency: Sociocultural diversity in the construction of action. In J. J. Berman & V. Murphy-Berman (Eds.), *Cross-cultural differences in perspectives on the self* (Vol. 49, pp. 18–74). Lincoln: University of Nebraska Press.

Markus, H. R., Mullally, P. R., & Kitayama, S. (1997). Selfways: Diversity in modes of cultural participation. In U. Neisser & D. A. Jopling (Eds.), *The conceptual self in context: Culture, experience, self-understanding* (pp. 13–61). Cambridge, UK: Cambridge University Press.

Mason, W. A., Capitanio, J. P., Machado, C. J., Mendoza, S. P., & Amaral, D. G. (2006). Amygdalectomy and responsiveness to novelty in rhesus monkeys (*Macaca mulatta*): Generality and individual consistency of effects. *Emotion*, *6*, 73–81.

Masuda, T., Ellsworth, P. C., Mesquita, B., Leu, J., Tanida, S., & Van de Veerdonk, E. (2008). Placing the face in context: Cultural differences in the perception of facial emotion. *Journal of Personality and Social Psychology*, *94*, 365–381.

Medin, D., & Ortony, A. (1989). Psychological essentialism. In S. Vosniadou & A. Ortony (Eds.), *Similarity and analogical reasoning* (pp. 179–195). New York: Cambridge University Press.

Meeren, H. K. M., van Heijnsbergen, C. C. R. J., & de Gelder, B. (2005). Rapid perceptual integration of facial expression and emotional body language. *Proceedings of the National Academy of Sciences USA*, *102*, 16518–16523.

Mesquita, B. (1993). *Cultural variations in emotions: A comparative study of Dutch, Surainamese, and Turkish people in the Netherlands*. Unpublished PhD thesis, University of Amsterdam.

Mesquita, B., & Markus, H. R. (2004). Culture and emotion: Models of agency as sources of cultural variation in emotion. In N. H. Frijda, A. S. R. Manstead, & A. H. Fischer (Eds.), *Feelings and emotions: The Amsterdam Symposium* (pp. 341–358). Cambridge, MA: Cambridge University Press.

Mischel, W. (1968). *Personality and assessment*. New York: Wiley.

Mischel, W. (2004). Towards an integrative science of the person. *Annual Review of Psychology*, *55*, 1–22.

Mischel, W., & Shoda, Y. (1995). A cognitive–affective system theory of personality: Reconceptualizing situations, dispositions, dynamics, and invariance in personality structure. *Psychological Review*, *102*, 246–268.

Nisbett, R. E. (2003). *The geography of thought: How Asians and Westerners think differently … and why*. New York: Free Press

Oliva, A., & Torralba, A. (2007). The role of context in object recognition. *Trends in Cognitive Sciences*, *11*, 520–527.

Palmer, S. E. (1975). The effects of contextual scenes on the identification of objects. *Memory and Cognition*, *3*, 519–526.

Prather, M. D., Lavenex, P., Mauldin-Jourdain, M. L., Mason, W. A., Capitanio, J. P., Mendoza, S. P., et al. (2001). Increased social fear and decreased fear of objects in monkeys with neonatal amygdala lesions. *Neuroscience, 106*, 653–658.

Proffitt, D. R., Stefanucci, J., Banton, T., & Epstein, W. (2003). The role of effort in perceiving distance. *Psychological Science, 14*, 106–112.

Reynolds, S. M., & Berridge, K. C. (2002). Positive and negative motivation in nucleus accumbens shell: Bivalent rostrocaudal gradients for GABA-elicited eating, taste "liking"/"disliking" reactions, place preference/avoidance, and fear. *Journal of Neuroscience, 22*(16), 7308–7320.

Reynolds, S. M., & Berridge, K. C. (2003). Glutamate motivational ensembles in nucleus accumbens: Rostrocaudal shell gradients of fear and feeding. *European Journal of Neuroscience, 17*(10), 2187–2200.

Reynolds, S. M., & Berridge, K. C. (2008). Emotional environments retune the valence of appetitive versus fearful functions in nucleus accumbens. *Nature Neuroscience, 11*(4), 423–425.

Righart, R., & de Gelder, B. (2008). Recognition of facial expressions is influenced by emotion scene gist. *Cognitive, Affective, and Behavioral Neuroscience, 8*, 264–278.

Russell, J. A., & Fehr, B. (1987). Relativity in the perception of emotion in facial expressions. *Journal of Experimental Psychology, 116*, 223–237.

Russell, J. A., & Widen, S. C. (2002). A label superiority effect in children's categorization of facial expressions. *Social Development, 11*, 30–52.

Savani, K., Markus, H. R., Naidu, N. V. R., & Kumar, S. (2009). *What counts as choice?: U.S. Americans are more likely than Indians to construe their actions as choices*. Unpublished manuscript, Stanford University.

Schwartz, C. E., Wright, C. I., Shin, L. M., Kagan, J., & Rauch, S. L. (2003). Inhibited and uninhibited infants "grown up": Adult amygdalar response to novelty. *Science, 300*, 1952–1953.

Schyns, P. G., & Oliva, A. (1999). Dr. Angry and Mr. Smile: When categorization flexibly modifies the perception of faces in rapid visual presentations. *Cognition, 69*(3), 243–265.

Serences, J. T., Ester, E. F., Vogel, E. K., & Awh, E. (2009). Stimulus-specific delay activity in human primary visual cortex. *Psychological Science, 20*, 207–214.

Sherman, M. (1927). The differentiation of emotion responses in infants. *Journal of Comparative Psychology, 7*, 265–284.

Shoda, Y., Mischel, W., & Wright, J. C. (1994). Intra-individual stability in the organization and patterning of behavior: Incorporating psychological situations into the idiographic analysis of personality. *Journal of Personality and Social Psychology, 65*, 674–687.

Shore, B. (1996). *Culture in mind: Cognition, culture, and the problem of meaning*. New York: Oxford University Press.

Shweder, R. A. (1991a). Cultural psychology: What is it? In *Thinking through cultures* (pp. 73–110). Cambridge, MA: Harvard University Press.

Shweder, R. A. (1991b). *Thinking through cultures.* Cambridge, MA: Harvard University Press.
Smith, E. R., & Semin, G. R. (2004). Socially situated cognition: Cognition in its social context. *Advances in Experimental Social Psychology, 36,* 53–117.
Steele, C. M. (1997). A threat in the air: How stereotypes shape intellectual identity and performance. *American Psychologist, 52*(6), 613–629.
Stefanucci, J. K., Proffitt, D. R., Clore, G., & Parekh, N. (2008). Skating down a steeper slope: Fear influences the perception of geographical slant. *Perception, 37,* 321–323.
Teachman, B. A., Stefanucci, J. K., Clerkin, E. M., Cody, M. W., & Proffitt, D. R. (2008). A new mode of fear expression: Perceptual bias in height fear. *Emotion, 8,* 296–301.
Trope, Y. (1986). Identification and inferential processes in dispositional attribution. *Psychological Review, 93,* 239–257.
Trope, Y., & Cohen, O. (1989). Perceptual and inferential determinants of behavior-correspondent attributions. *Journal of Experimental Social Psychology, 25,* 142–158.
Vallacher, R. R., & Wegner, D. M. (1987). What do people think they're doing?: Action identification and human behavior. *Psychological Review, 94,* 3–15.
Vazdarjanova, A., & McGaugh, J. L. (1998). Basolateral amygdala is not critical for cognitive memory of contextual fear conditioning. *Proceedings of the National Academy of Sciences, 95,* 15003–15007.
Weierich, M. R., Wright, C. I., Negreira, A., Dickerson, B. C., & Barrett, L. F. (in press). Novelty as a dimension in the affective brain. *NeuroImage.*
Wilson, F. A., & Rolls, E. T. (1993). The effects of stimulus novelty and familiarity on neuronal activity in the amygdala of monkeys performing recognition memory tasks. *Experimental Brain Research, 93,* 367–382.
Witt, J., Linkenauger, S., Bakdash, J., Augustyn, J., Cook, A., & Proffitt, D. (2009). The long road of pain: Chronic pain increases perceived distance. *Experimental Brain Research, 192,* 145–148.
Witt, J. K., Proffitt, D. R., & Epstein, W. (2005). Tool use affects perceived distance but only when you intend to use it. *Journal of Experimental Psychology: Human Perception and Performance, 31,* 880–888.
Wright, C. I., Martis, B., Schwartz, C. E., Shin, L. M., Fischer, H. H., McMullin, K., et al. (2003). Novelty responses and differential effects of order in the amygdala, substantia innominata, and inferior temporal cortex. *NeuroImage, 18,* 660–669.
Wright, C. I., Negreira, A., Gold, A. L., Britton, J. C., Williams, D., & Barrett, L. F. (2008). Neural correlates of novelty and face-age effects in young and elderly adults. *NeuroImage, 42,* 956–958.
Wright, C. I., Wedig, M. M., Williams, D., Rauch, S. L., & Albert, M. S. (2006). Novel fearful faces activate the amygdala in healthy young and elderly adults. *Neurobiology of Aging, 27,* 361–374.
Wright, J. C., & Mischel, W. (1988). Conditional hedges and the intuitive psy-

chology of traits. *Journal of Personality and Social Psychology, 55*, 454–469.

Wundt, W. (1998). *Lectures on human and animal psychology* (S. E. Creigton & E. B. Titchener, Trans.). New York: Macmillan. (Original work published 1894)

Xu, F., Cote, M., & Baker, A. (2005). Labeling guides object individuation in 12-month-old infants. *Psychological Science, 316*, 372–377.

Zhang, W., & Luck, S. J. (2009). Feature-based attention modulates feedforward visual processing. *Nature Neuroscience, 12*(1), 24–25.

PART I

GENES AND THE BRAIN

2

Epigenetic Inheritance

LAWRENCE V. HARPER

The issue to be addressed in this chapter is whether the outcomes of the interplay between individuals and their physical and social contexts can be passed from one generation to another. The idea that the experiences of prior generations might directly influence the behavior of subsequent generations has a long history in psychology (e.g., Weber & Depew, 2003). However, until recently, serious examination of the possibility that exigencies faced by one's ancestors could shape how one might react to or interpret events has seemed unnecessary because intergenerational similarities in responses to events could be explained plausibly in terms of the immediate context—the ways in which parents shaped the experiences of their offspring. However, a growing body of evidence now indicates that depending on the characteristics of the species' niche, adjustments made by prior generations might be transmitted directly to subsequent generations even in the absence of the conditions evoking these adjustments (see Jablonca & Lamb, 1995). For example, in inbred rats, early dietary restriction of the parental generation may alter not only the physical growth but also the maze learning performance of offspring and even grandoffspring, despite the fact that the latter were provided with ample nutrients throughout their lifetimes (Cowley & Griesel, 1966).

Thus, there is the possibility that behavioral reactions of humans—in terms of variations in responses to unfamiliar persons, or even the willingness to consider "the possible"—could be influenced by what has been called *transgenerational epigenetic inheritance*, the transmission of experientially induced response tendencies via alterations in the germ-cell chromosomal context for gene expression. The deoxyribonucleic acid (DNA) itself remains unchanged; however, the ways in which it is read out are constrained by the inheritance of adjustments made by (a) prior generation(s).

To provide framework for understanding such phenomena, I briefly describe what is known regarding the mechanisms underlying gene regulation during development and phenotypic adjustment to (current) conditions. With that as background, selected examples of the emerging evidence for transgenerational transmission of epigenetic adjustments in complex life forms are presented; the possible modes of transmission are considered, and the environmental conditions that would favor such transmission are discussed. Finally, I describe the kinds of evidence that would distinguish epigenetic from either Mendelian or cultural inheritance in humans, and suggest some aspects of human behavior that might be so influenced.

At the outset, I must emphasize that to understand the ontogeny of behavior—or any other aspect of growth—a rigid distinction between organismic and environmental influences is counterproductive. While what goes on "inside the skin" must be addressed to understand fully any biological function, such processes are dependent upon, and ultimately regulated by, the "external" context. Indeed, even within a single cell, the regulation of hereditary expression can only be understood in terms of the dynamic interplay between the nuclear materials and their cytoplasmic surroundings—as influenced by external conditions. Moreover, the organism's responses feed back to the environment in a dynamic interplay; the ultimate problem is to identify the elements involved and how they interact (Harper, 1989).

GENE REGULATION, DEVELOPMENT, AND ADJUSTMENT TO CONTEXT

Insofar as all terrestrial environments fluctuate to some degree (e.g., light–dark cycles, temporal variations in population density), all species must be able to adjust to the variations that are typical of their niches. Complex organisms, such as vertebrates, inherit the potentials to make adjustments to prevailing conditions that range from physical growth (Tanner, 1990) to social behavior (Lott, 1984). Most, if not all, of these phenomena may be understood in terms of the regulation of inherited potentials for (behavioral) development. For example, rats' adult responses to unfamiliarity vary according to the amount of time their mothers spent licking and grooming them during the preweaning period. This has been shown to be mediated in part by differential expression of genes producing receptors for adrenal corticosteroids in the hippocampus and thereby altering the dynamics of the hypothalamic–pituitary–adrenocortical (HPA) neuroendocrine feedback loop (e.g., Cameron et al., 2005; Holmes et al., 2005). Comparable findings have been reported for primates (Coplan et al., 2006). Therefore, an examination of what is known about the pathways underlying such adjustments provides a framework for conceptualizing how the outcomes of the interplay between environmental context and developmental process might be transmitted across generations.

As demonstrated by the fact that the nucleus from even a highly differentiated mammalian olfactory neuron can be induced to become the basis for a viable—and fertile—clone (Eggan et al., 2004), essentially all cells in an animal share the same DNA despite the fact that they have specialized to form different tissues. Tissue differentiation involves cell-specific selective activation and "silencing" of segments of the inherited chromosomal DNA. The process is progressive, in that each step provides the foundation for the next, until the basic structure of the organism is established (Davidson, 2006). Moreover, differentiated tissues must be able to maintain their specialized identities, while also adjusting to permit the organism to meet varying demands presented by the environment. For example, muscle cells can adjust their metabolism to perform aerobic or anaerobic work as a function of the pattern of activation received from motor neurons (Salmons & Streiter, 1976).

Thus, all development is a dynamic process of transaction among organismic components and their surroundings. Given that cloning typically is accomplished by transferring the nucleus of a differentiated cell into the cytoplasm of an egg, the latter can be said to provide a proximal context that controls gene expression. The cytoplasm of the fertilized egg, the zygote, provides initial, immediate context for development; it contains the "resources" necessary to support a number of cell divisions (Schier, 2007). In mammals, given the context provided by the female's reproductive tract, the conditions that regulate the earliest steps in development are thought to originate from variations in the distribution of the cytoplasmic contents of the fertilized egg as it divides—perhaps initially influenced by the point of entry of the sperm (Pedersen, 2001)—and chemical signals between the developing zygote and the maternal fallopian tube (Fazeli & Pewsey, 2008). These differences in the cytoplasmic environments of the dividing cells lead to alterations in the biochemical context for the chromosomes in the nuclei of the "daughter" cells and thereby give rise to tissue-specific patterns of gene expression. Further development is regulated by "cross talk" among the developing tissues (cf. Oliveri & Davidson, 2007).

Throughout this interplay, the conditions in the nucleus are altered in ways that permit each cellular lineage to maintain its specialized identity. In the nucleus, the DNA strands are coiled about and "packaged" among "histone" proteins, themselves products of the nuclear DNA. There are four basic types of these proteins, although some of these histone types may vary slightly depending on cell type. The locations of the histone proteins along the DNA strand help to determine the availability of the DNA for "transcription," and the degree to which they link to specific sites on a DNA strand can differ, among other things, as a result of the binding of small molecules, such as methyl or acetyl molecules, to the "tails" of certain of the histones' amino acid components. Other proteins either help to link the histones to one another or bind to additional sites on the chromosomal DNA. These components of the "chromatin" in the nucleus of the cell provide means for precisely "regulating" the readout of the DNA (Berger, 2007; Misteli, 2007). The products of transcription of the messages in the DNA are ribonucleic acids (RNAs), some of which are "translated" into enzymes and other proteins needed for the production of tissue-specific characteristics (Davidson, 2006); the other, untranslated RNAs, many of which are the products of what was previously considered "junk" DNA, often are involved in regulating the process (ENCODE Project Consortium, 2007; Hughes, 2006).

In mammals, perhaps partly mediated by histone modifications and RNAs, methyl molecules can also adhere directly to specific sites on the DNA strand, facilitating formation of inhibitory complexes (Berger, 2007). The dynamic conformations and locations of these DNA-associated elements and the resulting conformation of the chromosomes within this context (Misteli, 2007) are influenced both by extracellular signals, such as neurotransmitters or hormones, that are transmitted to the nucleus via receptors in the outer cellular membrane and, within the nucleus, by the "by-products" of the transcription process itself, non-(protein)-coding RNAs (Martianov, Ramadass, Barros, Chow, & Akoulitchev, 2007). Ultimately, it is this *nuclear context*—the result of the dynamic interplay between a cell and its surroundings—that determines which segments of the DNA strands are exposed for transcription by nuclear enzymes (RNA polymerases), and which genes or gene networks are (relatively) inaccessible to the polymerases as tissues and organs develop (Davidson, 2006; Misteli, 2007).

In summary, the *epigenetic commitment* of a cell to a specific, differentiated type as a result of complex exchanges with its surroundings is essentially a form of inheritance. What is inherited is not changes in the DNA itself, but alterations in the nature and locations on the DNA of proteins and other molecules, and in the resulting topological organization of the nuclear material that regulates protein production and leads to cellular specialization.

As mentioned earlier, there also must be flexibility of function within tissues and organs, permitting the organism to adjust to varying demands typical of the species' niche. Here, too, organismic functioning is altered by the same kinds of mechanisms by which intercellular signaling shapes the differentiation of specific tissues, by the above-mentioned factors regulating gene expression, a process that extends throughout the lifespan (e.g., human monozygotic twins' similarities in chromatin diverge progressively as a function of differential experiences as they age) (Fraga et al., 2005).

TRANSGENERATIONAL EPIGENETIC INHERITANCE

Observations in a wide range of species indicate that epigenetic adjustments to certain forms of environmental demands are in fact transmitted across generations (Jablonca & Lamb, 1995). Even though the young do not encounter the precipitating event(s), they display the same phenotypic adjustment made by their parent(s). Often, a defining feature of these traits is that in the absence of continued environmental challenge, their expression wanes across generations. In the field of evolutionary ecology, these phenomena, called *maternal effects*, are understood as evolutionary adaptations to environmental unpredictability that prepare the next generation to meet the conditions it is likely to encounter at some phase of its lifetime (e.g., Mousseau & Fox, 1998). That such adjustments can in fact provide the next generation with protection against exigencies that are likely to be encountered has been verified experimentally by Agrawal, Laforsch, and Tollrian (1999): Both an insect (water flea) and a plant (radish) that are subject to predation develop anatomical alterations (a heavy cuticle on the flea's head region and spines on the leaves of the radish, respectively) in response to the threat posed by the presence of a predator. In the case of the water flea, the threat is signaled by a waterborne chemical cue; for the radish, an insect predator's feeding on its leaves is the cue. Having been exposed to these challenges, not only do the adults develop defenses but also, once so exposed, even in the absence of concurrent signals relating to the presence of predators, the females produced eggs or seeds that, as they mature, without being exposed to predator-related cues, develop the same defensive characteristics. Moreover, as compared to offspring lacking these defenses, the young insects or seedlings that are so "prepared" are in fact less likely to be harmed when exposed to predators.

In mammals, experiments with rodents have shown that female young of nutrient-restricted mothers, despite having been provided with unrestricted nutrition from the postweaning period onward, had smaller offspring than untreated animals; that is, the grandmother's level of nutrition affected grandoffspring's growth even in the presence of adequate resources. These experiments also showed that undernourished rat young tended to have less brain DNA (Zamenhof, van Marthens, & Grauel, 1971) and performed more poorly in maze-learning tasks (Cowley & Griesel, 1966) than did controls. Just as with body size, the impacts on brain growth and behavior were manifest in the grandoffspring. It took several generations of unrestricted food availability for these changes to reverse themselves. In humans, similar transgenerational impacts of early nutrient levels on physical growth have been described, and the best predictors of neonatal offspring size were maternal birthweight (Stein & Lumey, 2000) or maternal height (Stein et al., 2003).

The latter findings leave open the possibility that, in mammals, the transgenerational restriction on fetal growth could be attributable to a correlated alteration in the uterine environment. However, in the case of rats, transgenerational effects of early restricted diets on metabolism have been demonstrated even after zygote transfers to untreated, same-strain foster mothers (Wu & Suzuki, 2006), and in humans, the effects of early malnutrition on subsequent generations' susceptibility to cardiovascular disease and diabetes in rural Sweden have been shown to be transmitted from both grandmothers and grandfathers to grandoffspring (Kaati, Bygren, & Edvinsson, 2002; Pembrey et al., 2006). Therefore, epigenetic inheritance is a viable explanation.

MODES OF TRANSMISSION

Until recently, existing knowledge of the processes underlying the development of multicellular organisms made such intergenerational transmission via the gametes seem unlikely. Insofar as the starting point for development is the fusion of sperm and egg, it seemed that these cells had to be clear of the constraints on the genome that defined differentiated somatic cells. Presumably, then, all epigenetic alterations of the nuclear context controlling DNA transcription had to be "reset" in order for the gametes to transmit the potential for the development of a new, fully differentiated organism (Kimmins & Sassone-Corsi, 2005). However, genetic *imprinting*, the selective expression of alleles depending upon the parent from whom they were inherited, and the effects of selective inactivation of one X chromosome (in female mammals) indicate that some constraints on gene expression can be transmitted across generations.

For example, in humans, girls with Turner syndrome (only one X chromosome) who inherited the paternal X (i.e., from the paternal grandmother) were rated as behaving typically for their age and gender, whereas those who inherited their X from their mothers were more impulsive and "boy-like" (Skuse et al., 1997). This may be a general mammalian pattern insofar as a somewhat similar gender-related, parent-of-origin, X-linked, pattern of differences in behavior has been demonstrated in mice (Davies, Isles, Smith, et al., 2005). Parent-of-origin effects on behavior are not limited to the X chromosome. For example, in rodents, imprinted, autosomal genes also have been implicated in early filial and parental behaviors (Plagge et al., 2004; see also Davies, Isles, & Wilkinson, 2005).

Several pathways for this transmission have been suggested. First of all, not all of the methyl molecules adhering to the DNA, presumably representing epigenetic modifications, are removed from mammalian gametes (Flanagan et al., 2006). Moreover, the gametes themselves are highly specialized cells, as is obvious from their differences in relative size and morphology, and they transmit more than just DNA. The egg carries unique histone variants, and its greater size reflects the fact that its cytoplasm provides the substrates for early metabolic functioning and cell division (even the mitochondria of the sperm are degraded, and only the maternal mitochondria are retained). Upon fertilization, the initial phase of cellular function is essentially under "maternal" control until one or more divisions have been completed, at which time the zygotic genome is expressed (Martin et al., 2006; Schier, 2007). Despite its smaller size, the sperm cell also transmits distinct signals. The sperm's nuclear chromosomes are packaged among specialized (sperm-specific) histone proteins (Kimmins & Sassone-Corsi, 2005), and although they have relatively little cytoplasmic volume, the sperm cells also transmit a number of distinctive RNAs (Krawetz, 2005). Insofar as methyl molecules at specific DNA sites affect the probability of transcription, and a number of (non-protein-coding) RNAs are intimately involved in regulation of DNA transcription and/or the fate of the "messenger" RNA that may be translated into protein (Hughes, 2006; Martianov et al., 2007), both mammalian gametes have the potential to transmit "additional" information across generations.

In summary, the gametes transmit more than "genes" as traditionally defined. At least a secondary layer of inherited information relating to parent of origin is transmitted across generations, and this provides a specific context for patterns of gene expression—and ultimately behavior—in the developing offspring. This being so, there would seem to be potential mechanisms whereby the adjustments made by prior generations to the then-prevailing environment could in some way lead to comparable "marks" that would influence the growth and behavior of subsequent generations.

While previously available evidence suggested that paternal transgenerational, epigenetic transmission of phenotypic variation was possible, a number of instances, such as the long-term effects of endocrine disruptors in rodents (e.g., Anway, Cupp, Uzumcu, & Skinner, 2005) might have been explained (away) in terms of toxic, pharmacological effects. Likewise, transgenerational transmission of metabolic risk for diabetes and cardiovascular disease in humans (Pembrey et al., 2006), might have been explained in terms of dietary or culinary custom or activity preferences. However, the relation, albeit somewhat complex, between grandparental nutrition and grandoffspring health found by Kaati and colleagues (2002) and Pembrey and colleagues (2006) suggests a pattern of transmission in which effects varied according to the gender of both the grandparent and the grandchild. Dietary, or culinary, preferences and activity patterns cannot easily explain the facts that the outcomes also varied as a function of the age at which (grand)parents were exposed to a period of limited food availability, and that there were gender differences in both the sensitive periods and the direction of response to dietary restriction. Instead, these results suggest transgenerational epigenetic inheritance, perhaps mediated by alterations in the regulation of imprinted genes, and highlight the importance of the timing of experience and the existence of gender-related effects.

In support of biparental transmission of epigenetic, phenotypic variation via the gametes, a study with mice has shown that the effects of a mutant parental genetic allele on the phenotype (white patches of fur) could be transmitted to offspring that did not inherit the allele itself—an example of what is known as a *paramutation*. In this case, it was also shown experimentally that RNA from the male sperm was a likely mediator of the paternal effect (Rassoulzadegan et al., 2006). Thus, there now is experimental evidence that both mammalian eggs and sperm can transmit information relating to ancestral patterns of gene regulation, in some cases in the form of RNA that affects gene expression across generations. Given that noncoding RNAs are differentially expressed in the brain (Makeyev & Maniatis, 2008), transgenerational epigenetic inheritance of behavior is possible in mammals, and, depending on the trait, it may be transmitted via the gametes from either parent.

CONTEXTS FAVORING TRANSGENERATIONAL EPIGENETIC INHERITANCE OF BEHAVIOR

If pathways exist for transgenerational epigenetic inheritance of metabolic or morphological adjustments in humans, then a number of questions must be addressed to guide the search for comparable effects on behavior. First, there is the issue of identifying the nature of the environmental contexts for which anticipatory adjustments might be advantageous.

Among the environmental variables identified by evolutionary ecologists (e.g., Tollrian & Harvell, 1999) as relevant for such transmission, the most fundamental one is whether the condition in question requires a significant organismic adjustment. However, for such conditions to be likely to lead to transmission of an anticipatory adjustment, the precipitating condition should be predictable only in the sense that at least a substantial proportion of a population is likely to face it at some point in a lifetime, and that the condition will also vary temporally in severity; that is, although having a real impact on the phenotype when encountered, the occurrence, timing, and severity of exposure should not be highly predictable within any one individual's lifetime. As in the case of the human studies mentioned earlier, extended periods of drought (and crop failure) are exigencies that could not be predicted with accuracy. Therefore, transgenerational, epigenetic transmission would be adaptive.

However, these variables also have to be considered against the backdrop of a species' biological "economy." If adjusting to a condition does not make a significant energetic demand on the organism or appreciably increase the likelihood of physical harm, there is little value in anticipating it. On the other hand, if the adjustment requires some sort of sacrifice, as in the case of restricted body or brain growth in the face of limited prenatal or early postnatal nutrient availability, it might be more advantageous to be prepared at the outset to "invest" less in growth in stature—to sacrifice physical size—and even risk limiting behavioral flexibility (cf. Zamenhof et al., 1971), than to be unable to meet the greater energy demands of a larger body in times of scarcity. In short, when adjusting "after the fact" is more costly, and the likelihood of exposure to an exigency is unpredictable, it can pay to anticipate the possibility of a challenge.

In mammals, the context provided by variations in maternal parenting style (e.g., the amount of pup licking/grooming performed by a rat mother) can serve as a signal indirectly reflecting the kinds of conditions that the young are likely to encounter only later, upon emergence from the nest (Cameron et al., 2005). Although there is no question that the ways people learn to interpret their experiences can shape the mental context that influences their choice of action, more indirect "environmental signs" (cf. Harper, 1989) comparable to maternal grooming in rodents are not irrelevant to the human condition. For example, Lieberman, Tooby, and Cosmides (2007) showed that the best predictors of attitudes associated with relatedness among siblings—including incest avoidance—was for firstborns the perinatal association with a younger sibling and, for those born later, the amount of time spent together in coresidence with the same mother figure. These contextual factors influenced attitudes toward siblings independently of the young adult respondents' declarative knowledge of kinship.

Although fully developed models are not yet available to predict where to find sensitivity to signs of environmental conditions with precision, in animals, at least two relevant elements have been demonstrated experimentally: The first is the degree to which conditions in the environment are consistent, or predictable, and, the second is the reliability of the sign (indirectly) related to an otherwise unpredictable condition. To the extent that the sign is a more reliable predictor of an event than one's prior experience, the sign can serve to guide behavior (McLinn & Stephens, 2006). An example can be drawn from the water flea: In late summer, the female cannot "know" that decreasing day length signals a nutrient-depleted environment in which her eggs must hatch; her own experience is limited to her (more brief) lifetime. However, she is sensitive to the light–dark cycle and on that basis modifies the content of her egg in ways that prepare her offspring to adjust to the coming season (Alekseev & Lampert, 2001). In short, then, in addition to direct cues relating to conditions in the environment, we should also be looking for reliable, detectable predictors of those conditions.

The next issue is to determine who might be affected. In several experimental studies with rodents (e.g., Huck, Labov, & Lisk, 1987) and naturalistic studies with humans (Kaati et al., 2002; Pembrey et al., 2006), the effects of the (grand)parental experience varied by gender. The human studies of transgenerational risk of cardiovascular disease and diabetes (probably reflecting differential metabolic "decisions" relating to the allocation of energy supplies) particularly highlight a need to identify likely contexts for gender differences in sensitivity and/or quality of response to environmental conditions. In the case of humans, one might expect gender differences in epigenetically transmitted response to an environmental challenge where, consistently over time, there has been a difference in the degree to which variable risks impact males and females and/or are associated with matrilocal or patrilocal residence.

These differences lead to the issue of when one might expect sensitivity for the transmission of anticipatory phenotypic adjustments to (future) offspring, and the mechanisms for transmission of such signals. Given that epigenetic transmission is via the gametes, the time windows would seem most likely to be the periods when the gametes themselves, and/or when the cells that provide the contexts for the final maturation of the gametes, are maturing. In the case of the human egg, differentiation of the primary oocytes occurs during gestation, and the granulosa cells that "nurse" the developing eggs in the ovarian follicles are thought to differentiate as distinct tissues at around the same time (Sathananthan et al., 2006). From the Pembrey and colleagues (2006) and the Stein and Lumey (2000) findings, it would seem that, at least for the control of allocation of energy resources, the most sensitive period for transmission via the egg would be from the last trimester of gestation through the end of the first year or two, perhaps reflecting interactions between oocytes and granulosa cells (Diaz, Wigglesworth, & Eppig, 2007).

Given the fact that DNA methylation of at least a number of genes in human sperm varies across individual sperm cells, and that this variation tends to increase with age, (Flanagan et al., 2006) predictable gametic transmission would seem to be more likely via RNA (cf. Rassoulzadegan et al., 2006). In the Swedish studies, conditions influencing gametic transmission of metabolic adjustment were primarily limited to the *slow growth period*, the phase of growth in the middle childhood years just before adolescence. Insofar as the stem cells that produce sperm differentiate prenatally, the data would implicate the Sertoli cells that provide the context for final maturation of the sperm as the pathways through which information is transmitted to the gametes. Although the history of the postnatal development of Sertoli cells in the human testis is not fully documented, the slow growth period represents a stage just prior to their final maturation under the influence of testosterone and follicle-stimulating hormone (FSH) (Petersen & Soder, 2006). Thus, current data suggest that there are sex differences in the periods of sensitivity for gametic transmission of epigenetic adjustments to environmental conditions to subsequent generations, and that the gametic alterations may be mediated by the gonadal environment.

At this point, the range of environmental exigencies that would meet the criteria for transgenerational epigenetic transmission in humans is open. The effects on growth of nutrient restriction are experimentally substantiated in several nonhuman species. Drought and famines have been common, if unpredictable, occurrences throughout human history, and the relatively protracted period of human growth would provide conditions favoring anticipation of hardship. Given the secular trends in more affluent societies with respect to both the onset of puberty and overall size among humans (e.g., Tanner, 1990) that are coincident with more reliable nutrient availability and disease prevention, it would seem that a fairly strong case has already been made for epigenetic transmission of the regulation of human growth. The Swedish data suggest that pathways related to energy metabolism are another area in which transgenerational transmission of epigenetic adjustments may be expected.

With respect to the effects of context on mental processing, although speculative, it is conceivable that the human tendency to reflect on "how things are done" and to entertain alternative scenarios—"what if?"—could be influenced by the experiences of prior generations. Given the wide range of habitats that humans occupy and the fact that, although migration is a frequent event, there is a tendency to remain in one's home territory, certain resource-related features of an environment could influence how individuals respond to available information. If the range of resources in a habitat is limited, and when resource acquisition involves risk and demands substantial expenditures of energy and time to yield just-adequate returns, this context might favor a bias against speculation or exploration of new ways to adjust—thinking of what "might be"—and favor a tendency toward doing things "the way it's always been done," thereby avoiding the risk of either immediate physical harm or of longer-term physiological challenge.

Another scenario, analogous to studies of early experience in animals, involves the effects of ancestral experience on affective responses to social encounters with strangers. In many species, messages transmitted via eggs prepare offspring for the probability of encountering predators (e.g., Agrawal et al., 1999). In vertebrates, prenatal signals to the developing young via maternal exposure to predators (Shine & Downes, 1999) or conspecific competitors (Dioniak, French, & Holekamp, 2006) also prepare offspring for appropriate postnatal responsiveness. In the case of humans, the most clearly documented, variable threats relate to confrontations by *nonkin conspecifics*—cycles of conquest and subjugation. Insofar as these cycles are not readily predictable and different populations may enjoy positions of power—or slavery— for multiple generations, this would seem a likely context for anticipatory behavioral adjustments, such as caution in social encounters. Thus, certain features of "temperament," such as cautiousness or boldness—tendencies to approach exchanges with strangers as hazardous or benign—are likely candidates for transgenerational, epigenetic transmission.

The facts that evidence of genetic allelic variation can account for (some) individual differences in temperament in humans (Van Gestel et al., 2002) and that there are strain differences in responses to early experience in rodents (Holmes et al., 2005) raise the issue of the criteria that can be used to distinguish individual differences inherited via epigenetic modifications from those attributable to allelic variation.

DISTINGUISHING EPIGENETIC FROM MENDELIAN INHERITANCE

Epigenetic inheritance can be distinguished from Mendelian inheritance and genetic imprinting in several ways: First, the pattern of inheritance should vary according to the historical experiences of parent(s): If a (grand)parent were exposed to a relevant exigency, then in the subsequent absence of the precipitating condition, the (same-sex) offspring of that individual should not only behave similarly, but, within the same population, (same-sex) grandoffspring should also differ consistently from (same-sex) children whose (grand)parent(s) were not so exposed. Second, epigenetically transmitted differences should be related to conditions affecting a (grand)parent during a restricted time window (e.g., for (grand)mothers, prenatally through the third year; for (grand)fathers, during the slow growth period).

To the extent that there are gender differences in adjustments—as long as there is outbreeding with individuals whose lineages were not so exposed—additional features will distinguish epigenetic inheritance: If transmission is maternal, via the egg, (same-sex) cousins in a matriline should be more alike than their counterparts in a patriline. Comparable gender-specific patrilineal similarities would be expected for male transmission, via sperm. Pembrey and colleagues' (2006) report indicates that the pathways may be complex: The message transmitted from (grand) mother to son may differ from the message transmitted from (grand) father to son and may be expressed only in (grand)daughters and (grand) sons, respectively.

Although imprinting might account for some transgenerational, gender-related variations in phenotype, uni- and biparental epigenetic transmission clearly differ further from Mendelian heredity in at least one key dimension: In most cases, insofar as they involve adjustments that can be "costly" under less threatening circumstances, these adjustments tend to diminish in intensity across generations in the absence of the precipitating conditions. Thus, they should be distinguishable from possibly imprinted traits, in that lineage-related differences would diminish or disappear after three or more generations.

Several points discussed earlier have potentially important implications for those seeking to overcome the effects of hardship or similar events on a (sub)population. First of all, as illustrated by the continuing secular trends in the onset of puberty, birthweights, and adult size of (advantaged) human populations, it is possible that some epigenetically transmitted, restrictive adjustments may, when conditions persist, accumulate in an "additive" manner. Thus, it may take amelioration across multiple generations to reverse a trend or condition fully. Second, from work with animals, there is the real possibility that the context provided by allelic variation in other loci may influence this effect; that is, there will be *epistatic* (genetic background) differences in the probability of epigenetic transmission (Rakyan et al., 2003). Thus, it is not realistic to expect everyone to react in the same way—or to overcome a condition equally rapidly. These considerations mean that in evaluating the effectiveness of attempts to compensate for, or to ameliorate, the sequelae of trauma or deprivation, follow-up may have to span more than one generation and also assess the number of prior generations for whom the conditions prevailed. Likewise, follow-up studies will need to be alert to not only individual differences in (Mendelian) inheritance but also the likelihood of gender differences in response to particular interventions.

REFERENCES

Agrawal, A. A., Laforsch, C., & Tollrian, R. (1999). Transgenerational induction of defences in animals and plants. *Nature*, *401*, 60–63.

Alekseev, V., & Lampert, W. (2001). Maternal control of resting-egg production in *Daphnia*. *Nature*, *414*, 899–901.

Anway, M. S., Cupp, A. S., Uzumcu, M., & Skinner, M. K. (2005). Epigenetic transgenerational actions of endocrine disruptors and male fertility. *Science*, *308*, 1466–1469.

Berger, S. (2007). The complex language of chromatin regulation during transcription. *Nature*, *447*, 407–412.

Cameron, N. M., Champagne, F. A., Parent, C., Fish, E. W., Ozaki-Kuroda, K., & Meaney, M. J. (2005). The programming of individual differences in defensive responses and reproductive strategies in the rat through variations in maternal care. *Neuroscience and Biobehavioral Reviews*, *29*, 843–865.

Coplan, J. D., Andrews, M. W., Rosenblum, L. A., Owens, M. J., Friedman, S., Gorman, J. M., et al. (2006). Persistent elevations of cerebrospinal fluid concentrations of corticotropin-releasing factor in adult non-human primates exposed to early-life stressors: Implications for the pathophysiology of mood and anxiety disorders. *Proceedings of the National Academy of Sciences USA*, *93*, 1619–1623.

Cowley, J. J., & Griesel, R. D. (1966). The effect on growth and behaviour of rehabilitating first and second generation low protein rats. *Animal Behaviour*, *14*, 506–517.

Davidson, E. H. (2006). *The regulatory genome*. New York: Academic Press.

Davies, W., Isles, A., Smith, R., Karunadasa, D., Burrmann, D., Humby, T., et al. (2005). *Xlr3b* is a new imprinted candidate for X-linked parent-of-origin effects on cognitive function in mice. *Nature Genetics*, *37*, 625–629.

Davies, W., Isles, A. R., & Wilkinson, L. S. (2005). Imprinted gene expression in the brain. *Neuroscience and Biobehavioral Reviews*, *29*, 421–430.

Diaz, F. J., Wigglesworth, K., & Eppig, J. J. (2007). Oocytes are required for the preantral granulosa cell to cumulus cell transition in mice. *Developmental Biology*, *305*, 300–311.

Dioniak, S. M., French, J. A., & Holekamp, K. E. (2006). Rank-related maternal effects of androgens on behaviour in wild spotted hyenas. *Nature*, *440*, 1190–1193.

Eggan, K., Baldwin, K., Tackett, M., Osborne, J., Gogos, J., Chess, A., et al. (2004). Mice cloned from olfactory sensory neurons. *Nature*, *428*, 44–49.

ENCODE Project Consortium. (2007). Identification and analysis of functional elements in 1% of the human genome by the ENCODE project. *Nature*, *447*, 799–816.

Fazeli, A., & Pewsey, E. (2008). Maternal communication with gametes and embryos: A complex interactome. *Briefings in Functional Genomics and Proteomics*, *7*, 111–118.

Flanagan, J. M., Popendikyte, V., Pozdniakovaite, N., Sobolev, M., Assadzadeh, A., Schumacher, A., et al. (2006). Intra- and interindividual epigenetic variation in human germ cells. *American Journal of Human Genetics*, *79*, 67–84.

Fraga, M. F., Ballestar, E., Paz, M. F., Ropero, S., Setien, F., Ballester, M. L., et al. (2005). Epigenetic differences arise during the lifetime of monozygotic twins. *Proceedings of the National Academy of Sciences USA*, *102*, 10604–10609.

Harper, L. V. (1989). *The nurture of human behavior.* Norwood, NJ: Ablex.

Holmes, A., le Guisquet, A. M., Vogel, E., Millstein, R. A., Leman, S., & Belzung, C. (2005). Early life genetic, epigenetic and environmental factors shaping emotionality in rodents. *Neuroscience and Biobehavioral Reviews*, *29*, 1335–1346.

Huck, U. W., Labov, J. B., & Lisk, R. D. (1987). Food-restricting first generation female hamsters (*Mesocricetus auratus*) affects sex ratios and growth of third generation offspring. *Biology of Reproduction*, *37*, 612–617.

Hughes, T. A. (2006). Regulation of gene expression by alternative untranslated regions. *Trends in Genetics*, *22*, 119–122.

Jablonca, E., & Lamb, M. J. (1995). *Epigenetic inheritance and evolution.* Oxford, UK: Oxford University Press.

Kaati, G., Bygren, L. O., & Edvinsson, S. (2002). Cardiovascular and diabetes mortality determined by nutrition during parents' and grandparents' slow growth period. *European Journal of Human Genetics*, *10*, 682–688.

Kimmins, S., & Sassone-Corsi, P. (2005). Chromatin remodelling and epigenetic features of germ cells. *Nature*, *434*, 583–589.

Krawetz, S. A. (2005). Paternal contribution: New insights and future challenges. *Nature Reviews Genetics*, *6*, 633–642.

Lieberman, D., Tooby, J., & Cosmides, L. (2007). The architecture of human kin detection. *Nature*, *445*, 727–731.

Lott, D. F. (1984). Intraspecific variation in the social systems of wild vertebrates. *Behaviour*, *88*, 266–325.

Makeyev, E. V., & Maniatis, T. (2008). Multilevel regulation of gene expression by microRNAs. *Science*, *319*, 1789–1790.

Martianov, I., Ramadass, A., Barros, A. S., Chow, N., & Akoulitchev, A. (2007). Repression of the human dihydrofolate reductase gene by a noncoding interfering transcript. *Nature*, *445*, 666–670.

Martin, C., Beaujean, N., Brochard, V., Audouard, V., Zink, D., & Debey, P. (2006). Genome restructuring in mouse embryos during reprogramming and early development. *Developmental Biology, 292*, 317–332.

McLinn, C., & Stephens, D. W. (2006). What makes information valuable?: Signal reliability and environmental uncertainty. *Animal Behaviour, 71*, 1119–1129.

Misteli, T. (2007). Beyond the sequence: Cellular organization of genome function. *Cell, 128*, 787–800.

Mousseau, T., & Fox, C. W. (Eds.). (1998). *Maternal effects as adaptations.* New York: Oxford University Press.

Oliveri, P., & Davidson, E. H. (2007). Built to run, not fail. *Science, 315*, 1510–1511.

Pedersen, R. A. (2001). Sperm and mammalian polarity. *Nature, 409*, 473–474.

Pembrey, M., Bygren, L. O., Kaati, G., Edvinsson, S., Northstone, K., Sjostrom, M., et al. (2006). Sex-specific, male-line transgenerational responses in humans. *European Journal of Human Genetics, 14*, 159–166.

Petersen, C., & Soder, O. (2006). The Sertoli cell: A hormonal target and "super" nurse for germ cells that determines testicular size. *Hormone Research, 66*, 153–161.

Plagge, A., Gordon, E., Dean, W., Boiani, R., Cinti, C., Peters, J., et al. (2004). The imprinted signaling protein XL alpha is required for postnatal adaptation to feeding. *Nature Genetics, 8*, 818–826.

Rakyan, V. K., Cong, S., Champ, M. E., Cuthbert, P. C., Morgan, H. D., Luu, K. V. K., et al. (2003). Transgenerational inheritance of epigenetic states at the murine *Axin*^{fu} allele occurs after maternal and paternal transmission. *Proceedings of the National Academy of Sciences USA, 100*, 2538–2543.

Rassoulzadegan, M., Grandjean, V., Gounon, P. Vincent, S., Gillot, I., & Cuzin, F. (2006). RNA-mediated non-Mendelian inheritance of an epigenetic change in the mouse. *Nature, 441*, 469–474.

Salmons, S., & Streiter, F. A. (1976). Significance of impulse activity in the transformation of skeletal muscle type. *Nature, 263*, 30–34.

Sathananthan, A. H., Selvaraj, K., Girijashankar, M. L., Ganesh, V., Selvaraj, P., & Trounson, A. O. (2006). From oogonia to mature oocytes: Inactivation of the maternal centrosome in humans. *Microscopy Research and Technique, 69*, 396–407.

Schier, A. F. (2007). The maternal–zygotic transition: Death and birth of RNAs. *Science, 316*, 406–407.

Shine, R., & Downes, S. J. (1999). Can pregnant lizards adjust their offspring phenotypes to environmental conditions? *Oecologica, 119*, 1–8.

Skuse, D. H., James, R. S., Bishop, D. V. M., Coppin, B., Dalton, P., Aanodt-Leeper, G., et al. (1997). Evidence from Turner's syndrome of an imprinted, X-linked locus affecting cognitive function. *Nature, 387*, 705–708.

Stein A. D., Barnhart, H. X., Hickey, M., Ramakrishnan, U., Schroeder, D. G., & Martorell, R. (2003). Prospective study of protein–energy supplementation early in life and growth in the subsequent generation in Guatemala. *American Journal of Clinical Nutrition, 78*, 162–167.

Stein, A. D., & Lumey, L. H. (2000). The relationship between maternal and offspring birth weights after maternal prenatal famine exposure: The Dutch Famine Birth Cohort Study. *Human Biology*, 72, 641–654.

Tanner, J. M. (1990). *Fetus into man*. Cambridge, MA: Harvard University Press.

Tollrian, R., & Harvell, C. D. (1999). *The ecology and evolution of inducible defenses*. Princeton, NJ: Princeton University Press.

Van Gestel, S., Forsgren, T., Claes, S., Del-Favero, J., van Duijn, C. M., Sluijs, S., et al. (2002). Epistatic effect of genes from the dopamine and serotonin systems on the temperament traits of novelty seeking and harm avoidance. *Molecular Psychiatry*, 7, 448–450.

Weber, B. H., & Depew, D. J. (Eds.). (2003). *Evolution and learning: The Baldwin effect reconsidered*. Cambridge, MA: MIT Press.

Wu, Q., & Suzuki, M. (2006). Parental obesity and overweight affect the body-fat accumulation in offspring: The possible effect of a high-fat diet through epigenetic inheritance. *Obesity Reviews*, 7, 201–208.

Zamenhof, S., van Marthens, E., & Grauel, L. (1971). DNA (cell number) in neonatal brain: Second generation (F2) alteration by maternal (F0) dietary protein restriction. *Science*, 172, 850–851.

3

Brain Networks and Embodiment

OLAF SPORNS

The functioning of the human mind is closely tied to the functioning of the brain, its neurons and connections. Modern neuroscience has made significant progress in unraveling the relationship between neural processes and behavior. Driven by powerful new technologies, the relatively new discipline of cognitive neuroscience is accumulating novel experimental findings at an ever-increasing pace, charting new connections between psychological and cognitive processes, and the activation and operation of specific brain systems. Nothing appears to stand in the way of a complete mechanistic understanding of the workings of the human brain/mind. Some, at one extreme end of the spectrum, have taken the strong philosophical position of *neuroreductionism*, a view that fully substitutes mental phenomena by neural mechanisms, summarized in the catch phrase "You are nothing but a pack of neurons" or, put more eloquently: " 'You,' your joys and your sorrows, your memories and your ambitions, your sense of personal identity and free will, are in fact no more than the behavior of a vast assembly of nerve cells and their associated molecules" (Crick, 1994, p. 3).

Yet the real picture turns out to be significantly more complex than that championed by neuroreductionists. Today, the severe limitations of reductionist approaches to complex systems, particularly those encountered in the life sciences, are felt everywhere. For example, a recent review (Sauer, Heinemann, & Zamboni, 2007) on cellular networks states that "the reductionist approach has successfully identified most of the components and many interactions but, unfortunately, offers no convincing concepts and methods to comprehend how system properties emerge" (p. 550). The authors continue to propose "the pluralism of causes and effects in biological networks is better addressed by observing, through quantitative measures, multiple components simultaneously, and by rigorous data integration with mathematical models" (p. 550), the research program of the emerging discipline of systems biology (Kitano, 2002). The highly interconnected, hierarchical, and dynamic nature of biological systems poses a significant experimental and theoretical challenge, one that is not addressed by the reductionist paradigm.

Nowhere else is the failure of reductionism more evident than in the case of the human mind and brain. The human brain has been called "the most complicated material object in the known universe" (Edelman, 1992, p. 17). In fact, the complexity of the brain extends much beyond that of the physical structure and metabolism of brain tissue. The brain grows and develops over time. The brain gives rise to complex neural dynamics. Furthermore, the brain is embodied. This last facet of brain complexity is particularly salient for the topic of this chapter. The nervous system is part of an organism that in turn is embedded in a physical and social environment. Interactions with this environment leave traces in brain and body that in turn shape future interactions, thus closely binding the organism to its surroundings and constructing its individual developmental and historical "lifeline" (Rose, 1997). A common theme that runs through most aspects of complexity as it relates to the brain is that of *integration*, of neural resources within the brain's many biological components, of information within neurocognitive networks, and of embodied cognition and action within the brain's environment. This chapter provides a brief systems-level perspective on the brain's many ways of achieving effective integration both within the brain itself and between brain and environment. First I examine our current state of knowledge on the architecture of brain networks and discuss briefly what brain networks might tell us about the neural basis of cognition, then sketch out a formal framework for integration that is rooted in statistical information theory, and look at how this framework can be used to understand the integration of information in the brain. Finally, I investigate the important linkages among brain, body, and environment, with a focus on how the framework of information theory might help in understanding embodied cognition.

THE ARCHITECTURE OF BRAIN NETWORKS

What are *brain networks*? Right at the outset, we encounter the difficult question of how *brain networks* or *brain connectivity* should be defined, and once defined, how it should be observed and measured. Connections in the brain have a physical basis in neuroanatomy, and it is this physical or structural aspect of brain networks that I focus on first. However, in addition we must also consider *networks of interactions*, the dynamic links between parts of the brain that are created as a result of brain activity. As we will see, such functional connections depend on structural anatomy, and they create a rich repertoire of functional patterns and context.

The anatomical structure of the brain, in particular the mammalian cerebral cortex, has been a major focus of research since the beginnings of modern neuroscience. Even a cursory look at the brain reveals its networks as intricately structured and shaped by development and evolution. In most nervous systems, particularly those that are more highly evolved, networks exist at multiple spatial scales, ranging from interconnections linking whole-brain regions to patterns of connections within a given brain region, for example, those between cell populations or individual cortical neurons (Swanson, 2003; Zeki, 1993). In the mammalian cerebral cortex, major building blocks are the *cortical column* and *minicolumn* (Mountcastle, 1978, 1997), local collectives or populations of cells that are coupled to each other and maintain connections to columns in other brain regions. Detailed anatomical and physiological studies have revealed many of the basic components and interconnections of cortical microcircuitry, linking a number of distinct cell types across different cortical layers (Douglas & Martin, 2004).

One of the most detailed and comprehensive studies designed to chart the architecture of the human cerebral cortex was carried out 100 years ago by Korbinian Brodmann (1909). Astonishingly, Brodmann's maps, derived from histological examination of human brain slices and resulting in the structural distinction of 44 brain regions (called *Brodmann areas*) remain in use today. Brodmann thought deeply about the functional implications of the existence of histologically distinct regions of cortex, and his own writings express the tension between localizationist and distributionist approaches to the brain. Brodmann saw structural differentiation as a basis for functional localization, but he also realized that segregated regions of the cortex do not operate in isolation. All such brain regions are interconnected by large numbers of neuronal fibers that relay signals over long distances. Although virtually nothing was known in Brodmann's time about how neurons communicate, his views of how mental function might map onto brain structure clearly went beyond those of simple-minded localizationism. Regarding complex mental faculties, he wrote that "one cannot think of their taking place in any other way than through an infinitely complex and involved interaction and cooperation of numerous elementary activities.

... We are dealing with a physiological process extending widely over the whole cortical surface and not a localised function within a specific region" (Brodmann, 1909, quoted in Garey's 1994 translation, p. 255). To paraphrase Brodmann's view in more modern terms, cognitive function emerges from the distributed activity and interaction of multiple cortical centers.

The tension between theories of brain function that focus either on localization or on distributed activity reflects the fact that both principles are in operation. Much experimental evidence suggests that cortical function requires both *segregation* and *integration*. Segregation is linked to specialization, as important correlates of specific functional brain states are found in localized changes of neuronal activity within specialized populations. However, segregated and specialized brain regions and neuronal populations must interact to generate function. Coherent perceptual and cognitive states require the coordinated activation (i.e., the functional *integration*) of very large numbers of neurons within the distributed system of the cerebral cortex (Friston, 2002, 2005; Tononi, Edelman, & Sporns, 1998; Tononi, Sporns, & Edelman, 1994). Segregation and integration are complementary and perhaps to some degree antagonistic principles. Gaining functional specialization through segregation carries the price of dividing up a limited architecture into a number of isolated communities, whereas the price of integration is the partial loss of specialization as communities are subjected to some degree of exogenous input or perturbation. This poses a major challenge for neural information processing, since these complementary demands need to be satisfied within a single and unified processing architecture.

What do we know about the structure of brain networks and their relationship to the workings of the human mind? Perhaps surprisingly, despite rapid progress in functional neuroimaging, the large-scale interregional networks of human cortex remain largely unmapped even today (Sporns, Tononi, & Kötter, 2005). While Brodmann's early histological studies have provided a simple parcellation of the human cortical surface into a small number of brain regions, mounting evidence suggests that the true number of anatomically distinct cortical areas is much greater, perhaps on the order of a few hundred. How these areas are interconnected is largely unknown, due to the lack of reliable, noninvasive fiber-tracing techniques and the sheer complexity and intricacy of cortical fiber pathways. Currently the most promising avenue is provided by diffusion imaging techniques, which are beginning to provide human connectivity maps (Hagmann et al., 2007, 2008; Iturria-Medina et al., 2007). While we do not currently have a map of brain connectivity (the "human connectome"), comprehensive descriptions of anatomical patterns of cortical connectivity have been collated for several other mammalian species (e.g., Felleman & Van Essen, 1991; Scannell, Burns, Hilgetag, O'Neil, & Young, 1999). These datasets offer a unique opportunity to characterize the structure of large-scale brain networks. Brain networks, once they are represented as *graphs* (a set of vertices linked by edges), are mathematical structures that can be analyzed using methods that have also been applied in parallel efforts to map and describe other biological networks (e.g., those of cellular metabolism, gene regulation, or ecology). Many of these methods have historical origins in the social sciences, especially in the analysis of social networks. The scope and sophistication of network analysis in neuroscience still lags far behind the rigorous and quantitative methods developed by social scientists decades ago.

A first series of analyses indicates that the cerebral cortex comprises clusters of densely and reciprocally coupled cortical areas that are globally interconnected (Hilgetag, Burns, O'Neill, Scannell, & Young, 2000; Sporns, Tononi, & Edelman, 2000). Importantly, large-scale cortical networks share some attributes of so-called small-world networks (Watts, 1999; Watts & Strogatz, 1998). *Small-world networks* have rather unique architectures that combine a high degree of local clustering among network elements, with short transmission paths across the network. High clustering indicates that there are coherent communities within the network, while short paths indicate that these communities can also exchange and integrate information effectively. Small-world attributes are found only in networks that are significantly different from random networks, and they appear to be ubiquitous within the natural, social, and technological world (e.g., Albert & Barabási, 2002; Strogatz, 2001). The two main features of small-world networks (high clustering and short path lengths) naturally support cortical segregation and integration (Sporns, Chialvo, Kaiser, & Hilgetag, 2004). A high degree of local clustering in small-world networks is consistent with a high level of local segregation, as high clustering points to the existence of dense local communities. In turn, the capacity to communicate among all their constituent vertices along short paths, measured as the characteristic path length, is consistent with global integration across the entire network. Small-world attributes are also associated with other structural characteristics, such as near-minimal wiring lengths often found in brain networks. Numerous studies (e.g., Chklovskii, Schikorski, & Stevens, 2002) have argued that wiring length must be conserved (perhaps minimized) in development and evolution, as only a limited amount of brain volume is available. Others have suggested that the actual "wiring diagram" found in present-day mammalian brains is actually not minimal but tends to preserve a number of costly long-range projections. Despite their wiring cost, these long-range projections may have been preserved, since they help to minimize the number of processing steps (i.e., the path length) between spatially distant brain regions (Kaiser & Hilgetag, 2006).

So far, we have considered brain networks only as structural entities, that is, networks of physical *wires* (axons, neuronal processes, fiber pathways) that link neurons and brain regions. How does this structural substrate shape the functional interactions as the brain becomes active, either in the course of spontaneous activity or in response to external perturbations that may correspond to stimuli or tasks? Here we must introduce a fundamental distinction among structural, functional, and effective connectivity (Figure 3.1). *Anatomical connectivity* (as discussed earlier) refers to physical or structural (synaptic) connections linking neurons within a network. Anatomical connectivity does not change on shorter timescales (seconds to minutes), but may be plastic or dynamic at longer timescales (hours to days), for example, during learning or development. *Functional connectivity* (Friston, 1994) captures deviations from statistical independence between distributed and often spatially remote neurons or brain regions, for example, by measuring their correlation/covariance, spectral coherence, or phase locking. Functional connectivity is highly time-dependent (on a scale of hundreds of milliseconds), and it typically exhibits characteristic changes between states of rest and functional (task-related) activation. *Effective connectivity* goes beyond functional connectivity, in that it forms a causal network (Büchel

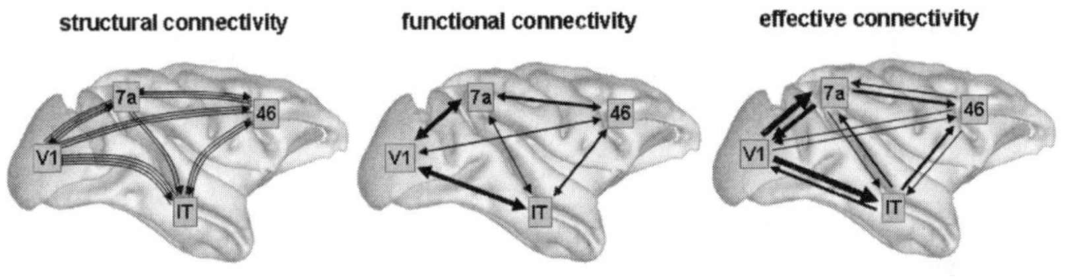

FIGURE 3.1. This diagram illustrates the distinction among structural, functional, and effective connectivity. The image of the brain in this and other figures in this chapter represents the surface of the macaque monkey cerebral cortex, and the boxes mark the positions of four specialized cortical regions: V1, primary visual cortex; 7a, visual cortex in the parietal lobe; IT, visual cortex in the inferior temporal lobe; and 46, an area of prefrontal cortex. In the "structural connectivity" panel these areas are shown to be linked by fiber pathways. In the "functional connectivity" panel these areas are dynamically coupled, indicated by undirected statistical relationships of varying strengths (bidirectional arrows). In the "effective connectivity" panel these areas are affecting each other along directed paths (directional arrows).

& Friston, 2000; Friston, 1994). Causality may be inferred experimentally through perturbations or from time series analysis, by exploiting the fact that causes must precede effects in time. It turns out that causality is a surprisingly slippery concept, and efforts at reconstructing causal effects on the basis of observations of a system's components are facing serious limitations. Nonetheless, some analysis techniques have proven useful in network studies, and I return to causal networks a little later in this chapter.

Functional connectivity is an expression of network interactions, and unlike structural connection patterns, the configuration of functional couplings across the brain changes rapidly over time (Figure 3.2). A growing body of evidence suggests that such network interactions are critical for the emergence of coherent cognitive states and organized behavior. Early experimental work in visual cortex revealed the existence of synchronous coupling both within and between brain regions (Singer & Gray, 1995), and led to numerous theoretical proposals for how such synchronous activity might underlie perceptual phenomena such as grouping, binding, and object segregation (Ross, Grossberg, & Mingolla, 2000; Sporns, Tononi, & Edelman, 1991). Synchrony is one way in which a functional connection may manifest itself, and synchronous or coherent patterns of activity have since been demonstrated across a broad range of cognitive functions, including sensorimotor coordination (Brovelli et al., 2004), attention (Steinmetz et al., 2000), working memory (Sarntheim, Petsche, Rappelsberger, Shaw, & von Stein, 1998), and awareness (Engel & Singer, 2001). Much of this work is carried out by simultaneously recording from multiple sites in the brain, while an animal or human subject is performing a task. Crucially, it has been

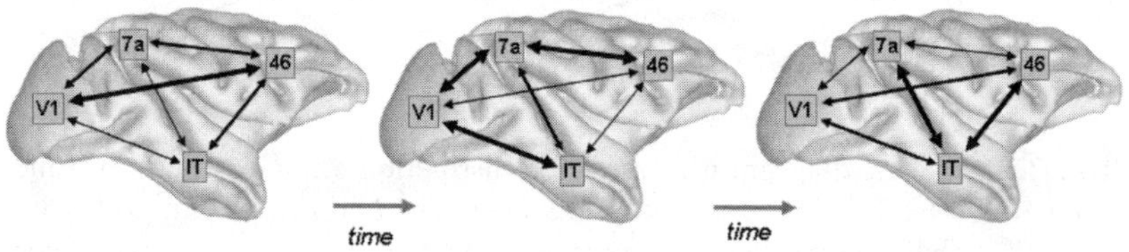

FIGURE 3.2. Functional connectivity (and effective connectivity, not shown) is dynamic and time-dependent. Even in the absence of external inputs, functional brain networks undergo fluctuations due to spontaneous coupling and uncoupling of brain regions, here represented by bidirectional arrows of different widths. This process occurs on multiple timescales, with a lower bound at around 100 milliseconds. In a sense, the dynamic context of each brain region undergoes continual reconfigurations.

shown in a number of experiments that synchrony or coherence is correlated with some measure of behavioral performance, or that the disruption of synchrony degrades a specific perceptual or cognitive task.

Noninvasive methods of observing large-scale brain activity, such as electroencephalography (EEG), magnetoencephalography (MEG), and functional magnetic resonance imaging (fMRI), allow the collection of datasets that cover large portions of the human brain as subjects are engaged in behavior. Functional connectivity analyses of such datasets produce patterns of cross-correlation, synchrony, or coherence that can be conceptualized as undirected graphs. The edges of these graphs represent the presence and absence or, in some cases, the strengths of the statistical relationships between the linked vertices. Studies of patterns of functional connectivity (based on coherence or correlation) among cortical regions have demonstrated that functional brain networks exhibit small-world (Achard, Salvador, Whitcher, Suckling, & Bullmore, 2006; Bassett, Meyer-Lindenberg, Achard, Duke, & Bullmore, 2007; Salvador et al., 2005; Stam, 2004) and scale-free properties (Eguiluz et al., 2005). Functional connectivity patterns change as task conditions are varied (Bassett et al., 2007), and they show often characteristic alterations in the course of brain dysfunction and disease (Stam, Jones, Nolte, Breakspear, & Scheltens, 2007). Characteristically, functional connectivity patterns measured for any given task or stimulus include a large portion of the brain and a wide range of brain regions, often going beyond those regions thought to be central for the task. This has led to the idea that functions of brain regions are partly defined by *neural context*, the pattern of activity elsewhere in the brain (McIntosh, 2000, 2004). This neural context is highly dynamic and variable, depending on endogenous brain activity (driven by internal causes), as well as external perturbations (e.g., sensory stimuli or varying task conditions).

Functional connectivity is of interest not just in association with behavioral or cognitive tasks. Numerous studies of functional connectivity in the human brain have revealed that the brain is continually active even “at rest” (i.e., when a human subject is awake and alert but does not engage in any specific cognitive or behavioral task (Buckner, Andrews-Hanna, & Schacter, 2008; Gusnard & Raichle, 2001). These observations raise the possibility that this “cortical resting state” may be much more than a “noisy background” that can and should be subtracted away, that it may contribute to cognitive processing. In this view, mental function may emerge from the interaction of exogenous perturbations (stimuli, motor activity) and endogenous spontaneous dynamics. The structural anatomy of the brain may play a unique role in shaping spontaneous dynamics, and individual differences in structural connections due to genetic factors and developmental history may contribute to individual differences in cognitive and behavioral performance. Systems-level modeling of the cortical resting state suggests that structural connections can shape functional connectivity patterns at multiple timescales (Honey, Kötter, Breakspear, & Sporns, 2007), and that variations in structural connections lead to changes in functional connectivity patterns.

To summarize this section of the chapter, the architecture of brain networks is highly nonrandom, expressing a variety of structural attributes that include high clustering and short path lengths indicative of small-world architectures. While individual brain regions may be specialized and segregated, their functional integration is essential to support human cognition. Small-world anatomical networks provide a structural substrate within which the interplay between segregation and integration can take place. As brain networks engage in endogenously or exogenously driven activity, they generate functional and effective connectivity patterns that are highly dynamic, even when the brain is seemingly at rest.

FROM NETWORKS TO INFORMATION

Earlier I defined *functional* and *effective connectivity* as patterns of statistical dependencies between variables. Statistical dependencies directly relate to shared information. Thus, functional and effective connectivity essentially quantify how information is distributed and integrated within a network. Most measures of functional connectivity (i.e., patterns of statistical dependence between often remote neural units or brain regions; Friston, 1994) build on statistical information theory (Cover & Thomas, 1991; Papoulis, 1991). I argue in this chapter that information theory can provide a formal framework for mapping network and contextual influences across a broad range of applications, including networks within and between brains. At this point I need to introduce a few core notions of information theory to provide a foundation for the last sections of the chapter.

For the following definitions, let us consider a system X that comprises a set of units, which could represent brain regions or single neurons, that is generating observable dynamics. Let us further assume that we can record their activity, and that we possess a way to calculate the entropies of the units. This last assumption is rather crucial, as the calculation of valid entropies from real-world data presents numerous, often insurmountable, challenges. Entropy is the very foundation of information theory, and all informational measures defined here build on it. As defined by Shannon and Weaver (1949; based on the earlier definition by Boltzmann), entropy is high if a variable occupies many states in its available state space with equal probability: In that case, an observation of the variable in one state provides high amounts of information. In this formulation, entropy is a statistical concept, its estimation from observed data is subject to sampling problems, and it is sensitive to the choice of state space. While entropy may be hard to estimate, this does not undermine its fundamental importance for physical and informational systems (doubters are referred to the second law of thermodynamics).

Mutual information between two units *A* and *B* is defined as the difference between the sum of their individual entropies and their joint entropy. Mutual information will be zero if no statistical relationship exists between *A* and *B* (i.e., if *A* and *B* behave statistically independently). Mutual information expresses the amount of information that the observation of one unit conveys about the other unit. In the case of statistical independence, observing the state of one unit provides no information about the state of the other. Mutual information is, in some sense, a generalized correlation. Unlike correlation, which is a linear measure of association between variables, mutual information captures all linear and nonlinear relationships.

Importantly, mutual information does not capture causal effects between variables. Such causal effects can be estimated with a related measure, *transfer entropy* (Schreiber, 2000), which is designed to detect "directed" information exchange or coupling between two elements or parts of a system. Essentially, transfer entropy captures the degree to which observation of one variable improves the prediction of the time evolution of another variable. Numerous other approaches to extracting causality exist (cf. Lungarella, Ishiguro, Kuniyoshi, & Otsu, 2007), each with its own set of strengths and weaknesses.

While mutual information captures the degree of statistical dependence between two units (or subsets of units), the integration of a system measures the total amount of statistical dependence among an arbitrarily large set of units (Tononi et al., 1994). Integration can be viewed as the *multivariate generalization of mutual information*, defined as the difference between the sum of the entropies of the individual units and their joint entropy. Similar to mutual information, integration may be viewed as the error one makes given the assumption of independence between all variables. Note further that like mutual information, integration is always positive. If all elements are statistically independent, their joint entropy is exactly equal to the sum of the elements' individual entropies. Any amount of statistical dependence between the elements will express itself in a reduction of the elements' joint entropy and thus in a positive value for integration.

Integration can be used to quantify the amount of statistical structure present at multiple scales within a given system. This would allow us to measure the extent to which a system is both functionally segregated (small subsets of the system tend to behave independently) and functionally integrated (large subsets tend to behave coherently). A statistical measure, called *neural complexity*, that combines segregation and integration was proposed by Tononi and colleagues (1994). The complexity of a system is high when, on average, the mutual information between any subset of the system and its complement is high. High mutual information between a subset and a complementary part of the system may be interpreted as a *meaningful context*, a contextual relation across different portions of an integrated system. To say it differently, the context for any given subset is not disconnected (zero mutual information) but rather is integrated (high mutual information)—by inference, the subset is sensitive to changes that occur in other parts of the system rather than forming an isolated module. Thus, complexity emerges when rich and dynamic contextual influences prevail, and complexity is low when context is either unrelated (as in systems that engage in random activity) or homogenous (as in systems that are highly regular; see Figure 3.3). The hierarchical nature of this measure of complexity spanning all levels of scale within the system is inherently well suited for a system such as the brain, which is characterized by "granularity" at several different levels, ranging from single neurons to brain regions. Extensions of complexity take into account the relation of internal patterns to external (environmental) statistics (e.g., Tononi, Sporns, & Edelman, 1996).

The definition of these measures of information opens up an interesting perspective on how structural and functional connectivity may be related. If we fix key aspects of the dynamics (e.g., by enforcing a high value of integration or complexity) and then search for structural connection patterns that give rise to this type of dynamics, what relationship, if any, do we find? For example, what kinds of structural connection patterns are associated with high values for integration or complexity? What is the role of context in generating high complexity? One way to address this question is to use information-theoretical measures of functional connectivity, such as entropy, integration, or complexity, as cost functions in simulations designed to optimize network architectures. As it turns out, networks that are optimized for high complexity develop structural motifs that are very similar to those observed in real cortical connection matrices (Sporns et al., 2000; Sporns & Tononi, 2002), whereas networks that are optimized for entropy or integration do not resemble the brain. Networks optimized for complexity exhibit an abundance of reciprocal (reentrant) connections, a strong tendency to form clusters, and they have short characteristic path lengths. While it is

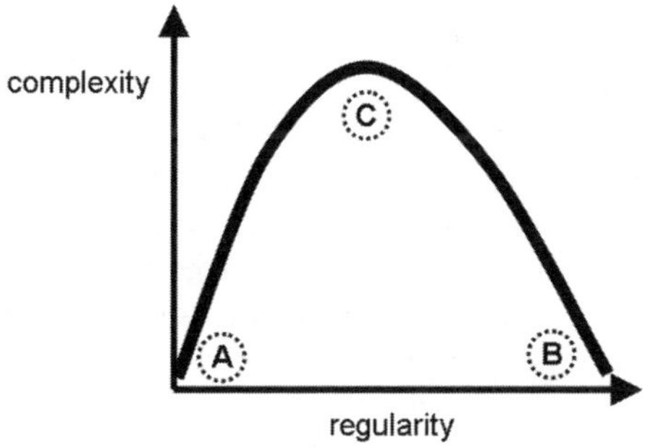

FIGURE 3.3. A schematic diagram of how complexity, as defined by Tononi and colleagues (1994), depends on the degree to which elements of a system are expressing regular patterns. Systems that exhibit no regularities whatsoever (A; i.e., display random dynamics) have low complexity. Their internal mutual information tends to be very low because in random systems, one part of the system cannot have any information about the present or future state of any other part. In other words, there is no contextual influence on the state of a part of the system by way of any other part. A system (B) that is in lockstep (i.e., completely regular in its dynamical evolution) will display some mutual information, but this information will be identical across all partitions. All parts of the system are copies of each other, and their contextual influence is therefore highly stereotypical. The complexity of such a system is low. Finally, a system (C) that combines some degree of local specialization with a degree of global integration will display a mixture of randomness (or variability) and regularity. Here, mutual information will be high across many partitions, and the context will be rich and differentiated. Many parts of the system influence many other parts in many different ways.

computationally expensive to employ most types of nonlinear dynamics in the context of such optimizations, a closer examination of specific connection topologies (sparse, uniform and clustered, or cortex-like) that are simulated as nonlinear systems has shown that the association of small-world attributes and complex functional dynamics can hold for more realistic models of cortical architectures as well (Sporns & Zwi, 2004). Thus, high complexity, a measure of global statistical features and of functional connectivity, appears to be strongly and uniquely associated with the emergence of small-world networks (Sporns, 2006; Sporns et al., 2004).

Evolutionary algorithms for growing connectivity patterns have been used in evolving motor controllers (Psujek, Ames, & Beer, 2006), as well as in the context of sensorimotor coordination (Seth, 2005; Seth & Edelman, 2004). While many current applications, for example, those used in evolutionary robotics, rely on small networks with limited connectivity patterns (due to constraints requiring the convergence of evolutionary algorithms in finite computational time), the gap to larger, more brain-like networks is rapidly closing. An exciting future avenue for computational research in this area involves the evolution of behaviorally capable architectures that incorporate features of biological organization. Results from this research may ultimately contribute to resolving long-standing controversies, such as whether biological evolution inherently tends toward biological structures of greater and greater complexity. Initial studies of evolving connectivity patterns embedded in simulated creatures within a computational ecology (Yaeger & Sporns, 2006) suggest that as econiches become more demanding, neural architectures evolve toward greater structural elaboration, elevated levels of plasticity, and with functional activity patterns of higher neural complexity.

Finally, it has been suggested that the capacity of networks to integrate information, which, as I discussed earlier, is associated with high levels of complexity, is a necessary prerequisite for the emergence of consciousness (Tononi & Edelman, 1998). Tononi (2004) has developed a theoretical framework and a set of explicit measures (Tononi & Sporns, 2003) that in principle allows the quantification of the capacity of a network to integrate information, provided its connectivity structure is known. The measure evaluates maximal causal information flow within the network by charting the effects of perturbations on subsets of the network. The theory makes a range of predictions about the different degrees to which neural architectures are capable of integrating information. Here again, distributed and contextual influences of parts of a system on other parts are crucial: High levels of integration of information require that the state of any subset of a system be sensitive to changes in the state of the system elsewhere (i.e., sensitive to context).

In summary, network interactions can be formally described by using concepts from statistical information theory, for example, mutual information, integration, and complexity. Some of these measures allow us to characterize statistical interactions in a network as a whole. When structural connections are arranged in such a way as to maximize some of these informational quantities, it appears that complexity is uniquely associated with structural patterns that resemble those of brain networks. This result is consistent with the theoretical idea that brain networks balance *segregation* and *integration*, which we defined as complexity. High complexity allows networks to integrate efficiently large amounts of information, a capacity that has been linked to consciousness.

INFORMATION AND EMBODIMENT

So far, I have discussed the architecture of brain networks and how this architecture might be linked to informational processes carried out within and between brain regions. I have taken a large-scale view, looking at the whole brain at once, and attempting to characterize networks of interactions between the brain's components. The ubiquity of interactions among brain regions and their empirically documented central role in cognition naturally leads to a view of brain function in which global context is equally as important as local functionality.

In this final section, I expand this view further to take into account the interactions between brain, body, and environment. This leads into a very brief discussion of embodied cognition. Most theories of *embodied cognition* are based on the notion that brain, body, and environment are dynamically interactive, and that coherent, coordinated, or intelligent behavior is at least in part the result of this interaction (Chiel & Beer, 1997; Iida, Pfeifer, Steels, & Kuniyoshi, 2004; Sporns, 2003). According to embodied cognition, cognitive function, including its development, cannot be understood without making reference to interactions between brain, body, and environment (Thelen & Smith, 1994; Varela, Thompson, & Rosch, 1991). Body morphology and sensorimotor activity have special roles to play in this process. For example, sensor morphology has a direct role to play in the way a nervous system receives and processes information. Sensorimotor activity, and the specific patterns by which an agent interacts with its environment, has been shown to introduce into the agent's sensory input constraints and patterns that can be exploited for learning (Lungarella, Pegors, Bulwinkle, & Sporns, 2005; Nolfi, 2002; Scheier, Pfeifer, & Kuniyoshi, 1998). Experiments have shown that the active manipulation of objects by adult human subjects can promote perceptual learning and object recognition (Harman, Humphrey, & Goodale, 1999). In the nervous system, it is known to be easier for neural circuits to process and learn about sensory data containing informational regularities, by stabilizing neural connections that capture recurrent statistical features. This important aspect of embodiment becomes even more salient from a developmental perspective. Embodiment of an agent can generate correlations and redundancies across multiple sensory modalities that lead to a disambiguation of the sensory input and to a reduction of the effective dimensionality of the sensory space, supporting concept formation, categorization, and other high-level cognitive processes (Thelen & Smith, 1994). Embodied intelligence in humans develops as children grow in and interact with the environment through a sensory-rich body that is particularly adapted to recognize statistical regularities (Smith & Gasser, 2005). Despite the central importance of brain–body–environment interactions, little has been done to develop a theoretical and quantitative framework that would allow the identification and mapping of dynamic brain–body–environment interrelationships. In the remainder of this chapter, I outline some initial steps toward such a framework. Essentially, I adopt some of the theoretical concepts that were originally developed for studying brain networks and apply them to networks of interactions among sensory, neural, and motor variables.

One way to approach embodiment is through the use of computational models or robotic implementations. Numerous such models have been constructed to help identify principles of autonomous development in embodied agents (reviewed in Lungarella, Metta, Pfeifer, & Sandini, 2003). For example, robotic models have been employed to study the role of embodiment in the development of neural circuits involved in object recognition (Almassy, Edelman, & Sporns, 1998; Wyss, Konig, & Verschure, 2006), learning (Verschure, Voegtlin, & Douglas, 2003), and reward conditioning (Alexander & Sporns, 2003). In all these studies, environmental context turned out to provide important constraints that guided the formation of neural connections and units that were optimally adapted for operating within their surroundings. These contextual effects were not well captured in simulations that did not include actual interactions between the agent and the environment (i.e., simulations that did not explicitly include continuous sensorimotor coupling).

The importance of coupling sensory inputs, neural signals, and motor outputs in a single system pointed to a fundamental principle of embodied cognition. The dynamical coupling between brain, body, and environment in an embodied system has consequences for the structure of information *within* the agent's *control architecture* (its brain). More precisely, embodied interactions actively shape inputs (i.e., statistical patterns that serve as inputs to the agent's brain). To say it even more simply, outputs shape inputs just as much as inputs shape outputs, and for this simple reason the brain is not autonomous, but depends on embodied interactions for structured information. Embodied systems are informationally bound to their surroundings, and the statistical interactions within their brain networks are subject to influences that result from these network's actions in the real world.

To approach this issue from a modeling perspective and to evaluate appropriate formal frameworks, Max Lungarella and I investigated the role of embodied interactions in actively structuring the sensory inputs of embodied agents (robots) (Lungarella et al., 2005; Lungarella & Sporns, 2006; for related approaches, see also Klyubin, Polani, & Nehaniv, 2005; Philipona, O'Regan, & Nadal, 2003). We found that coordinated and dynamically coupled sensorimotor activity induced quantifiable changes in sensory information, including decreased entropy and increased mutual information, integration, and complexity within specific regions of sensory space. We were able to plot these changes by comparing two different sets of systems. In one set, sensorimotor coupling was unperturbed, "naturally" leading to well-coordinated behavior. In the other set, we disabled the link between sensory inputs and motor outputs by substituting motor time series from another experiment, thus decoupling motor outputs from their sensory consequences. When comparing these two sets of systems, we found that intact sensorimotor coupling led to greater amounts of information in most sensors, which in turn could benefit the operation of brain networks. This additional information was not contained in the stimulus itself; it was created by the sensorimotor interaction—effectively allowing the system to go "beyond the information given." On the basis of these studies, we proposed that active structuring of sensory information may be a fundamental principle of embodied systems, supporting a range of psychological processes, such as perceptual categorization, multimodal sensory integration, and sensorimotor coordination.

The notion of brain–body–environment interaction implicitly (or explicitly) refers to causal effects. Somewhat simplistically, we may take a minimally but effectively embodied system as one in which sensory inputs causally affect motor outputs, and these motor outputs in turn causally affect sensory inputs. Such *perception–action loops* may be viewed as fundamental building blocks for learning and development in embodied systems. As dynamic structures, we would expect such loops to be intermittent and transient, waxing and waning in the course of behavior, and linking sensory and motor events at specific timescales. Thus, mapping causal relations between sensory and motor states is likely to uncover networks that involve specific subsets of sensory and motor units localized in time.

We applied a set of measures designed to extract undirected and directed informational exchanges among coupled systems, such as brain, body, and environment (Lungarella & Sporns, 2006). We found that there exist patterns of noncausal, as well as causal, relations that can be mapped between a variety of sensory and motor variables sampled by two morphologically different robotic platforms (a humanoid robot and a mobile quadruped). We demonstrated that causal information structure can be measured at various levels of the robots' control architectures, and that the extracted causal structure can be a useful quantitative tool to reveal the pattern and strength of embodied interactions. We also examined the relation of information to body morphology. Using a simulated system, and varying the spatial arrangement and density of photoreceptors on a simulated retina, we found that different morphological arrangements resulted in different patterns and quantities of information flow. This indicates that information processing within the control architecture (e.g., the brain) depends on not only sensorimotor interactions but also body morphology, for example, the physical arrangement of sensory surfaces and motor structures.

In this section I have argued that embodiment is not only a crucial ingredient in development and cognition but it is also capable of structuring information that is available to the brain, and hence capable of shaping information processing and brain dynamics. This view leads to the prediction that internal functional couplings between brain regions are subtly influenced by perturbations generated via inputs from the environment, which in turn may be the result of embodied sensorimotor activity (Figure 3.4). Brain processes are thus not only dependent on other brain processes but also are crucially shaped by embodiment, which generates a rich set of perturbations across multiple timescales, from immediate effects due to motor activity to much more complex effects, for example, those due to social interactions.

MIND IN CONTEXT

Many complex systems comprise large numbers of components that engage in dynamic interactions and give rise to emergent phenomena (Sporns, 2007). The brain is no exception: One could argue that the nested hierarchical structure of brain systems, their propensity for spon-

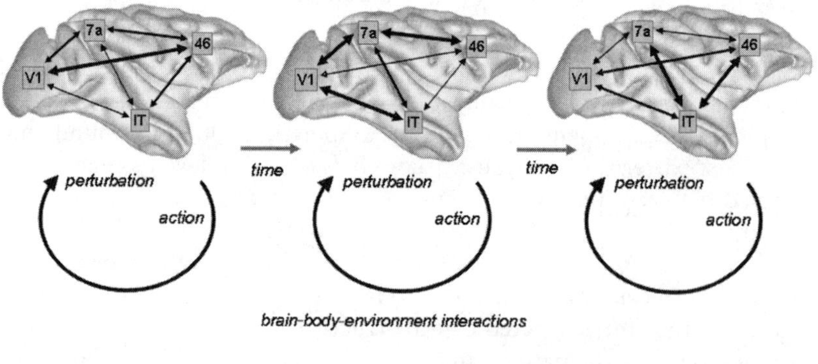

FIGURE 3.4. Functional connectivity can change as a result of external perturbations. Such perturbations, in turn, may be generated via brain–body–environment interactions.

taneous and exogenously driven nonlinear dynamics, and their embeddedness within a behaving organism, presents unique challenges to our attempts to understand how the brain/mind works. The reductionist paradigm, while providing much-needed information on individual components and processes, cannot succeed in formulating a viable theory of how nervous systems function. Key ingredients of such a theory must address how mental or cognitive processes emerge from the interactions of large populations of neurons in distributed brain regions *and* how these interactions are shaped by the dynamic interplay of brain, body, and environment.

Clearly, the notion of context is crucial in this endeavor. We encounter powerful contextual influences everywhere in the brain/mind system. Neural context shapes the operation of individual brain regions, defining their functionality at least as much as their intrinsic circuitry. Embodiment creates its own set of contextual influences, as sensorimotor activity regulates and structures information flow from the environment to the brain. A promising formal framework for contextual influences in complex systems is provided by statistical information theory. Applications of information theory are gaining momentum in the analysis of recordings of large-scale brain activity, in models of information integration and consciousness, and in new empirical approaches to embodied cognition.

If the brain/mind is fundamentally (and not merely coincidentally) contextual in nature, then our approach to such a system through empirical research and modeling may need revision. For example, autonomous behavior is marginalized in much of cognitive neuroscience, in particular in functional neuroimaging because of technical requirements that essentially immobilize all subjects. In neural modeling, very few approaches target the integrated behavior of neural systems at the large scale, or take into account the embodied perspective, for example, by allowing for continuity in inputs and outputs via sensorimotor coupling. Novel integrative approaches are needed to help elucidate the many ways in which context shapes the structure and function of the human brain and mind.

REFERENCES

Achard, S., Salvador, R., Whitcher, B., Suckling, J., & Bullmore, E. (2006). A resilient, low-frequency, small-world human brain functional network with highly connected association cortical hubs. *Journal of Neuroscience*, *26*, 63–72.

Albert, R., & Barabási, A.-L. (2002). Statistical mechanics of complex networks. *Reviews of Modern Physics*, *74*, 47–97.

Alexander, W., & Sporns, O. (2003). An embodied model of reward conditioning. *Adaptive Behavior, 11*(2), 143–159.

Almassy, N., Edelman, G. M., & Sporns, O. (1998). Behavioral constraints in the development of neuronal properties: A cortical model embedded in a real-world device. *Cerebral Cortex, 8*, 346–361.

Bassett, D. S., Meyer-Lindenberg, A., Achard, S., Duke, T., & Bullmore, E. (2006). Adaptive reconfiguration of fractal small-world human brain functional networks. *Proceedings of the National Academy of Sciences USA, 103*, 19518–19523.

Brovelli, A., Ding, M., Ledberg, A., Chen, Y., Nakamura, R., & Bressler, S. L. (2004). Beta oscillations in a large-scale sensorimotor cortical network: Directional influences revealed by Granger causality. *Proceedings of the National Academy of Sciences USA, 101*, 9849–9854.

Büchel, C., & Friston, K. J. (2000). Assessing interactions among neuronal systems using functional neuroimaging. *Neural Networks, 13*, 871–882.

Buckner, R. L., Andrews-Hanna, J. R., & Schacter, D. L. (2008). The brain's default network: Anatomy, function, and relevance to disease. *Annals of the New York Academy of Sciences, 1124*, 1–38.

Chiel, H. J., & Beer, R. D. (1997). The brain has a body: Adaptive behaviour emerges from interactions of nervous system, body, and environment. *Trends in Neurosciences, 20*, 553–557.

Chklovskii, D., Schikorski, T., & Stevens, C. (2002). Wiring optimization in cortical circuits. *Neuron, 34*, 341–347.

Cover, T. M., & Thomas, J. A. (1991). *Elements of information theory.* New York: Wiley.

Crick, F. (1994). *The astonishing hypothesis: The scientific search for the soul.* New York: Scribner's.

Douglas, R., & Martin, K. (2004). Neuronal circuits of the neocortex. *Annual Review of Neuroscience, 27*, 419–451.

Edelman, G. M. (1992). *Bright air, brilliant fire.* New York: Basic Books.

Eguiluz, V. M., Chialvo, D. R., Cecchi, G. A., Baliki, M., & Apkarian, A. V. (2005). Scale-free brain functional networks. *Physical Review Letters, 94*, 018102.

Engel, A. K., & Singer, W. (2001). Temporal binding and the neural correlates of sensory awareness. *Trends in Cognitive Sciences, 5*, 16–25.

Felleman, D. J., & Van Essen, D. C. (1991). Distributed hierarchical processing in the primate cerebral cortex. *Cerebral Cortex, 1*, 1–47.

Friston, K. J. (1994). Functional and effective connectivity in neuroimaging: A synthesis. *Human Brain Mapping, 2*, 56–78.

Friston, K. J. (2002). Beyond phrenology: What can neuroimaging tell us about distributed circuitry? *Annual Review of Neuroscience, 25*, 221–250.

Friston, K. J. (2005). Models of brain function in neuroimaging. *Annual Review of Psychology, 56*, 57–87.

Garey, L. J. (1994). *Brodmann's localization in the cerebral cortex.* London: Smith-Gordon.

Gusnard, D., & Raichle, M. E. (2001). Searching for a baseline: Functional imaging and the resting human brain. *Nature Reviews Neuroscience, 2*, 685–694.

Hagmann, P., Cammoun, L., Gigandet, X., Meuli, R., Honey, C. J., Wedeen, V.J., et al. (2008). Mapping the structural core of human cerebral cortex. *PLoS Biology, 6*, e159.

Hagmann, P., Kurant, M., Gigandet, X., Thiran, P., Wedeen, V. J., Meuli, R., et al. (2007). Mapping human whole-brain structural networks with diffusion MRI. *PLoS ONE, 2*(7), e597.

Harman, K. L., Humphrey, G. K., & Goodale, M. A. (1999). Active manual control of object views facilitates visual recognition. *Current Biology, 9*, 1315–1318.

Hilgetag, C. C., Burns, G. A., O'Neill, M. A., Scannell, J. W., & Young, M. P. (2000). Anatomical connectivity defines the organization of clusters of cortical areas in the macaque monkey and the cat. *Philosophical Transactions of the Royal Society of London B, 355*, 91–110.

Honey, C. J., Kötter, R., Breakspear, M., & Sporns, O. (2007). Network structure of cerebral cortex shapes functional connectivity on multiple time scales. *Proceedings of the National Academy of Sciences USA, 104*, 10240–10245.

Iida, F., Pfeifer, R., Steels, L., & Kuniyoshi, Y. (Eds.). (2004). *Embodied artificial intelligence*. Berlin: Springer-Verlag.

Iturria-Medina, Y., Canales-Rodriguez, E. J., Melia-Garcia, L., Valdes-Hernandez, P. A., Martinez-Montes, E., Aleman-Gomez, Y., et al. (2007). Characterizing brain anatomical connections using diffusion weighted MRI and graph theory. *NeuroImage, 36*, 645–660.

Kaiser, M., & Hilgetag, C. C. (2006). Nonoptimal component placement, but short processing paths, due to long-distance projections in neural systems. *PLoS Computational Biology, 2*, e95.

Kitano, H. (2002). Systems biology: A brief overview. *Science, 295*, 1662–1664.

Klyubin, A. S., Polani, D., & Nehaniv, C. L. (2005). Empowerment: A universal agent-centric measure of control. *Proceedings of the Congress on Evolutionary Computation 2005*, 128–135.

Lungarella, M., Ishiguro, K., Kuniyoshi, Y., & Otsu, N. (2007). Methods for quantifying the casual structure of bivariate times series. *International Journal of Bifurcation and Chaos, 17*(3), 903–921.

Lungarella, M., Metta, G., Pfeifer, R., & Sandini, G. (2003). Developmental robotics: A survey. *Connection Science, 15*, 151–190.

Lungarella, M., Pegors, T., Bulwinkle, D., & Sporns, O. (2005). Methods for quantifying the information structure of sensory and motor data. *Neuroinformatics, 3*(3), 243–262.

Lungarella, M., & Sporns, O. (2006). Mapping information flow in sensorimotor networks. *PLoS Computational Biology*, 2e144.

McGill, W. (1954). Multivariate information transmission. *Psychometrika, 19*, 97–116.

McIntosh, A. R. (2000). Towards a network theory of cognition. *Neural Networks, 13*, 861–870.

McIntosh, A. R. (2004). Contexts and catalysts. *Neuroinformatics, 2*, 175–181.

Mountcastle, V. B. (1978). An organizing principle for cerebral function. In G. M. Edelman & V. B. Mountcastle (Eds.), *The mindful brain* (pp. 7–50). Cambridge, MA: MIT Press.

Mountcastle, VB (1997). The columnar organization of the neocortex. *Brain, 120*, 701–722.

Nolfi, S. (2002). The power and limit of reactive agents. *Neurocomputing, 49*, 119–145.

Papoulis, A. (1991). *Probability, random variables, and stochastic processes.* New York: McGraw-Hill.

Philipona, D., O'Regan, J. K., & Nadal, J.-P. (2003). Is there something out there?: Inferring space from sensorimotor dependencies. *Neural Computation, 15*(9), 2029–2050.

Psujek, S., Ames, J., & Beer, R. D. (2006). Connection and coordination: The interplay between architecture and dynamics in evolved model pattern generators. *Neural Computation, 18*, 729–747.

Rose, S. (1997). *Lifelines: Biology beyond determinism.* New York: Oxford University Press.

Ross, W. D., Grossberg, S., & Mingolla, E. (2000). Visual cortical mechanisms of perceptual grouping: Interacting layers, networks, columns, and maps. *Neural Networks, 13*, 571–588.

Salvador, R., Suckling, J., Coleman, M., Pickard, J. D., Menon, D. K., & Bullmore, E. T. (2005). Neurophysiological architecture of functional magnetic resonance images of human brain. *Cerebral Cortex, 15*, 1332–1342.

Sarntheim, J., Petsche, H., Rappelsberger, P., Shaw, G. L., & von Stein, A. (1998). Synchronization between prefrontal and posterior association cortex during human working memory. *Proceedings of the National Academy of Sciences USA, 95*, 7092–7096.

Sauer, U., Heinemann, M., & Zamboni, N. (2007). Genetics: Getting closer to the whole picture. *Science, 316*, 550–551.

Scannell, J. W., Burns, G. A. P. C., Hilgetag, C. C., O'Neill, M. A., & Young, M. P. (1999). The connectional organization of the cortico-thalamic system of the cat. *Cerebral Cortex, 9*, 277–299.

Scheier, C., Pfeifer, R., & Kuniyoshi, Y. (1998). Embedded neural networks: exploiting constraints. *Neural Networks, 11*, 1551–1569.

Schreiber, T. (2000). Measuring information transfer. *Physical Review Letters, 85*, 461–464.

Seth, A. K. (2005). Causal connectivity analysis of evolved neural networks during behavior. *Network Computation in Neural Systems, 16*, 35–54.

Seth, A. K., & Edelman, G. M. (2004). Environment and behavior influence the complexity of evolved neural networks. *Adaptive Behavior, 12*, 5–20.

Shannon, C. E., & Weaver, W. (1949). *The mathematical theory of communication.* Chicago: University of Illinois Press.

Singer, W., & Gray, C. M. (1995). Visual feature integration and the temporal correlation hypothesis. *Annual Review of Neuroscience, 18*, 555–586.

Smith, L., & Gasser, M. (2005). The development of embodied cognition: Six lessons from babies. *Artificial Life, 11*, 13–30.

Sporns, O. (2003). Embodied cognition. In M. Arbib (Ed.), *Handbook of brain theory and neural networks* (pp. 395–398). Cambridge, MA: MIT Press.

Sporns, O. (2006). Small-world connectivity, motif composition, and complexity of fractal neuronal connections. *BioSystems, 85*, 55–64.

Sporns, O. (2007). Complexity. *Scholarpedia, 2*, 1623.

Sporns, O., Chialvo, D., Kaiser, M., & Hilgetag, C. C. (2004). Organization, development and function of complex brain networks. *Trends in Cognitive Sciences, 8*, 418–425.

Sporns, O., & Kötter, R. (2004). Motifs in brain networks. *PLoS Biology, 2*, 1910–1918.

Sporns, O., & Tononi, G. (2002). Classes of network connectivity and dynamics. *Complexity, 7*, 28–38.

Sporns, O., Tononi, G., & Edelman, G. (1991). Modeling perceptual grouping and figure–ground segregation by means of active reentrant connections. *Proceedings of the National Academy of Sciences USA, 88*, 129–133.

Sporns, O., Tononi, G., & Edelman, G. M. (2000). Theoretical neuroanatomy: Relating anatomical and functional connectivity in graphs and cortical connection matrices. *Cerebral Cortex, 10*, 127–141.

Sporns, O., Tononi, G., & Kötter, R. (2005). The human connectome: A structural description of the human brain. *PLoS Computational Biology, 1*, 245–251.

Sporns, O., & Zwi, J. (2004). The small world of the cerebral cortex. *Neuroinformatics, 2*, 145–162.

Stam, C. J. (2004). Functional connectivity patterns of human magnetoencephalographic recordings: A "small-world" network? *Neuroscience Letters, 355*, 25–28.

Stam, C. J., Jones, B. F., Nolte, G., Breakspear, M., & Scheltens, P. (2007). Small-world networks and functional connectivity in Alzheimer's disease. *Cerebral Cortex, 17*, 92–99.

Steinmetz, P. N., Roy, A., Fitzgeerald, P. J., Hsiao, S. S., Johnson, K. O., & Niebur, E. (2000). Attention modulates synchronized neuronal firing in primate somatosensory cortex. *Nature, 404*, 131–133.

Strogatz, S. H. (2001). Exploring complex networks. *Nature, 410*, 268–277.

Swanson, L. W. (2003). *Brain architecture.* Oxford, UK: Oxford University Press.

Thelen, E., & Smith, L. B. (1994). *A dynamic systems approach to the development of cognition and action.* Cambridge, MA: MIT Press.

Tononi, G. (2004). An information integration theory of consciousness. *BMC Neuroscience, 5*, 42.

Tononi, G., & Edelman, G. M. (1998). Consciousness and complexity. *Science, 282*, 1846–1851.

Tononi, G., Edelman, G. M., & Sporns, O. (1998). Complexity and coherency: Integrating information in the brain. *Trends in Cognitive Science*, 2, 474–484.

Tononi, G., & Sporns, O. (2003). Measuring information integration. *BMC Neuroscience, 4*, 31.

Tononi, G., Sporns, O., & Edelman, G. M. (1994). A measure for brain complexity: relating functional segregation and integration in the nervous system. *Proceedings of the National Academy of Sciences USA, 91*, 5033–5037.

Tononi, G., Sporns, O., & Edelman, G. M. (1996). A complexity measure for selective matching of signals by the brain. *Proceedings of the National Academy of Sciences USA, 93*, 3422–3427.

Varela, F. J., Thompson, E., & Rosch, E. (1991). *The embodied mind: Cognitive science and human experience*. Cambridge, MA: MIT Press.

Verschure, P. M. F. J., Voegtlin, T., & Douglas, R. J. (2003). Environmentally mediated synergy between perception and behavior in mobile robots. *Nature*, *425*, 620–624.

Watts, D. J. (1999). *Small worlds*. Princeton, NJ: Princeton University Press.

Watts, D. J., & Strogatz, S. H. (1998). Collective dynamics of "small-world" networks. *Nature*, *393*, 440–442.

Wyss, R., Konig, P., & Verschure, P. F. M. J. (2006). A model of the ventral visual system based on temporal stability and local memory. *PLoS Biology*, *4*, e120.

Yaeger, L., & Sporns, O. (2006). Evolution of neural structure and complexity in a computational ecology. In L. M. Rocha, L. S. Yager, M. A. Bedau, D. Floreano, R. L. Goldstone, & A. Vespignani (Eds.), *Artificial life X* (pp. 330–336). Cambridge, MA: MIT Press.

Zeki, S. (1993). *A vision of the brain*. London: Blackwell.

4

Social Modulation of Hormones

SARI M. VAN ANDERS

SOCIAL NEUROENDOCRINOLOGY

Though it is an advance in many ways to conceptualize the mind as operating with biological and socioenvironmental spheres, contextualization of the mind's function should not end there. Rather than employing a unidirectional hierarchical perspective whereby only the mind is understood to be sensitive to biology in exclusion to the converse, with biology thus positioned at the top of an artificial chain of command, contextualizing the mind within biology should be more nuanced. Hierarchies that include social context and biology are dynamic, continually in flux, and mutually influencing.

In this chapter, I specifically argue that social context in various forms can fundamentally alter and influence endocrine function, and that these hormonal changes can be best discussed within an evolutionary framework of adaptation and functionality—a research approach known as *social neuroendocrinology* (van Anders & Watson, 2006b). This approach represents a truly interactionist perspective that requires attention to both social context and biology, and a conscious move away from biological determinism or assumptions of evolutionarily "hardwired" effects. As I discuss more thoroughly in the following sections, we can reasonably expect evolution to "select" for endocrine responses to sexual contexts, since hormones are related to many sexual processes. For example, sperm need to be produced after ejaculation, and hormones are involved in sperm production. To test evolutionary questions of hormones influenced by social and sexual context, one first needs context;

that is, we could not logically expect to see evidence for evolved sexual modulation of hormones in the absence of sexual context of some kind. Additionally, many processes we reasonably consider to be influenced by evolution are influenced by past context, as when previous parenting experience modulates present hormonal responses to parenting. As such, *social neuroendocrinology*, by definition, attends to the joint and mutual influences of social context and hormones.

The endocrine system is a paramount exemplar of the need for a nuanced situating of the mind contextualized within biology: Hormone cascades "begin" with the hypothalamus (but see Kriegsfeld, 2006, for a review of upstream neuroendocrine controls of hypothalamic hormone releasers), but the hypothalamus receives converging inputs with socially relevant information. Hypothalamic function therefore is sensitive to social context, and hormonal function resultingly is as well. Hormones can also serve as a context for other hormonal actions, as when some hormones have inhibitory effects on other hormones, but this has received little empirical attention in social neuroendocrinology.

Social neuroendocrinology addresses hormonal function as situated within social context, and the research agenda is to examine social modulation of hormones (which is the focus of this chapter), bidirectional influences, and feedback–feedforward effects. The examination of how social context affects hormones is not a unidirectional endeavor, however, as the implicit and explicit goal is largely oriented to questions of effect (e.g., What are the sequelae of social context modulating hormones?) and function (e.g., Why does social context modulate hormones?) As I argue in this chapter, social neuroendocrinology represents a fundamentally important perspective in understanding the mind in context; the mind does not sit quietly in a corner, waiting for biology to tell it what to do. Social neuroendocrinology helps to reinforce a dynamic contextualization of the mind.

In this chapter, I review how social context modulates endocrine function. I focus on social contexts—parenting and sexuality—that are evolutionarily significant and have received empirical attention. Studying how social context modulates hormones necessitates an evolutionary framework, as there is no other way to examine *why* social context modulates hormones except through an evolutionary lens. By social context, I include the following:

1. Contextual cues that can be transferred from one individual to another (and therefore are socially communicated information); the information in these cues and/or their transmission can be physiological, behavioral, and so forth.
2. Social behaviors of selves or others.

3. Perceptions and anticipation of cues relevant to social context.
4. Information related to social contexts that have been transmitted intergenerationally. As such, social contexts can be immediate (e.g., infants crying) and/or in the past (e.g., past parental experience), brief (e.g., sexual anticipation) and/or longer-lasting (e.g., pregnancy), and modulatory (e.g., stage of pregnancy) or a cue itself (e.g., erotic films).

PARENTING AND PREGNANCY STIMULI AND HORMONES

Pregnancy as a Social Influence on Expectant and New Fathers

Conceptualizing social contexts, by definition, necessitates envisioning individuals embedded within perceived social networks. As such, social influences on endocrine function could include addressing how the social contexts of some individuals affect the endocrine states of others. States of one individual that would affect endocrine states in another should be evolutionarily relevant, like reproductive states. Reproductive states should have a highly potent social context; as such, the pregnancy status of a woman can be thought of as an extremely salient, evolved social signal—especially to those who are fundamentally invested in the outcome of the pregnancy. Humans tend to form pair-bonds, and human fathers are part of a small number of mammalian species with relatively high paternal investment and involvement (Wynne-Edwards, 2001). Though a mother can provide the gestating fetus and resulting baby with nutritional resources, additional support and resources from other figures (e.g., coparents, family) are likely necessary to support a woman through pregnancy, birth, and childrearing (Hrdy, 1997). As such, it would be adaptive if endocrine changes in a coparent co-occur with a woman's pregnancy, to potentate and facilitate parental responsivity. Research has focused on fathers and paternal endocrine responses to infant and pregnancy stimuli, but could (and should!) be extended to examine any persons taking on a coparenting role.

Expectant fathers do show endocrine changes alongside their female partners' pregnancies. Various changes occur in men over the early and late prenatal stages (i.e., when their female partners are pregnant), in the immediate period surrounding parturition (birth), and in the postnatal period. For example, prolactin (PRL) increases in fathers over the pregnancy (Storey, Walsh, Quinton, & Wynne-Edwards, 2000), cortisol (C) increases near birth and decreases afterwards (Berg & Wynne-Edwards,

2001, 2002; Storey et al., 2000), and testosterone (T) shows an opposite pattern to C, with decreases near birth and increases afterward (Berg & Wynne-Edwards, 2001, 2002; Storey et al., 2000). The decline in fathers' T is actually consistent with decreases in males of other species that show extensive paternal care (see, e.g., Wynne-Edwards, 2001, for discussion).

Pheromones/chemosignals are one possible mechanism by which this occurs (i.e., chemosignals passing between individuals). Chemosignals from pregnant women may increase sexual desire and fantasy in nonpregnant women (Spencer et al., 2004), buttressing the possibility that pregnant women could affect male partners through chemosignals, and that pregnancy states have social effects on others. Consideration of pheromones as social modulators of hormones adds an important perspective to this discussion; pheromones *are* social context, since they pass between individuals as social signals.

Why would T decline in new fathers? Possible speculations include decreased sexual desire, as T has been related to desire (e.g., Alexander, Sherwin, Bancroft, & Davidson, 1990), which could be adaptive in directing new fathers' focus away from sexuality and toward the mother and baby in caring ways. Another speculation is energy redistribution from reproductive and anabolic processes to stress processes, which may be important in attending to the newborn infant. In many species, T inhibits forms of paternal care (e.g., Wingfield, Hegner, Dufty, & Ball, 1990). In humans, men with lower T exhibit better paternal responsiveness (Fleming, Corter, Stallings, & Steiner, 2002) and better father–child relationships (Julian & McKenry, 1989), so decreased T around birth may facilitate paternal care.

Infants as Social Cues on Hormones, and Modulation by Pregnancy

In addition to pregnancy states, cues from offspring should provide an extremely salient social context relevant to endocrine systems because offspring are crucial to reproductive fitness. Infants can themselves be social cues via visual, chemical, and vocal signals or direct contact. Studies have examined effects of the context of having an infant on parental hormones, again, most often looking at fathers. Researchers generally use not only aversive auditory stimuli (e.g., pain or hunger cries) but also videos of pregnancy stimuli or ask men to hold baby dolls. Some have used all three in a likely attempt to maximize the "infant" experience without the difficulty and lack of control that could accompany the presence of real, live infants.

Fathers' hormones are significantly altered after exposure to infant stimuli, and this socially modulated change in hormones can further be influenced by female partners' stage of pregnancy. For example, men show larger decreases in C in response to infant cues in the late prenatal phase relative to other phases (Storey et al., 2000). PRL does not appear to change in response to infant cries (Fleming, Corter, et al., 2002), but T does show a significant increase in expectant fathers after some infant cues (Storey et al., 2000), with the largest increase occurring in the early postnatal phase (Storey et al., 2000).

Increased T upon infant cues seems counterintuitive given the possible functionality of low T described, evidence that T inhibits some parental behaviors in other species (Wingfield et al., 1990), and research showing that T is negatively associated with paternal–child bonding (Julian & McKenry, 1989). However, an increase in T specific to the early postnatal phase may reflect some evolutionary history of the need for infant defense in this phase. Parental behavior should not be understood to be a monolithic phenomenon, and I have theorized elsewhere (van Anders & Gray, 2007) that infant cues associated with close intimacy should be classified as *bond maintenance* and thus predictably lead to decreased T. In contrast, infant cues that might signal need for interventions such as protection or defense should be classified as *competitive* and lead to increased T. Since many of the infant cues in these studies include aversive baby cries, it may be that these cued a competitive rather than a bond-maintenance response. Additionally, evidence in other species suggests that the largest increases in T in response to social stimuli are seen during phases of lower T, and that androgen sensitivity to social contexts such as challenge are greatest during times of high parental care, and not times of regular social challenge, as counterintuitive as this may seem (Wingfield et al., 2000). Similarly, in human studies, the largest increases in men's T in response to infant cues are seen during the phases when they have the lowest T (i.e., around birth). Fascinatingly, fathers' current T levels can thus serve as a context for socially modulated changes in T.

Perhaps ironically, given societal conflation of mothers and infants, fewer researchers have studied effects of infant stimuli on maternal endocrine function (apart from lactation; see Ellison, 2001), though it should be noted that, overall, research on the modulation of infant stimuli on paternal hormones is also limited. Still, some studies have examined infant modulation of maternal endocrine function, and expectant and new mothers show increases in PRL after holding babies (Delahunty, McKay, Noseworthy, & Storey, 2007). Women's endocrine response to infant contextual cues can also differ depending on their own parturition status and context; after exposure to infant cues, PRL shows significant increases in pregnant but not in nonpregnant women (Storey et al., 2000). This is likely adaptive, since pregnant women's bodies should be ramping up the ability to respond to infants with lactation, and PRL is involved in this milk letdown.

Previous Infant Experience and Infant Cues on Hormones

Behavioral neuroendocrine research with animals often focuses on priming of the endocrine system, and previous parenting experience has been used as a possible context for or modulator of the endocrine axes in response to subsequent infant stimuli. In humans, researchers have thus examined how social context involving previous parenting experiences affects present social modulation of hormones.

For example, new, but not experienced, fathers show elevated C in response to cry stimuli (Fleming, Corter, et al., 2002). The social salience of baby cries may change depending on past experience, and this difference in social salience may elicit parallel changes in endocrine responses. In contrast to C responses, experienced fathers show a larger increase in PRL after hearing cries than do new fathers (Fleming, Corter, et al., 2002), and a similar pattern holds for fathers holding babies after birth, with experienced fathers showing increases in PRL and new fathers showing decreases (Delahunty et al., 2007). Men with younger siblings also show an increase in PRL in response to infant stimuli, but men with none show a decrease in PRL (Storey et al., 2000). These parallel findings suggest that the context of previous bond-maintenance experience with infants/children (whether with offspring or siblings) influences subsequent endocrine responses to infant stimuli. Which aspects of experience with infants might sensitize the brain to respond to subsequent infant stimuli with characteristic hormone responses is unclear at present because humans have received little empirical attention.

Transgenerational Effects of Parenting on Offspring Endocrine Axes

Research examining the effects of parental context on infant endocrine function and subsequent parenting has generally been carried out in nonhuman species (e.g., rats, mice) exposed to experimentally or naturally varied amounts and patterns of maternal care. Research with nonhuman species (e.g., rats) shows profound effects of parenting context on offspring endocrine function and behavior, especially in terms of hypothalamic–pituitary–adrenocortical (HPA) axis function in general situations, and HPA responsivity to stress (see, e.g., Fleming, Kraemer, et al., 2002). And, these effects show intergenerational transmission (e.g., Meaney, Szyf, & Seckl, 2007). Research with primates in cross-fostering studies has shown that maternal behavior of individuals is altered by the maternal behavior these individuals received as infants, and that changes in neurotransmitters (e.g., serotonin and dopamine), as well as HPA hormones (e.g., epinephrine), are implicated (Maestripieri, Lindell, & Higley, 2007). Therefore, influences of social contexts on hormones are likely to be long lasting, transmittable to subsequent generations, and of high import in future human research.

SEXUALITY AND HORMONES

Like pregnancy and parental/nurturant behavior, sexuality and reproductive behaviors should be a prime site for evolutionary pressures. Sexuality-related context should exert strong effects on endocrine function (e.g., van Anders & Watson, 2006b) because of the prime importance of sexuality in both fitness and sexual selection. Hormones have strong and direct influences on fertility in terms of ovulation and sperm production, menstruation, and also on morphological sexual differentiation. Social context can include sexual anticipation, in which the expectation of sexual activity might affect hormones, and these can be direct or embodied expectations. Sexual context can also include sexual stimuli (e.g., erotic movies) or sexual activity with another partner.

Sexual Anticipation Influences on Hormones

Though we might conceptualize effects of sexual activity on endocrine function as limited to actual sexual activity, expectation of sexuality should be also a highly salient signal. It could be adaptive for the body to expect and/or prepare for sexuality, since sexual activity involves a number of potentially hormonally mediated processes and cognitions. Of the few studies relevant to anticipatory effects of sexuality on hormones, most have found supporting evidence. Thus, the anticipation of a sexual context, or even the experience of a psychologically (but not physically) sexual context, can lead to endocrine alterations.

One of the most widely known and earliest reports of anticipatory effects of sexuality on physiology is by Anonymous (1970), who reported on his experience as a researcher on a deserted island; he was alone except when he traveled back to the mainland to visit his female romantic partner and engage in sexual activity. During his island stay, he collected his beard clippings and measured their weight (odd, but perhaps not that odd for a bored empirical scientist on a deserted island). His beard clippings were heavier on the days prior to the mainland visits, and Anonymous suggested that his androgens were increased prior to the visits by anticipation of sexual activity with his partner, since beard growth can be a bioassay for androgenic function.

More recent research has provided supportive evidence using direct assays. Researchers who examined correlations between sexual activity diaries and hormone levels from regularly repeated assays in men found that there is some indication of increased T immediately preceding sexual activity (Knussmann, Christiansen, & Couwenbergs, 1986). A study with women showed that T is significantly higher immediately prior to intercourse than prior to cuddling or exercise (van Anders, Hamilton, Schmidt, & Watson, 2007). Neither of these studies explicitly measured "anticipation" using a self-report or questionnaire measure, but it remains unclear what terms other than *anticipation* are appropriate for describing how knowledge of specific future behavior might affect hormones.

Research with abstinence and hormones might also be conceptualized as falling under the broad rubric of anticipation. Abstinence denotes a period of time without sexual activity; when randomly assigned, individuals know they will be engaging in sexual activity again at the conclusion of the abstinent period. Intriguingly, experimental assignment of sexual abstinence could thus conflate abstinence with sexual anticipation. If so, or if abstinence is generally associated with increased sexual anticipation, abstinence might be expected to be associated with increased T. Evidence supports this, as men exhibit higher T after periods of abstinence (Exton et al., 2001), and lower frequency of orgasmic experience has also been associated with higher T in men (Kraemer et al., 1976) but not women (cf. van Anders et al., 2007). Thus, researchers need to attend to which factors of social situations are relevant (e.g., abstinence vs. anticipation).

What functional aspects would exist for endocrine changes in response to anticipation of sexual activity? Increased T (in female rats: Traish, Kim, Stankovic, Goldstein, & Kim, 2007) and estradiol (E2) (in ewes: Brown & Mattner, 1977) increase blood flow to the genitals. Genital vasocongestion is a key contributor to genital sexual arousal and lubrication; anticipatory increases in T and E2 may facilitate physiological responses that make sexual activity more pleasurable and/or conducive to conception. In addition, since sexual activity in men generally involves ejaculation, increased T likely reflects upregulation of hormones to stimulate sperm production in anticipation of sperm depletion.

Effects of Sexual Cues on Hormones

Unlike sexual anticipation, sexual cues involve transmission of information. For example, people may view sexual stimuli, though engagement with two-dimensional stimuli lacks many of the social cues inherent to interaction with a live person. Still, the evolutionary development of the neuroendocrine system might be seen as unlikely to reflect this distinction.

Visual sexual cues from videos do lead to changes in hormones. Men's T is increased following sexual movies compared to neutral and/or aggressive films (Hellhammer, Hubert, & Schürmeyer, 1985; Pirke, Kockott, & Dittmar, 1974; Rowland et al., 1987; Stoleru, Ennaji, Cournot, & Spira, 1993). However, nongonadal steroids, such as C or PRL, have not been found to increase following sexual stimuli in men (Exton et al., 2000). Interactions with live women also alter heterosexual men's hormones, as shown when men's T and C are increased following conversations with women (Roney, Lukaszewski, & Simmons, 2007; Roney, Mahler, & Maestripieri, 2003). Conversations should not be understood as sexual interactions; more specifically, Roney and colleagues (2003) found that men's T increases were correlated with their flirtatious behaviors. This suggests that the social perception of a context as potentially sexual and/or romantic and performing relevant behaviors are associated with T increases.

Hormone changes in response to sexual context might be functional in similar ways to sexual anticipation; that is, increased T may facilitate sperm production or genital vasocongestion, influencing fertility parameters or sexual pleasure. Increases in C may reflect stress responses, but Roney and colleagues (2007) noted that participants' C was uncorrelated with perceptions of situational stress. Increased C may thus be more related to attention to arousal or social stimuli, such as facial emotions (Roelofs, Bakvis, Hermans, van Pelt, & van Honk, 2007). Additionally, C has been shown to facilitate pair-bonding in species that regularly form monogamous pair-bonds (e.g., corticosterone in prairie voles: DeVries, DeVries, Taymans, & Carter, 1996), so increased C in a sexual context may be facilitory for pair-bonding.

Sexual Activity Effects on Hormones

Engaging in sexual activity with a partner should also have endocrine effects, but whether this context should be stronger than sexual anticipation and cues, because it involves live people and their concomitant social cues, has not really been tested. Since sexual activity generally involves ejaculation on the male's part, whereas anticipation or cues do not always, sexual activity may be a stronger sexual cue to the endocrine system. Humans often engage in sexual activity within the context of some sort of relationship or pair-bond, so sexual activity with others may influence hormones in ways that are relevant to promotion or maintenance of the pair-bond. Indeed, sexual activity itself can facilitate pair-bond formation in prairie voles (Young, Murphy Young, & Hammock, 2005). And women feel more intimate with their partners the morning following partnered sexual activity compared to partnered exercise (van Anders et al., 2007). Fewer studies have examined how partnered sexual activity might affect oxytocin (Ot) in humans, but Carter (1998) notes that mating and especially vaginocervical stimulation in females of other species both increases Ot and facilitate pair-bond promotion.

Studies examining the immediate effects of sexual activity on men's T have generally not found empirical support (e.g., Stearns, Winter, & Faiman, 1973), though one more recent study has (Dabbs & Mohammed, 1992). However, studies have found that men's T is increased at a latency following sexual activity (Knussmann et al., 1986; Kraemer et al., 1976), with especially large increases the morning following sexual activity with multiple or unfamiliar partners (Hirschenhauser, Frigerio, Grammer, & Magnusson, 2002). And Knussman and colleagues (1986) found higher T in 48-hour periods surrounding orgasm in men.

Researchers have also examined the effects of sexual stimuli and masturbation to orgasm, finding significant increases in PRL following orgasm in both women and men, with elevations remaining for at least 1 hour (Exton et al., 2001). This increase in PRL appears to be orgasm-dependent, and is thought to be a sexual satiety signal. And solitary masturbation increases men's T (Purvis, Landgren, Cekan, & Diezfalusy, 1976; cf. Krüger et al., 1998), even with no latency, whereas sexual activity with a partner does not. Could the social presence of a female partner inhibit immediate T releases in response to sexuality? Since partnered men tend to have lower T (e.g., van Anders & Watson, 2006a) and T may inhibit pair-bonding in other species (Wingfield et al., 1990), this seems a possible though speculative conclusion.

T levels are increased in women immediately following intercourse with male partners, but no significant increases are apparent as yet in longer-term measures (e.g., the next morning) (van Anders et al., 2007). However, the social cues leading to increased T are not limited to partnered sexual involvement, since women also show significant increases in T following cuddling. In fact, the increase in T after cuddling was larger (though nonsignificantly) than the increase following intercourse. One interpretation is that the close physical intimacy of both activities leads to increases in T. Another interpretation is that cuddling leads to sexual anticipation, and because sexual anticipation is associated with increased T in women, postcuddling increases in T might be mediated by anticipation of partnered sexual activity.

CONCLUSIONS

Social Modulation of Hormones via Parental and Sexual Context

Social contexts that are especially relevant to evolution and reproductive fitness are the best candidates for examining social modulation of hormones; these influences, in turn, are interpretable only when evolutionary considerations are taken into account. Thus, social neuroendocrinology is inherently evolutionary, regardless of the home disciplines of its practitioners. As is evident in the preceding sections, examining the effects of social context on hormones is also an inherently interactionist endeavor and can only be accomplished with the explicit recognition that evolved responses occur only within specific social contexts. As such, social neuroendocrinology is perhaps uniquely situated to challenge biological determinism; evolved physiological responses—by definition—require social context to occur. And given the modulatory effects of past context (e.g., parenting experience) on the influences of current context (e.g., infant exposure) on hormones (e.g., increased PRL), there are many points at which considerations of social contexts are prerequisites to understanding potentially evolved mechanisms.

Sexuality-related stimuli are particularly relevant to social neuroendocrinology because of their importance in reproduction and the involvement of hormones in processes such as fertility, sexual development, and sexual morphology. The extensive research foundation on sexuality and hormones in nonhuman species provides an experimental literature resource from which human researchers can draw. As described, sexual context does affect endocrine function in a multitude of ways that can be understood to exist under a monolithic *sexuality* category or a subdivided group of avenues of influence. However, setting sexuality up as a monolithic, undivided category is unlikely to provide for the level of detail needed to make key insights. For example, how do social cues inherent to interaction with people, viewing sexual stimuli, or solitary sexual pursuits differentially affect endocrine responses?

The functional implications of endocrine changes in response to sexual stimuli range from fertility to physiological preparations for intercourse (e.g., lubrication), but all remain speculative, since little research has actually examined the possible sequelae of sexuality-stimulated endocrine changes. Empirical investigations into functionality, and not just presentations of convincing speculations, are needed and important for understanding basic questions of hormone–sexuality associations, in addition to furthering the social neuroendocrinology research agenda. Understanding the actual, as opposed to attractive, sequelae will increase the relevance of social neuroendocrinology to other disciplines, including clinical practice with sexual therapy or infertility.

Like sexuality, parenting-related contexts are prime targets for social neuroendocrinology because of their key association with reproductive fitness and survival, and because hormones are already implicated in known parental processes (e.g., lactation). Similarly, parenting has been extensively studied in nonhuman species, with comprehensive linkages among neural circuits, hormones, and maternal behavior. The focus on intergenerational transmission of socially modulated endocrine function has provided exceedingly important insights in the nonhuman literature, and a major challenge and opportunity is to examine these issues in humans (daunting though the timescales might appear). Additionally, the elision of subcategories within *infant stimuli* likely undermines the development of a solid empirical and theoretical foundation. Researchers need to examine how different contextual modalities (e.g., live baby vs. vocal only vs. visual only) and contextual valences (e.g., crying vs. happy) differentially elicit endocrine changes.

Challenges and Future Directions

Like most newly emerging disciplines, social neuroendocrinology faces both a challenging and promising future. A major initiative involves incorporating a focus on the functionality of social neuroendocrinology (van Anders & Watson, 2006b); researchers allude to tantalizing and interesting possible adaptive functions of socially induced endocrine alterations but need to conduct empirical studies. As noted earlier, the elements of social context need to be more closely examined. What social cues in social context elicit (which) hormone changes? The use of "sexual" or "parental" or even "social" context needs to allow for and provide opportunities to determine how individuals engage with these stimuli (perception, etc.), and how this engagement then influences hormones. A major challenge lies in the need for independent replication of results, which can be a difficult premise given that human researchers often focus on idiosyncratic though overlapping questions. A major advantage is that social neuroendocrinology allows for transdisciplinary collaborations to examine questions of the evolved physiology of social behavior rather than parallel work using different methodologies.

Methodological issues have been and will likely continue to be a challenge. Analyses are not really that expensive, until researchers think about the inclusion of multiple hormones, multiple sampling points, and sufficient sample sizes with women and men. Attending to all of these is as yet an unreached ideal. For example, some studies have pointed to the importance of time of day (another context in itself), with sociality–hormone associations apparent in the afternoon but not the morning (e.g., Roney et al., 2007). Other studies have pointed to latency between context and sampling, with delays needed after some types of social contexts but not others, which can lead to "null" findings despite significant associations (if only hormones were measured later or earlier). Fortunately, important insights have already been gleaned with these introductory methodologies; as the field matures, methodological insights and improvements are certain to follow as researchers are able actually to test both methodological and conceptual questions that are crucial to social neuroendocrine research.

Social neuroendocrinology provides a novel but powerful approach to understand the evolved physiology of social behavioral contexts. Hormones may influence social behaviors and perceptions, and brain areas may develop as substrates for specific kinds of social behavior (e.g., sexuality- or parenting-related), but the mind should not just be contextualized as lying within a larger biological sphere of influences. Instead, the mind should be understood to be an active component within this larger physiological sphere, as social context and hormones actively engage in a complex and dynamic relationship, affecting each other with degrees and direction of influence that change in response to specific social contexts—a socially apt process for the social modulation of hormones.

REFERENCES

Anonymous. (1970). Effects of sexual activity on beard growth in men. *Nature*, *226*, 869–870.

Alexander, G. M., Sherwin, B. B., Bancroft, J., & Davidson, D. W. (1990). Testosterone and sexual behavior in oral contraceptive users and nonusers: A prospective study. *Hormones and Behavior*, *24*(3), 388–402.

Berg, S. J., & Wynne-Edwards, K. E. (2001). Changes in testosterone, cortisol, and estradiol levels in men becoming fathers. *Mayo Clinic Proceedings*, *76*(6), 582–592.

Berg, S. J., & Wynne-Edwards, K. E. (2002). Salivary hormone concentrations in mothers and fathers becoming parents are not correlated. *Hormones and Behavior*, *42*, 424–436.

Brown, B. W., & Mattner, P. E. (1977). Capillary blood flow in the genital tracts of conscious ewes: Cyclic changes the effect of ovarian hormones. *Journal of Endocrinology*, *74*(2), 185–191.

Carter, C. S. (1998). Neuroendocrine perspectives on social attachment and love. *Psychoneuroendocrinology*, *23*(8), 779–818.

Dabbs, J. M., Jr., & Mohammed, S. (1992). Male and female salivary testosterone concentrations before and after sexual activity. *Physiology and Behavior, 52*, 195–197.

Delahunty, K. M., McKay, D. W., Noseworthy, D. E., & Storey, A. E. (2007). Prolactin responses to infant cues in men and women: Effects of parental experience and recent infant contact. *Hormones and Behavior, 51*(2), 213–220.

DeVries, A. C., DeVries, M. B., Taymans, S. E., & Carter, C. S. (1996). The effects of stress on social preferences are sexually dimorphic in prairie voles. *Proceedings of the National Academy of Sciences USA, 93*, 11980–11984.

Ellison, P. T. (2001). *On fertile ground.* Cambridge, MA: Harvard University Press.

Exton, M. S., Kruger, T. H., Bursch, N., Haake, P., Knapp, W., Schedlowski, M., et al. (2001). Endocrine responses to masturbation-induced orgasm in healthy men following a 3-week sexual abstinence. *World Journal of Urology, 19*(5), 377–382.

Exton, M. S., Tryong, T. C., Exton, M. S., Wingenfeld, S. A., Leygraf, N., Saller, B., et al. (2000). Neuroendocrine response to film-induced sexual arousal in men and women. *Psychoneuroendocrinology, 25*(2), 187–199.

Fleming, A. S., Corter, C., Stallings, J., & Steiner, M. (2002). Testosterone and prolactin are associated with emotional responses to infant cries in new fathers. *Hormones and Behavior, 42*, 399–413.

Fleming, A. S., Kraemer, G. W., Gonzalez, A., Lovic, V., Rees, S., & Melo, A. (2002). Mothering begets mothering: The transmission of behavior and its neurobiology across generations. *Pharmacology Biochemistry and Behavior, 73*(1), 61–75.

Hellhammer, D. H., Hubert, W., & Schürmeyer, T. (1985). Changes in saliva testosterone after psychological stimulation in men. *Psychoneuroendocrinology, 10*, 77–81.

Hirschenhauser, K., Frigerio, D., Grammer, K., & Magnusson, M. S. (2002). Monthly patterns of testosterone and behavior in prospective fathers. *Hormones and Behavior, 42*, 172–181.

Hrdy, S. B. (1997). Raising Darwin's consciousness: Female sexuality and the prehominid origins or patriarchy. *Human Nature, 8*, 1–49.

Julian, T., & McKenry, P. C. (1989). Relationship of testosterone to men's family functioning at mid-life: a research note. *Aggressive Behavior, 15*, 281–289.

Knussmann, R., Christiansen, K., & Couwenbergs, C. (1986). Relations between sex hormone levels and sexual behavior in men. *Archives of Sexual Behavior, 15*(5), 429–445.

Kraemer, H. C., Becker, H. B., Brodie, H. K. H., Doering, C. H., Moos, R. H., & Hamburg, D. A. (1976). Orgasmic frequency and plasma testosterone levels in normal human males. *Archives of Sexual Behavior, 5*, 125–132.

Kriegsfeld, L. J. (2006). Driving reproduction: R Famide peptides behind the wheel. *Hormones and Behavior, 50*, 655–666.

Krüger, T., Exton, M. S., Pawlak, C., von zur Mühlen, A., Hartmann, U., & Schedlowski, M. (1998). Neuroendocrine and cardiovascular response to sexual arousal and orgasm in men. *Psychoneuroendocrinology*, *23*, 401–411.

Maestripieri, D., Lindell, S. G., & Higley, J. D. (2007). Intergenerational transmission of maternal behavior in rhesus macaques and its underlying mechanisms. *Developmental Psychobiology*, *49*(2), 165–171.

Meaney, M. J., Szyf, M., & Seckl, J. R. (2007). Epigenetic mechanisms of perinatal programming of hypothalamic–pituitary–adrenal function and health. *Trends in Molecular Medicine*, *13*(7), 269–277.

Pirke, K. M., Kockott, G., & Dittmar, F. (1974). Psychosexual stimulation and plasma testosterone in man. *Archives of Sexual Behavior*, *3*, 577–584.

Purvis, K., Landgren, B.-M., Cekan, Z., & Diczfalusy, E. (1976). Endocrine effects of masturbation in men. *Journal of Endocrinology*, *70*, 439–444.

Roelofs, K., Bakvis, P., Hermans, E. J., van Pelt, J., & van Honk, J. (2007). The effects of social stress and cortisol responses on the preconscious selective attention to social threat. *Biological Psychology*, *75*(1), 1–7.

Roney, J. R., Lukaszewski, A. W., & Simmons, Z. L. (2007). Rapid endocrine responses of young men to social interactions with young women. *Hormones and Behavior*, *52*(3), 326–333.

Roney, J. R., Mahler, S. V., & Maestripieri, D. (2003). Behavioral and hormonal responses of men to brief interactions with women. *Evolution and Human Behavior*, *24*, 365–375.

Rowland, D. L., Heiman, J. R., Gladue, B. A., Hatch, J. P., Doering, C. H., & Weiler, S. J. (1987). Endocrine, psychological and genital response to sexual arousal in men. *Psychoneuroendocrinology*, *12*, 149–158.

Spencer, N. A., McClintock, M. K., Sellergren, S. A., Bullivant, S., Jacob, S., & Mennella, J. A. (2004). Social chemosignals from breastfeeding women increase sexual motivation. *Hormones and Behavior*, *46*(3), 362–370.

Stearns, E. L., Winter, J. S., & Faiman, C. (1973). Effects of coitus on gonadotropin, prolactin and sex steroids in man. *Journal of Clinical Endocrinology and Metabolism*, *37*, 687–691.

Stoleru, S. G., Ennaji, A., Cournot, A., & Spira, A. (1993). LH pulsatile secretion and testosterone blood levels are influenced by sexual arousal in human males. *Psychoneuroendocrinology*, *18*, 205–218.

Storey, A. E., Walsh, C. J., Quinton, R. L., & Wynne-Edwards, K. E. (2000). Hormonal correlates of paternal responsiveness in new and expectant fathers. *Evolution and Human Behavior*, *21*, 79–95.

Traish, A. M., Kim, S. W., Stankovic, M., Goldstein, I., & Kim, N. N. (2007). Testosterone increases blood flow and expression of androgen and estrogen receptors in the rat vagina. *Journal of Sexual Medicine*, *4*(3), 609–619.

van Anders, S. M., & Gray, P. B. (2007). Hormones and human partnering. *Annual Review of Sex Research*, *18*, 60–93.

van Anders, S. M., Hamilton, L. D., Schmidt, N., & Watson, N. V. (2007). Associations between testosterone secretion and sexual activity in women. *Hormones and Behavior*, *51*(4), 477–482.

van Anders, S. M., & Watson, N. V. (2006a). Relationship status and testosterone in North American heterosexual and non-heterosexual men and women: Cross-sectional and longitudinal data. *Psychoneuroendocrinology, 31*(6), 715–723.

van Anders, S. M., & Watson, N. V. (2006b). Social neuroendocrinology: Effects of social contexts and behaviors on sex steroids in humans. *Human Nature, 17,* 212–237.

Wingfield, J. C., Hegner, R. E., Dufty, A. M., Jr., & Ball, G. F. (1990). The "challenge hypothesis": Theoretical implications for patterns of testosterone secretion, mating systems, and breeding strategies. *American Naturalist, 136,* 829–846.

Wynne-Edwards, K. E. (2001). Hormonal changes in mammalian fathers. *Hormones and Behavior, 40*(2), 139–145.

Young, L. J., Murphy Young, A. Z., & Hammock, E. A. (2005). Anatomy and neurochemistry of the pair bond. *Journal of Comparative Neurology, 493*(1), 51–57.

PART II

COGNITION AND AFFECT

5

Emoting

A Contextualized Process

BATJA MESQUITA

Psychological research has treated emotions such as anger, happiness, and fear as properties of the individual. In many experiments, participants seated in a laboratory cubicle are exposed to a stimulus that triggers the emotion, which is then measured in some individual response modality. For example, respondents are exposed to a movie or slide, or alternatively are asked to recall some emotional episode, after which their brain activity, muscular changes in the face, voice intonation, skin conductance, or self-reported experience are registered. The idea is that individuals' emotions can be fruitfully studied when they are by themselves. In fact, I suspect that an unspoken assumption is that the real or the purest form of emotions is best studied when "social noise" is kept at bay.

In this chapter, I want to argue the contrary, that emotions are first and foremost a type of connection with our social worlds, and that all other features follow this basic fact. Emotions represent types of engagements with the world (Frijda, 2007) that aim to change relationships in a certain direction, or alternatively, maintain their current state. "The point is that an emotion is not merely a 'feeling,' as, say, pain is a feeling. It is ... a reaching out to the world" (Solomon, 2003, p. 49). Thus, having an emotion means that one has a relationship with the world or, put more sharply, a strategy or a goal in the world (Solomon, 1978). This conceptualization of emotions as engagements with the world is more than just that emotions *can* be and *may* be communicated with others, and that emotions *can* and often *do* occur in social situations. It is rather that emotions themselves are social phenomena that in the moment constitute a relationship and are constituted by it.

My proposal to view emotions as contextualized acts fits the *Zeitgeist*. Parallel to developments in personality (see Mischel & Shoda, Chapter 8, this volume) and cognition (see Smith & Collins, Chapter 7, this volume), the shift is from representing emotion as a static entity within the person to viewing it as a dynamic process that emerges from interaction with the environment. Consistent with the paradigm shifts in other domains of psychology, I thus propose that the object of study should be action in context, *emoting*, rather than a static entity, *emotion*. Emoting is different from emotion in that it is a property of the relationship rather than the individual; that it is a process rather than an entity; and that it is embedded in the structure of relationships as they occur in the wider cultural context rather than invariant states with fixed properties (see Figures 5.1 and 5.2). By contextualizing emotions, it becomes clear that (1) emoting is not easily reduced to merely individual-level processes, (2) emotions themselves may vary according to contexts, and (3) emotions are functional to the cultural context in which they occur.

Taking *emoting* as the starting point for research means to acknowledge that emotional processes emerge in dynamic interaction between individuals and their social contexts. The question about "the nature of emotion" (Ekman & Davidson, 1994) would be replaced by an interest in the "dynamics of emoting" or, at the very least, in "the contextualized nature of emoting." Concretely, the focus of research shifts to how a given emotion is produced by and materializes in a concrete context. Research should focus on relationship contexts and examine the multiple ways in which these contexts may constitute emotion, rather than measure emotion in the isolation of a cubicle.

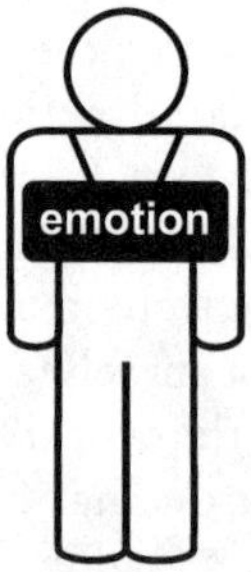

FIGURE 5.1. Emotion as a static property of the individual.

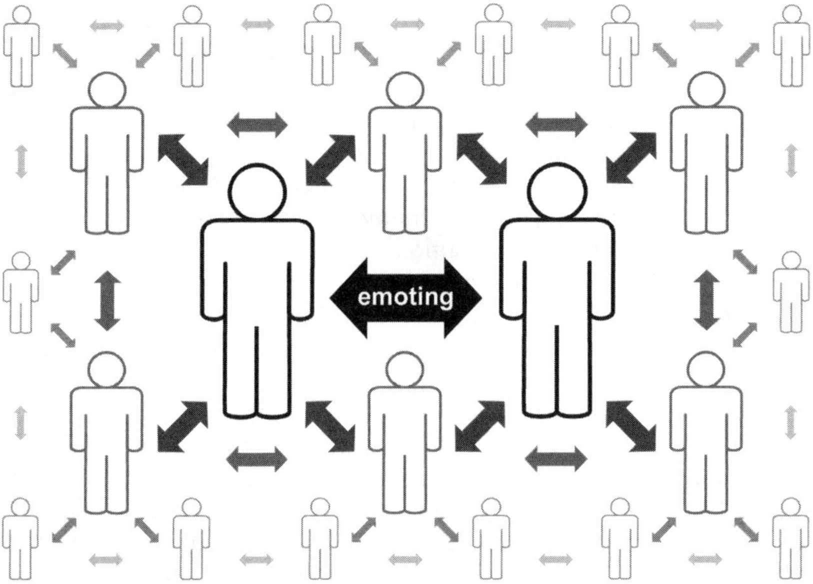

FIGURE 5.2. Emoting as a contextualized, dynamic process within relational engagements.

DEVELOPMENT OF EMOTING

It is certainly beyond the scope of this chapter to give an exhaustive review of the developmental research on emotions. However, it is this literature that perhaps most convincingly shows that emoting is a dynamic, relational process. If we understand emoting primarily as relational action, then emoting is present from the beginning of life (cf. Parkinson, Fischer, & Manstead, 2005).

Infant Emoting

Very early on in life, human infants share affect with their caregivers. Infants' understanding of emotions originates from this relationship. There is now ample evidence that infants emote in the actual context of the relationship—which means they understand and reciprocate emotions—long before they have abstract concepts or representations of emotions, and also well before they have adult-like experiences of emotions. In other words, emoting precedes anything that we could call emotion.

An important strand of evidence comes from infant perception of emotions. Very young infants understand the affective meaning of rich, multimodal, affective displays, especially in their caregivers, and they respond reciprocally to that information (Walker-Andrews, 2008). Infants have been shown to discriminate between anger, happiness, and sadness when in real interactions with their caregivers, before they have abstract representations of these emotions in separate modalities (face, voice). Infant recognition of emotions is helped by the time dynamics of different modes of emotional expression. In other words, abstract, internal representations of emotions emerge well after the capacity of understanding emotions *in situ*, that is, in the actual relationships formed by infants early in life.

Infants *communicate* affective messages to their caregiver, in addition to *responding* to them. Behaviors such as fussing, crying, and smiling communicate to the caregiver that adjustments to the environment need to be made, or conversely, that the interaction is going well (Oatley & Jenkins, 1992; Oatley, Keltner, & Jenkins, 2007). Thus, from a very early age on, expressive behaviors on the part of infants have emotional meaning within the relationship with the caregiver, at least from the point of view of the caregivers who respond to them. This is not to say that infant emotional displays are associated with adult-like emotions: They are not (e.g., Camras, Meng, & Ujie, 2002; Hiatt, Campos, & Emde, 1979). However, the way caregivers act upon infant displays imbues these displays with emotional meaning. Caregivers either reduce or increase stimulation, such that good feeling states of the baby are recognized and sustained, and bad feeling states are taken into account and discontinued (Oatley et al., 2007). For example, mothers were found to maintain babies' positive states by mirroring babies' positive emotions and ignoring or responding with surprise to their babies' negative expressions. The caregiver's behavior thus renders the baby's behaviors emotionally meaningful.

This may be a good model of the path of emotional development generally.

> Infants may have a sense of themselves as participants in an interaction. Infants' responses during interactions are coordinated, multimodal actions involving vocalizations, gaze, facial expressions, body movements, and gestures, which relay information to the others as well as themselves about internal states, and which regulate the behavior of both partners. Affective arousal may mediate [the] associations among [the different modes] of infants' [actions]. (Walker-Andrews, 2008, p. 372)

In other words, babies' behaviors acquire emotional meaning by their caregivers' responses to them as affectively meaningful. It is also the case that social interactions create a correspondence between multi-modal responses that in and of itself affords sense making in babies. "Babies' behaviors are both entrained by the mother's pattern and educated by the multi-modal correspondences that interactions create" (Smith, 2005, p. 294). Emotional development thus consists of "a series of accumulated changes that reflect past opportunities for learning emotion-laden meaningful connections, but that only become manifest or expressed in the context of the moment" (Saarni, 2008, p. 334).

The relationship with the caregiver can also provide meaning to objects outside the infant–caregiver relationship, as is the case in social referencing (Hertenstein & Campos, 2004; Mumme & Fernald, 2003). Children as young as 11 to 12 months will appraise a novel object by referencing the emotions of a nearby adult, usually the caregiver, and infer from these emotions the significance of the object. Social referencing has been shown to influence both the infant's expressions and emotional responses to the novel object. Thus, for instance, a caregiver's disgust expressions both increase the chances of an infant's crying and make the infant less likely to touch or approach the new toy. There is also some evidence that social referencing in the case of negative emotion changes the infant's behavior vis-à-vis the caregiver. Infants tend to stay closer to the mother (Carver & Vaccaro, 2007). Yet, again, emotional appraisal of an object or event is not the result of an internal mental assessment by the infant; rather, it is inferred in the context of the relationship with the caregiver.

Early Childhood Emoting

Relationships with caregivers (and peers) are also an important context of emotional development in the childhood years, during which emotions are often the object of communication between caregivers and children (Dunn, 2004). Interesting in the current context is that children learn about observable aspects of emotions before they learn to talk about mentalistic states (Harris, 2008); that is, toddlers can talk about situations eliciting emotions and emotional behaviors ("He cries because he bumped his head") before they can talk about desires, values, and preferences that would underlie certain emotional states ("He cries because he did not get the ice cream he wanted"). Although different interpretations are possible, one possible way to read this development is that a child's initial understanding of emotions is based not so much on his or her own internal experiences, but on observable facts in the environment. Mentalistic inferences are made only later. They are thus a development beyond the first representations of emotions based in the external environment.

Caregivers label, interpret, and evaluate emotions. They do so in two ways. First, caregivers explicitly talk about emotions, communicating rules and beliefs. Furthermore, caregivers' own emotional responses may lend meaning to their children's emotions, too (Saarni, 2008). One way of looking at caregivers' (verbal, as well as emotional) communications is that they teach children about the propriety of certain ways of emoting—that is, certain ways of relational engagement—in particular contexts. Consistent with this interpretation is the finding that parental talk about emotions is an important predictor of children's social adroitness (Dunn, Brown, & Beardsall, 1991; Harris, 2008). For example, the frequency with which preschool children discuss emotions with caregivers predicts their later ability to understand other people's feelings.

Parental talk about emotions varies across cultural contexts (Cole, Tamang, & Shrestha, 2006; Miller, Fung, & Mintz, 1996), and reflects cultural ideas and practices about valued and devalued types of relational engagements. Thus, one study compared conversations of American and Taiwanese moms with their 2½-year-olds. Consistent with the American cultural model that emphasizes the importance of high self-esteem and independence, American moms emphasized children's independent achievements that had evoked happiness and pride. On the other hand, Taiwanese moms drew attention to children's transgressions, and how these transgressions had burdened and saddened them, thus shaming the children (Cole et al., 2006; Miller et al., 1996). The latter is consistent with the East Asian model of being, in which the individual's accommodation to the needs of the relationship and the avoidance of norm violation are central. Parents thus draw attention to those types of relational engagement—that is, those types of emotion—that are most likely to render the children into well-socialized individuals in their culture.

Similarly, Cole and colleagues (2006; Cole, Bruschi, & Tamang, 2002) found different socialization practices in two Nepalese groups, the Tamang and the Brahman. The Tamang—Tibetan Buddhists—value self-effacement and compassionate tolerance. In this group, anger is viewed as destructive to social harmony, but shame is seen as a valuable emotion by which an individual subjects him- or herself to the larger group. On the other hand, the Brahman—high-caste Hindus—conceive of anger as a way to establish dominance and competence, assuming it gets properly regulated. On the other hand, shame is seen as a sign of weakness. Consistently, adult responses to anger and shame episodes in 3- to 5-year-olds were very different in these two groups. Whereas Tamang caregivers responded to children's shame with teaching and nurturing, children's anger aroused teasing and rebuking. Conversely, Brahman adults ignored signs of shame in their children but gave their angry children attention, teaching them proper ways of expressing anger. Caregivers' responses to given emotions thus function to enhance and moderate culturally valued emotions, and suppress culturally devalued emotions. In other words, caregivers assist their children in selection of rewarding relational engagements, and suppression of unrewarding ones.

Thus, in each interaction with the parent, certain forms of emotion are modeled or encouraged, while others are not. These interactions produce successive (not end-point oriented) changes in emoting (Saarni, 2008) that enhance functionality to the particular social context. The different ways of emoting—or relationship engagements—that are rewarding vary across contexts, particularly cultural contexts. Consistently, the modal caregiver–infant transactions vary across cultural contexts and afford variability both in the patterns of emotion and in emotional understanding. Emoting belongs to the relationship first, and articulated emotional experience, as well as mental representations, emerge later in development. Quoting Vygotsky:

> It is necessary that everything internal in higher [mental functions] was external, that is, for others it was what it now is for oneself. Any higher mental function necessarily goes through an external stage in its development because it is initially a social function. When we speak of a process, "external" means "social." Any higher function was first external because it was social at some point before becoming an internal, truly mental function. (cited in Wertsch, 1985, p. 62)

Emoting in the Adult Context

Though some aspects of emotions may get internalized during adult life (Holodynski & Friedlmeier, 2006), the process of *emoting* is still best described as a dynamic engagement in the relationships in which it occurs. *Emoting* can be viewed to consist of "ongoing adjustments attuned to unfolding transactions with the practical and social world" (Parkinson, 2008, p. 24). Although emoting presumably requires some form of cognitive mediation, no conscious cognitive representations of the events are needed. Rather, representations may be embodied, more like "perceptual affordances that provide action guidance" (Frijda, 2007, p. 108). Emoting, then, is afforded by the interactions with others or, more precisely, interactions with others as rendered meaningful by cultural meanings and practices. In other words, given social interactions as understood increase the likelihood of some forms of emoting and render others less likely. This conceptualization of emoting as based in action—often, social interaction—focuses attention on their dynamics in context. It highlights the conditions of emoting and renders the connection between different instances of emoting more transparent.

Not many studies are attuned to the question of emoting in context, but research on marital dispute provides an interesting exception. Several of these studies have established meaningful couple patterns of emoting (Gottman, Swanson, & Murray, 1999). One study found, for instance, that some couples' emotional patterns consisted of reciprocal negative emotions (contempt, anger), with one spouse's negative emotions predicting the other's on the next interaction turn (even when researchers controlled for the first spouse's own emotions on previous turns). Other couples' dynamics did not show the same reciprocity because one of the spouses would have a *negativity threshold*, meaning that the hostility of the other partner had to be much more pronounced for the first partner to respond in kind on the next turn (Gottman et al., 1999). The negativity threshold was predicted by not only the partner's hostility on the previous turn but also earlier hostility in the interaction. One partner's negative emoting during the first half of the discussion predicted a higher negativity threshold in the other partner during the latter half. One possible interpretation is that those who received too many messages of disapproval from their spouses stop engaging in the relationship. This interpretation fits with the finding that a negativity threshold predicted failure of the marriage 1 year later.

The important point here is that emotions of the spouses mutually afford or constrain each other, as it may be, even in the course of *one* interaction. One can only imagine how emotional patterns of partners afford each other in the course of a long-term relationship. We suggest, therefore, that the context of the relationship may be powerful in accounting for individual instances of emoting.

Another example of the mutual constitution of emotion comes from research with undergraduates selected to have either very high or very low social anxiety (Heerey & Kring, 2007). Nonanxious respondents were paired with nonanxious peers, or alternatively, with socially anxious counterparts. Partners in each pair were instructed to "get to know" each other. Highly anxious participants engaged in more self-talk, asked fewer questions, reciprocated genuine smiles more often with polite smiles and less often with pleasant genuine smiles, and sought more reassurance than the nonanxious participants in either type of dyad. Central to the current argument is that this emotional behavior constituted the emotions of the nonanxious participants who were paired with anxious conversation partners. These nonanxious participants comprised the only group that did *not* report an increase in positive affect as a result of the interaction. Moreover, they offered more empathy and support to conversation partners than did members of any other group in the study. Finally, both interaction partners in the socially anxious–nonanxious pair perceived lower quality of interaction and fidgeted more than the partners of nonanxious pairs. Fidgeting tended to be started by the socially anxious partner, and seemed to be transmitted across interaction partners. Again, although the study was not meant to provide an example of online emoting, it illustrates how emotions are meaningfully described as interactive patterns. Moreover, describing emotions this way renders it much more apparent how the emotions of one (i.e., the nonanxious) partner in the interaction are prompted by the emotions of the other (i.e., the anxious person)—and perhaps vice versa as well.

In a recent article, Algoe, Haidt, and Gable (2008) described how gratitude on the part of one person instills positive feelings about the relationship in the other. Although the study itself does not describe emoting as acts in context, I suggest that this conceptualization would fit the data. The researchers followed the development of the relationship between little and big sisters of a sorority: Little sisters had just joined the sorority, whereas big sisters had been members of the sorority since the prior year. During little sister week, when big sisters anonymously surprised their little sisters, little sisters' gratitude was measured. This gratitude was associated with little sisters' appreciation of the relationship with their anonymous big sisters. Thus, gratitude can be framed as the act of valuing the particular relationship. One month later, a little sister's gratitude predicted the quality of the relationship and the amount of time spent together, as reported by the big sister. Though the exact way in which gratitude on the part of the little sister constituted the positive feelings on the part of the big sister is unknown, the data fit the model of gratitude as an act in context that constitutes the emotions in the partner and thus the relationship. This is another example where emotions and relationships dynamically constitute each other, a process that is not captured by the representation of emotions as mental phenomena, isolated from the context.

In summary, mapping the dynamics of emoting in interaction yields insights not provided by the description of individual emotions only. It shows effectively how emotions are in fact relational engagements. In the previous examples, emoting in one partner equaled the act of disapproval, of claiming to have received coping assistance, or of appreciating and investing in the relationship. Each instance of emoting should thus be conceived of as either a *move* or a *countermove* in the dyadic relationship. Of making a claim on receiving coping assistance from the partner, they become "rational" in ways they would not be without consideration of the relational context.

Note that this focus on emoting does more than describe within-person-level phenomena at the higher level of the relationship. It goes beyond the claim that emoting is either socially influenced or embedded. Rather, emoting itself is a social act that derives its meaning and predictability from the relationship in which it takes place. Adopting a contextualized perspective on emoting enhances our insight into why and when emoting occurs. It renders apparent the connections between different instances of emoting, as well as between instances of emoting and the relationship in which they occur.

CONVERGENT EMOTIONS

Emotions of the members of dyads and groups converge over time. This is another illustration that the emotional processes of interest exceed the boundaries of the individual person.

The first demonstration of emotional convergence came from a study by Robert Zajonc and his colleagues, showing that married couples look more alike after 25 years of marriage that they did at their first anniversary (Zajonc, Adelmann, Murphy, & Niedenthal, 1987). Relationship closeness and marriage satisfaction predicted how much better the couples were recognized after 25 years than after just 1 year by students asked to match the faces. The authors postulated imitation as the underlying process. Relationship closeness might lead to empathy, and to the mimicking of emotions. Twenty-five years of mimicking one's partner, thus using similar facial muscles, would account for the resemblance between partners' faces.

Not only partners start looking alike emotionally, so do roommates in college, dating couples, groups, and cultures (Anderson & Keltner, 2004; Anderson, Keltner, & John, 2003; Kim, Mesquita, & Gomez, 2008; Smith, Seger, & Mackie, 2007). In all cases, people who belong together become more emotionally similar over time, or are so at the time of measurement.

Anderson and colleagues (2003) reported two experimental studies in which the emotions of roommates and romantic couples were measured at the beginning of the academic year, then 6 or 9 months later in the year. Emotions were measured both by self-reports and facial coding, and were elicited in a number of different ways (conversations about topics with different valence, watching emotion-eliciting movies). In all cases, convergence of emotions was higher at the second measurement point than at the first. Emotional convergence was related to relationship satisfaction and liking of the partner/roommate, and this was true even when researchers controlled for personality similarities. A third study showed that after 7 months of sharing a room, the emotions of roommates were more similar to each other than to randomly chosen students, even when roommates separately watched emotion-eliciting movies to prevent contagion. Thus, living together may lead to similarity in emotional reactivity, and whatever the mechanism, it develops in a relatively short time.

In two different studies, Smith and colleagues (2007) showed that members of ingroups converge on group-level emotions. In these studies, respondents were asked to rate their own personal emotions, as well as their emotions as a group member (e.g., American, Democrat, or Republican) on 12 emotion scales (e.g., anger, happiness). The scores on those 12 scales constituted their emotion profiles. Group emotions produced significantly different profiles than did individual emotions. Furthermore, an individual's group emotion (e.g., happiness as an American) was predicted by the average group member's group emotion (e.g., the level of happiness averaged across all Americans) when controlling for the individual emotion (e.g., happiness reported by the individual). Thus, emotions of group members converged. The authors suggest that group emotions are thus seen as "true, objective, and externally driven in a type of social construction of emotional reality. ... The emotions, because they are shared, come to be seen as true and objective" (p. 442).

A final example of convergence comes from a study with U.S. natives and Korean immigrants (Kim et al., 2008). In a between-subject design, respondents reported emotional events from their own lives that varied along the dimensions of valence and social engagement (Kitayama, Mesquita, & Karasawa, 2006). They subsequently reported how they had felt by rating 30 different emotion scales. Individual emotion profiles were calculated for each type of situation. Individual profiles were then compared with the average American profile. Consistent with the finding of ingroup convergence, Americans' emotion profiles were more similar to the American average emotion profile than were Koreans' emotion profiles. Furthermore, Koreans who scored higher on acculturation scales, and thus felt closer to American culture, had profiles more similar to the average American emotion profile than did those with low acculturation scores.

Convergence of emotions has been established, therefore, for roommates, couples, ingroups, and cultural groups in contact. Convergence is particularly pronounced for those whose connection is a close, happy, or identified one. The mechanism by which convergence emerges is not clear (see Anderson et al., 2003, and Smith et al., 2007, for similar observations), but one way of thinking about convergence is that agreement on normative and desirable ways of engagement grows over time. Alternative explanations have been proposed. Regardless of the precise mechanisms underlying convergence, its occurrence makes a case for conceiving of emoting as a process that exceeds the individual mind.

SOCIOCULTURAL FUNCTIONALITY OF EMOTIONS

Emoting may, and often does, change the relationship with others. Anger may force concessions, as was shown in a virtual negotiation experiment, in which participants made more concessions when they negotiated with someone who was made to look angry than when they negotiated with a neutral person (van Kleef, De Dreu, & Manstead, 2004). Consistently, angry politicians in another study were considered more worthy of power than sad ones, and employees in an information technology (IT) company, who were described by their peers as more easily angered, received more promotions (Tiedens, 2001). Anger may be a claim, an expression of entitlement that, in these cases, was being met.

However, the meaning of emotions appears to be dependent on the context. This context may be defined by different types of relationship arrangements, depending on culture, power differential, or gender roles. Emoting is thus an engagement that derives meaning from the specific relationship context in which it occurs. Emoting may represent claims that are successful and justified in one context but not in another.

When the claim of anger is considered to be justified by one's environment, anger brings about an improvement of position. However, the strategic bid of anger may also be countered or challenged. Gender contexts appear to affect the legitimacy of anger. In a recent study, respondents watched a video of either a man or a woman displaying anger or sadness. Respondents conferred less power on angry women than on angry men, and on angry women than on sad women (Brescoll & Uhlmann, 2008). Furthermore, participants explained anger in a woman by making negative, internal attributions ("She is not in control"), but they justified anger in men by external circumstances. Thus, women do not gain from being angry, whereas men make a successful claim to status. Hence, gender is a constituting context for the interactive meaning of anger.

The meaning of emotional engagements may also vary according to the cultural meanings of certain relationship arrangements. This is clear for shame, an emotion that may be seen as aligning oneself with the social rules and expectations. Whether this act is condoned by others seems to depend on the specific cultural models (Mesquita & Karasawa, 2004). Shame in East Asian cultures tends to be condoned, as it is consistent with interdependent goals of accommodating to others. It fits the values and practices of modesty and self-criticism that are prevalent in East Asian cultures. But shame in Western contexts is an uneasy, painful, and often *invisible* (Scheff, 1988) emotion. It signals that one has failed to achieve the central tasks of an independent self, namely, self-esteem and positive independence.

In some cultures, emotions are more literally taken as bids that can be negotiated, if unreasonable. Shame and anger were described as the currency for power negotiations among the Kaluli in Papua New Guinea (Schieffelin, 1983). In the Kaluli cultural model, nearly every reason to be angered, "any loss, wrong, injury, insult, or disappointment, is interpreted in the scheme of reciprocity. ... A person who is angry is in some sense owed something: He has a legitimate expectation that he is due redress" (pp. 186–187). Legitimacy can be challenged by shaming the angry person, implying that he is overasking. Shaming is basically undermining the legitimacy of the appeal that anger makes. *Shame* is "a situation, or a state of powerlessness and rejection. The legitimacy of one's basic posture of assertion or appeal has been removed" (p. 189). But shaming requires an assessment of power: "A person does not try to shame another if he does not think he can dominate the situation. If one tries to shame a stronger opponent without proper social support, his opponent may become provoked, override shame, and dominate him by intimidation" (p. 190). Thus, the legitimacy of anger in a Kaluli context also seems dependent on the social power of the person who is angry.

Lest I give the impression that only negative emotions are strategic bids or relational engagements, there are many examples of positive emotions in negotiating or establishing relationships as well. Love, for example, involves redefining oneself as a part of a couple (Solomon & Higgins, 1991); gratitude is the currency of many intimate relationships and plays an important role in the negotiation of what is valued in a relationships (Fields, Copp, & Kleinman, 2006). Hochshield (1989, cited in Fields et al., 2006) found that, as gender culture shifted, with more women participating in the labor market, the marital baseline against which women measured, received, and appreciated gifts, shifted as well, but often men did not follow these changes. Women may consider their paychecks as gifts, but men may find their wives' financial success shaming. Therefore, women may expect that men are doing their fair share in the household (their spouses folding the laundry is not considered a gift), whereas men may wash the dishes as a gift. Gratitude, or the abstinence from it, may be considered moves in the relationship.

In summary, emotions are directed engagements with the social environments, relationship alignments, or strategic bids. They position an individual in a relationship. Emotions may make an appeal on others to conform to the strategic bid, to accept the relationship alignment, or to welcome or reject the changed (or, alternatively, sustained) relationship engagement. The meaning of the bid depends on the contextual meanings of certain relationship arrangements.

If emotions are moves in interactions or strategic bids, one may expect that the prevalence of a given emotion is contingent on its fit with the prevalent relationship goals in that context. In other words, if emoting is largely strategic, then it should be functional to the sociocultural environment in which it occurs. There is much evidence that this is in fact the case. Examples of this principle can be found at the level of both social roles and culture.

For example, low- and high-status contexts are associated with different rates of emotions. In one study (Tiedens, Ellsworth, & Mesquita, 2000), business students from a Midwestern university read a vignette in which a boss and an employee formed a sales team that failed in its mission and did not reach the customer on time with the product. Responsibility for this bad outcome could not be inferred from the description. Respondents inferred that the level of anger was higher for the boss, and levels of sadness and guilt for the employee. Thus, the emotion that expressed rightfulness and power was associated with the boss, and the emotions of powerlessness and regret, to the employee. Status roles render certain emotions more appropriate and therefore more likely. Interestingly, when emotions rather than status roles were given in the same vignettes, respondents recognized the boss in the angry person, and the employee in the sad or guilty person. Emoting thus engages in status roles, and from status roles people can predict which emotions are likely. Emotions are functional to these status roles.

Furthermore, and consistent with Western gender schemas that prescribe strength and independence for men, and emotional expressiveness and connectedness for women, crying is more prevalent in women than in men (Vingerhoets & Scheirs, 2000). There is some evidence that crying is more rewarding for women than for men: Crying men are helped and comforted less often than are crying women (Hendriks, Nelson, Cornelius, & Vingerhoets, 2008).

The most prevalent emotions in given cultural contexts also appear to be the ones that are consistent with the culturally preferred relationship arrangements (Kitayama et al., 2006; Mesquita & Leu, 2007). For example, Kitayama and his colleagues (2006) found that socially engaging emotions, such as friendly feelings or shame, were more prevalent in Japanese interdependent than in the American independent cultural contexts; the reverse was true for socially disengaging emotions, such as pride and anger. Engaging emotions underline and reinforce the relatedness between people and thus fit the interdependent model. This is obviously the case with friendly feelings, but an emotion of shame also signals the acknowledgment of social rules, as well as preparedness to submit to those rules. Socially disengaging emotions tend to signal and contribute to the boundedness and independence of an individual, and thus fit the goals in independent contexts. Data from several studies converged. In one experience sampling study, both positive and negative engaged emotions were more frequent than disengaged emotions in Japanese contexts, whereas the reverse was true in independent European American contexts (Kitayama et al., 2006). In these studies, Japanese and European American students rated both engaged and disengaged emotions subsequently in a daily experience sampling study, and in response to 22 very diverse emotional events. In these studies, the largest differences appeared in the disengaged emotions. Whereas Japanese and European American students appraised situations similarly with regard to their implications for relational engagement, European American students reported significantly higher levels of disengaged emotions for both the positive and the negative situations. Thus, the combined work on power and culture contexts suggests that emotions that have the greatest strategic benefits in the context are those most likely to occur. In other words, the reinforcement structure of the context predicts the likelihood of an emotion to occur. A finding in the same study by Kitayama and colleagues corroborates this idea. Not only were disengaged emotions relatively more frequent in the European American samples, and engaged emotions more frequent in the Japanese samples, but also self-reported well-being in European Americans was better predicted by disengaged emotions, and in the Japanese by engaged emotions. Thus, the most frequent emotions may in fact have been the most rewarding, if rewards can be assumed to translate into well-being.

In summary, the studies here discussed suggest that contextualized relationship arrangements may account for the types of emotions that occur. The contextualized norms, habits, or reward structures affect which emotions occur most frequently. Note that these features of the context help us understand the regularities of an individual's emotional life. Thus, what emotions a person is likely to experience can be inferred from the contexts in which his or her emotional life is embedded.

CULTURAL DIFFERENCES IN EMOTING

Emoting is thus embedded in relationships, which are organized according to cultural models, that is, the meanings and practices of relationships in a given culture. For example, North American cultural models highlight the boundaries of each individual, whereas Japanese interdependent models assume the mutual interdependence of people in relationships (Markus & Kitayama, 2003; Triandis, 1995). Consistently, emoting in independent, American contexts seems to highlight the individual as bounded, autonomous, and self-sufficient, and often entails influencing relationships in ways that reinforce the individual's autonomy. On the other hand, emoting in interdependent, Japanese contexts highlights and expresses the relatedness between people, and furthers action that leads to a strengthening of interpersonal bonds (Kitayama et al., 2006; Markus & Kitayama, 1994; Mesquita & Karasawa, 2002).

Emotional affordances vary according to different cultural models. This was beautifully illustrated in a series of studies by Cohen, Nisbett, Bowdle, and Schwarz (1996) in which they examined differences between the meaning of emotions in several regions of the United States rather than making a cross-national comparison. Cohen and colleagues studied the ways Southerners and Northerners of the United States emoted in situations of offense. Southerners were more likely than Northerners to be aggressive after an insult. In the South, insults afford aggression because the target of offense is perceived as weak and will be subject to bullying, unless he restores his honor by violent retaliation; insult in the North does not in the same way necessitate aggression. Aggression, by force, refers to a very different type of relational engagement in the South than in the North. Southerners consider the problem to be mitigated after aggression; aggression evens the bill and solves the insult. On the other hand, aggression in the North is seen to aggravate the conflict further (Nisbett & Cohen, 1996). Aggression thus counts as a different relational move in these two contexts. Many other examples of culture-specific emotional affordances are available in the literature.

Cultural differences in emoting go beyond differences in either affordance or the meaning of certain ways of emoting. Emotions themselves may differ in ways that fit the cultural models; that is, emoting in different cultural contexts may consist of significantly different actions and be associated with very different meanings (Mesquita, 2001; Mesquita et al., 2006). In one study, we interviewed Japanese and American respondents about experiences of offense. This situation type was associated with the emotion of anger in both groups. However, the most prevalent actions reported in both cultures were rather different in ways that can be understood from the cultural models. Seventy percent of American respondents and only 30% of Japanese respondents reported being assertive or aggressive. On the other hand, 60% of Japanese and only 40% of Americans reported doing nothing. The prevalent actions can be understood from the cultural models.

Assertiveness and aggression are actions that fit well with an American, independent model that foregrounds the individual and promotes the maintenance of self-esteem (Kitayama & Markus, 2000; Markus, Mullally, & Kitayama, 1997). On the other hand, doing nothing is a response that is consistent with the Japanese cultural model, which emphasizes the central importance of relationship harmony. These cultural models seem to imply different meanings of offense, as an event in which an individual needs to protect his or her rights and maintain self-esteem or, alternatively, as one in which the relationship needs attention. In fact, the appraisals of offense reported in the Japanese and American narratives were consistent with the respective cultural models.

Importantly, emotions themselves are conceived of differently, in ways that can be understood from the respective cultural models. For example, North American folk theory conceives of emotions as psychological events that occur within a single individual (Uchida, Townsend, Markus, & Bergsieker, 2009), and that reflect the individual's wishes, goals, and preferences in ways that uniquely define the person. In contrast, many other cultures, such as Japan and several small, indigenous Asian cultures, characterize emotions as primarily social and moral processes (Levenson, Ekman, Heider, & Friesen, 1992; Lutz, 1987; Rosaldo, 1980; Uchida et al., 2009), as properties of the relationship and the community.

These different folk theories are consequential in the sense that they govern the ways people recognize emotions in themselves and in others (Levenson et al., 1992; Uchida et al., 2009). While Westerners read emotions in people who are alone (including themselves), people from Asian cultures assume that emotions require people in relationship. Moreover, while Westerners read emotion from the face or the behavior of an individual, Japanese have been shown to infer the emotional experience of an individual from the faces and behaviors of several people in the same context (Masuda, Ellsworth, Mesquita, Leu, & Veerdonk, 2008).

It is no coincidence, then, that the psychology of emotions has started from the cultural assumption in the West that emotions are confined to the individual. Emotion psychology is a product of Western culture that focuses on facets of reality highlighted in Western contexts. It is our Western cultural model that may have blinded psychology from the important relational and social quality of emotions.

In summary, emotions are relational engagements. Cultural differences exist with respect to the desirable and normative engagements. This has been shown in studies that compare the valence of certain emotions. An example was that shame is more positively regarded in interdependent than independent cultures. However, in this section I have suggested that emotions themselves may be differently constituted in ways that fit culturally normative relationship goals. These data are consistent with the evidence from the infant and childhood literature that emotions develop across many successive interactions with others. Modeling, emotional feedback, and explicit labeling and interpretation of emotions may all amount to the development of emotions into culturally functional packages. Children learn in the course of development to emote in ways that promote culturally desirable relationships. Finally, I have suggested that the dominant approach of emotions as entities within the individual also reflects Western cultural models, and the ensuing Western folk model of emotions.

CONCLUDING REMARKS

In this chapter, I have suggested that emotions are productively viewed as social relationship acts. They develop from interactions with the caregiver, and are rooted in observable situations and acts. Only later in development do these observable aspects of emotions become associated with meanings and adult-like experiences. But even in adult life, the view of emotions as behavioral intentions, or even acts, in social relationship is a productive one. This view can explain (1) that emotions that are functional to the relationship goals in a given (cultural) context tend to be more prevalent, (2) that emotional responding of the partners in a dyad can be understood in connection to one another, and (3) that there may be convergence in the emotions of people who are identified as roommates, couples, groups, and cultures.

This view of emotions as rooted in interaction would affect the research agenda in some profound ways. First, it suggests that emotions should be studied in more action-relevant contexts. This means that a change of paradigm is needed, in which emoting is measured in real-time interactions rather than, for instance, as a response to contexts that hardly require action at all (slides, movies, scenario prompts). Second, research should focus on the actual emotional meaning as relevant to action, and should therefore study emoting in relevant, complex social contexts, considering the cultural models that feed emotional interpretation. Third, we should focus on the ways in which emoting of members of dyads and groups are intertwined. What are the interactive processes of emotions? How do the emotions of one person affect the emotions of the others? What mechanisms account for the mutual affordance of emotions? In all, a contextualized view of emotions calls for much more *in situ* research, with attention to the dynamic, social, and cultural processes that constitute emoting. Describing the properties of the internal emotional experience in a static experimental situation will not be enough to allow us to gain perspective on the contextualized nature of emoting.

REFERENCES

Algoe, S.-B., Haidt, J., & Gable, S.-L. (2008). Beyond reciprocity: Gratitude and relationships in everyday life. *Emotion*, *8*(3), 425–429.

Anderson, C., & Keltner, D. (2004). The emotional convergence hypothesis: Implications for individuals, relationships, and cultures. In L. Z. Tiedens

& C. W. Leach (Eds.), *The social life of emotions* (pp. 144–163). Cambridge, UK: Cambridge University Press.

Anderson, C., Keltner, D., & John, O. P. (2003). Emotional convergence between people over time. *Journal of Personality and Social Psychology, 84*(5), 1054–1068.

Brescoll, V. L., & Uhlmann, E. L. (2008). Can an angry woman get ahead?: Status conferral, gender, and expression of emotion in the workplace. *Psychological Science, 19*, 268–275.

Camras, L., Meng, Z., & Ujie, T. (2002). Observing emotion in infants: Facial expression, body behavior, and rater judgments of responses to an expectancy-violating event. *Emotion, 2*, 179–193.

Carver, L. J., & Vaccaro, B. G. (2007). 12-month-old infants allocate increased neural resources to stimuli associated with negative adult emotion. *Developmental Psychology, 43*, 54–69.

Cohen, D., Nisbett, R. E., Bowdle, B. F., & Schwarz, N. (1996). Insult, aggression, and the Southern culture of honor: An "experimental ethnography." *Journal of Personality and Social Psychology, 70*(5), 945–960.

Cole, P. M., Bruschi, C. J., & Tamang, B. L. (2002). Cultural differences in children's emotional reactions to difficult situations. *Child Development, 73*(3), 983–996.

Cole, P. M., Tamang, B. L., & Shrestha, S. (2006). Cultural variations in the socialization of young children's anger and shame. *Child Development, 77*, 1237–1251.

Dunn, J. (2004). Individual differences in understanding emotion and mind. In A. S. R. Manstead, N. H. Frijda, & A. H. Fischer (Eds.), *Feelings and emotions: The Amsterdam Symposium* (pp. 303–320). New York: Cambridge University Press.

Dunn, J., Brown, J., & Beardsall, L. (1991). Family talk about feeling states and children's later understanding of others' emotions. *Developmental Psychology, 27*(3), 448–455.

Ekman, P., & Davidson, R. J. (1994). *The nature of emotion: Fundamental questions.* New York: Oxford University Press.

Fields, J., Copp, M., & Kleinman, S. (2006). Symbolic interactionism, inequality, and emotions. In J. E. Stets & J. H. Turner (Eds.), *Handbook of the sociology of emotions* (pp. 155–178). New York: Springer.

Frijda, N. H. (2007). *The laws of emotion.* Mahwah, NJ: Erlbaum.

Gottman, J., Swanson, C., & Murray, J. (1999). The mathematics of marital conflict: Dynamic mathematical nonlinear modeling of newlywed marital interaction. *Journal of Family Psychology, 13*(1), 3–19.

Harris, P. L. (2008). Understanding emotion. In M. Lewis, J. M. Haviland-Jones, & L. F. Barrett (Eds.), *The handbook of emotions* (3rd ed., pp. 320–331). New York: Guilford Press.

Heerey, E. A., & Kring, A. M. (2007). Interpersonal consequences of social anxiety. *Journal of Abnormal Psychology, 116*(1), 125–134.

Hendriks, M. C. P., Nelson, J. K., Cornelius, R. R., & Vingerhoets, A. J. J. M. (2008). *Why crying improves our well-being: An attachment-theory perspective on the functions of adult crying.* New York: Springer Science + Business Media.

Hertenstein, M. J., & Campos, J. J. (2004). The retention effects of an adult's emotional display on infant behavior. *Child Development*, *75*, 595–613.

Hiatt, S., Campos, J. J., & Emde, R. N. (1979). Facial patterning and infant facial expression: Happiness, surprise, and fear. *Child Development*, *50*, 1020–1035.

Holodynski, M., & Friedlmeier, W. (2006). *Development of emotions and emotion regulation*. New York: Springer Science + Business Media.

Kim, H., Mesquita, B., & Gomez, G. (2008). *Emotional concordance: A cultural psychology perspective on acculturation*. Unpublished manuscript, University of California, Santa Barbara.

Kitayama, S., & Markus, H. R. (2000). The pursuit of happiness and the realization of sympathy: Cultural patterns of self, social relations, and well-being. In E. Diener & E. Suh (Eds.), *Subjective well-being across cultures* (pp. 113–161). Cambridge, MA: MIT Press.

Kitayama, S., Mesquita, B., & Karasawa, M. (2006). Cultural affordances and emotional experience: Socially engaging and disengaging emotions in Japan and the United States. *Journal of Personality and Social Psychology*, *91*(5), 890–903.

Levenson, R. W., Ekman, P., Heider, K., & Friesen, W. V. (1992). Emotion and autonomic nervous system: Activity in the Minangkabu of West Sumatra. *Journal of Personality and Social Psychology*, *62*(6), 972–988.

Lutz, C. (1987). Goals, events, and understanding in Ifaluk emotion theory. In N. Quinn & D. Holland (Eds.), *Cultural models in language and thought* (pp. 290–312). Cambridge, UK: Cambridge University Press.

Markus, H. R., & Kitayama, S. (1994). The cultural construction of self and emotion: Implications for social behavior. In S. Kitayama & H. R. Markus (Eds.), *Emotion and culture: Empirical studies of mutual influence* (pp. 89–130). Washington, DC: American Psychological Association.

Markus, H. R., & Kitayama, S. (2003). Models of agency: Sociocultural diversity in the construction of action. In J. J. Berman & V. Murphy-Berman (Eds.), *Cross-cultural differences in perspectives on the self* (Vol. 49, pp. 18–74). Lincoln: University of Nebraska Press.

Markus, H. R., Mullally, P. R., & Kitayama, S. (1997). Selfways: Diversity in modes of cultural participation. In U. Neisser & D. A. Jopling (Eds.), *The conceptual self in context: Culture, experience, self-understanding* (pp. 13–61). Cambridge, UK: Cambridge University Press.

Masuda, T., Ellsworth, P. C., Mesquita, B., Leu, J., & Veerdonk, E. (2008). Putting the face in context: Cultural differences in the perception of emotions from facial behavior. *Journal of Personality and Social Psychology*, *94*, 365–381.

Mesquita, B. (2001). Emotions in collectivist and individualist contexts. *Journal of Personality and Social Psychology*, *80*(1), 68–74.

Mesquita, B., & Karasawa, M. (2002). Different emotional lives. *Cognition and Emotion*, *16*(1), 127–141.

Mesquita, B., & Karasawa, M. (2004). Self-conscious emotions as dynamic cultural processes. *Psychological Inquiry*, *15*, 161–166.

Mesquita, B., Karasawa, M., Haire, A., Izumi, S., Hayashi, A., Idzelis, M., et al. (2006). *What do I feel?: The role of cultural models in emotion representations*. Unpublished manuscript, Wake Forest University.

Mesquita, B., & Leu, J. (2007). The cultural psychology of emotion. In S. Kitayama & D. Cohen (Eds.), *The handbook of cultural psychology* (pp. 734–759). New York: Guilford Press.

Miller, P. J., Fung, H., & Mintz, J. (1996). Self-construction through narrative practices: A Chinese and American comparison of early socialization. *Ethos*, *24*, 237–280.

Mumme, D. L., & Fernald, A. (2003). The infant as onlooker: Learning from emotional reactions observed in a television scenario. *Child Development*, *74*, 221–237.

Nisbett, R. E., & Cohen, D. (1996). *Culture of honor: The psychology of violence in the South*. Boulder, CO: Westview Press.

Oatley, K., & Jenkins, J. H. (1992). Human emotions: Function and dysfunction. *Annual Review of Psychology*, *43*, 55–85.

Oatley, K., Keltner, D., & Jenkins, J. M. (2007). *Understanding emotions* (2nd ed.). Malden, MA: Blackwell.

Parkinson, B. (2008). Emotions in direct and remote social interaction: Getting through the spaces between us. *Computers in Human Behavior*, *24*, 1510–1529.

Parkinson, B., Fischer, A. H., & Manstead, A. S. R. (2005). *Emotion in social relations: Cultural, group, and interpersonal processes*. New York: Psychology Press.

Rosaldo, M. Z. (1980). *Knowledge and passion: Ilongot notions of self and social life*. Cambridge, UK: Cambridge University Press.

Saarni, C. (2008). The interface of emotional development with social context. In M. Lewis, J. M. Haviland-Jones, & L. F. Barrett (Eds.), *The handbook of emotions* (3rd ed., pp. 332–347). New York: Guilford Press.

Scheff, T. J. (1988). Shame and conformity: The deference–emotion system. *American Sociological Review*, *53*, 395–406.

Schieffelin, E. L. (1983). Anger and shame in the tropical rainforest: On affect as a cultural system in Papua New Guinea. *Ethos*, *11*(3), 181–209.

Smith, E. R., Seger, C. R., & Mackie, D. M. (2007). Can emotions be truly group level?: Evidence regarding four conceptual criteria. *Journal of Personality and Social Psychology*, *93*(3), 431–446.

Smith, L. B. (2005). Cognition as a dynamic system: Principles from embodiment. *Developmental Review*, *25*, 278–298.

Solomon, R. B., & Higgins, K. (1991). *The philosophy of (erotic) love*. Lawrence: University Press of Kansas.

Solomon, R. C. (1978). Emotions and anthropology: The logic of emotional world views. *Inquiry*, *21*, 181–199.

Solomon, R. C. (2003). The politics of emotion. In *The joy of philosophy* (pp. 38–63). New York: Oxford University Press.

Tiedens, L. (2001). Anger and advancement versus sadness and subjugation: The effect of negative emotion expression on social status conferral. *Journal of Personality and Social Psychology*, *80*, 86–94.

Tiedens, L., Ellsworth, P. C., & Mesquita, B. (2000). Sentimental stereotypes: Emotional expectations for high- and low-status group members. *Personality and Social Psychology Bulletin, 26*, 560–574.

Triandis, H. C. (1995). *Individualism and collectivism.* Boulder, CO: Westview Press.

Uchida, Y., Townsend, S., Markus, H. R., & Bergsieker, H. B. (2009). Emotions as within or between people?: Cultural variation in lay theories of emotion expression and inference. *Personality and Social Psychology Bulletin, 35*, 1427–1439.

van Kleef, G. A., De Dreu, C. K. W., & Manstead, A. S. R. (2004). The interpersonal effects of anger and happiness in negotiations. *Journal of Personality and Social Psychology, 86*(1), 57–76.

Vingerhoets, A., & Scheirs, J. (2000). *Sex differences in crying: Empirical findings and possible explanations.* New York: Cambridge University Press.

Walker-Andrews, A. S. (2008). Intermodal emotional processes in infancy. In M. Lewis, J. M. Haviland-Jones, & L. F. Barrett (Eds.), *Handbook of emotions* (3rd ed., pp. 364–375). New York: Guilford Press.

Wertsch, J. V. (1985). *Vygotsky and the social formation of mind.* Cambridge, MA: Harvard University Press.

Zajonc, R. B., Adelmann, P. K., Murphy, S. T., & Niedenthal, P. M. (1987). Convergence in the physical appearance of spouses. *Motivation and Emotion, 11*(4), 335–346.

6

Meaning in Context

Metacognitive Experiences

NORBERT SCHWARZ

As psychologists have long been aware, human cognition is highly context sensitive. How we perceive simple objects, comprehend texts and utterances, form evaluative judgments, make sense of others' behavior, and perform myriad other tasks is profoundly influenced by the immediate context in which the respective tasks are situated. To account for such influences, researchers commonly assume that the context influences the accessibility of applicable knowledge, which is brought to bear on the task at hand (for reviews, see Förster & Liberman, 2007; Higgins, 1996). Under most natural conditions, this context sensitivity is adaptive by privileging information that is relevant in the current situation at the expense of other information that may be less germane given current circumstances (for discussions, see Schwarz, 2007; Smith & Collins, Chapter 7, this volume). However, the common focus on knowledge accessibility misses the fact that there is more to thinking than *what* comes to mind.

Thinking is accompanied by a host of subjective experiences, from metacognitive feelings of ease or difficulty to affective reactions and bodily sensations. As Higgins (1998) noted, people commonly assume that any thoughts that come to mind, and any feelings they experience while thinking about something, bear on what they are thinking about—or why else would they have these thoughts and feelings now, at this moment? Hence, people draw on their feelings as a source of information, unless they become aware that their feelings may be due to an irrelevant source, thus undermining their feelings' perceived relevance to the task at hand (for a review, see Schwarz & Clore, 2007). Accordingly, we cannot predict a person's judgments or decisions by merely knowing *what* came to mind, without taking the accompanying subjective experiences into account. Adding further complexity, the meaning of subjective experiences is itself malleable, and the same experience can convey different information in different contexts.

This chapter addresses a particular type of subjective experience, namely, the metacognitive feelings that arise from monitoring one's own cognitive processes. Not surprisingly, processing new information, retrieving information from memory, and generating thoughts can be experienced as easy or difficult. Because numerous different variables—from environmental conditions and the information's presentation format to the nature of the task and the person's knowledge and bodily state—can make processing easy or difficult, the specific meaning of the experience is ambiguous and requires interpretation: Is this text difficult to make sense of because I'm distracted, because I know little about the topic, because the print font is hard to read, or because the argument is utter nonsense? How people interpret their metacognitive experiences depends on which of many potentially relevant variables they attend to and which of many potentially applicable naive theories of mental processes they bring to bear. In most cases, an applicable theory, entailing a specification of relevant variables, is brought to mind by the task they face; if not, it may be constructed on the spot to make sense of the experience in the given context. As in other domains of judgment, people are likely to rely on the most accessible theory, without considering plausible alternatives, unless the first interpretation fails to yield a plausible result. This limited exploration of plausible alternatives is consistent with the assumption that our feelings are "about" whatever is the focus of attention. As a result, the meaning of metacognitive experiences is itself highly malleable and context sensitive.

As this discussion indicates, the role of contextual influences in judgment is more complex than the common focus on knowledge accessibility suggests. At the first level, contextual variables such as previous exposure, primes, or task characteristics influence *what* comes to mind, as assumed by knowledge accessibility models. At the second level, contextual variables also influence the metacognitive experience, that is, how *easily* information can be retrieved from memory, thoughts can be generated, or novel material can be processed, giving rise to differential inferences from the same declarative inputs. At the third level, contextual variables further influence how the metacognitive experience is *interpreted*, giving rise to differential inferences from the same experience, with differential downstream implications for inferences from declarative inputs.

The interplay among these different levels is the topic of this chapter. The first section addresses the fluency with which new information can be processed, whereas the second addresses the fluency of recall and thought generation. Both sections highlight how metacognitive experiences give rise to different inferences from declarative inputs and how naive theories of the mind change the conclusions drawn from a given experience. The third section illustrates how metacognitive experiences can affect individuals' choice of processing strategies. I conclude the chapter by noting parallels between the use of metacognitive experiences and other feelings as a source of information, placing the findings in the context of a general feelings-as-information approach to the interplay of declarative and experiential information (Schwarz, 1990; Schwarz & Clore, 2007). Throughout, the review is illustrative rather than exhaustive.

THE EASE OF PROCESSING NEW INFORMATION: PROCESSING FLUENCY

Numerous variables can influence the ease or difficulty with which new information can be processed. Some of these variables affect the speed and accuracy of low-level processes concerned with the identification of a stimulus's physical identity and form; they influence *perceptual fluency* (e.g., Jacoby, Kelley, & Dywan, 1989). Relevant variables include figure–ground contrast, the clarity with which a stimulus is presented, the duration of its presentation, or the amount of previous exposure to the stimulus. Other variables influence the speed and accuracy of high-level processes concerned with the identification of stimulus meaning and its relation to semantic knowledge structures; these variables influence *conceptual fluency* (e.g., Whittlesea, 1993). Relevant variables include semantic predictability, the consistency between the stimulus and its context, and the availability of appropriate mental concepts for stimulus classification. Empirically, both types of fluency tend to show parallel influences (for a review, see Winkielman, Schwarz, Fazendeiro, & Reber, 2003) and can be subsumed under the general term *processing fluency*.

What Does the Experience Mean?

Because the diverse variables that influence processing fluency result in similar phenomenological experiences of fluent processing, the meaning of the experience is open to interpretation. Which interpretation people choose, and which inferences they draw from their experience, depends on which of many applicable naive theories is brought to mind by the current context, most notably, by the task posed. Some of these theories pertain to characteristics of the stimulus and presentation conditions, whereas others pertain to one's own state of knowledge.

Stimulus-related theories include, for example, that it is easier to perceive a stimulus when it is shown with high rather than low clarity and for a long rather than short duration. These assumptions affect judgments of clarity and duration, even when the fluency experience is due to some other variable, such as previous exposure to the stimulus. Hence, people who saw the stimulus before infer that the current presentation lasted longer, or had higher clarity, than people who were not previously exposed to the stimulus (e.g., Whittlesea, Jacoby, & Girard, 1990; Witherspoon & Allan, 1985). Similarly, Masson and Caldwell (1998) observed that participants inferred that a target word was presented for a longer duration, or with higher visual clarity, when a preceding semantic task (e.g., complete the sentence, "An archer shoots a bow and ____") had rendered the target word (*arrow*) highly accessible. In these cases, fluency resulting from previous exposure to the stimulus or related concepts gave rise to erroneous inferences about physical characteristics of the stimulus once the physical judgment task brought an applicable theory to mind (see Kelley & Rhodes, 2002, for a review).

Other naive theories relate processing fluency to one's own state of knowledge. The most important one holds that familiar (previously seen) material is easier to process than novel material. Accordingly, people erroneously conclude that novel material is familiar when it is easy to process due to the influence of other variables. For example, Whittlesea and colleagues (1990) exposed participants to a study list of rapidly presented words. Subsequently, participants completed a recognition test that manipulated the fluency with which test words could be processed through differential visual clarity. As expected, test words shown with higher clarity seemed more familiar and were hence more likely to be "recognized" as having appeared on the previous list. This effect was eliminated when participants were aware that the clarity of the visual presentation was manipulated and hence attributed their fluency experience to this source, rendering it uninformative for the recognition task.

Fluency and Familiarity: Judgments of Risk, Consensus, and Truth

Fluency-based impressions of familiarity have important implications for a wide range of judgments that are relevant in daily life, including assessments of risk, social consensus, and truth.

Judgments of Risk

Not surprisingly, familiarity figures prominently in intuitive assessments of risk: If a stimulus is familiar and elicits no negative memories, then it presumably has not hurt us in the past. Accordingly, incidental variables that affect processing fluency may influence people's risk assessments. Confirming this prediction, Song and Schwarz (2009) observed that ostensible food additives were rated as more likely to be hazardous when their names were difficult (e.g., Fluthractnip) rather than easy (e.g., Magnalroxate) to pronounce. Moreover, the effect of ease of pronunciation on risk ratings was mediated by the perceived novelty of the stimuli.

Highlighting the real-world implications of this observation, Alter and Oppenheimer (2006) found that initial public offerings on the New York Stock Exchange provided a higher return on investment when their ticker symbol was easy (e.g., KAR) rather than difficult to pronounce (e.g., RDO). This effect was most pronounced on the first day of trading, when investing $1,000 in a basket of stocks with fluent ticker symbols would have yielded an excess profit of $85.35 over a basket with dysfluent ticker symbols; this advantage was reduced to a still impressive $20.25 by the end of the first year of trading, as more information about the companies became available.

In addition to the mediating role of perceived familiarity observed by Song and Schwarz (2009), intuitive assessments of risk may be further affected by perceivers' positive affective response to fluently processed stimuli (addressed below), consistent with the observation of mood effects on judgment of risk (e.g., Johnson & Tversky, 1983) and the beneficial influence of sunny weather on the stock market (e.g., Hirshleifer & Schumway, 2003). Future research may fruitfully address the relative contributions of familiarity and affect in mediating the observed fluency effects.

Social Consensus and Truth

When the objective truth of a statement is difficult to evaluate, people often draw on social consensus information to arrive at a judgment, based on the assumption that what many people believe is probably true (Festinger, 1954). To determine whether they "heard it before," people may assess the apparent familiarity of the information, drawing on the fluency with which it can be processed as a relevant input (e.g., Weaver, Garcia, Schwarz, & Miller, 2007). If so, variables that increase processing fluency should increase the perceived truth value of the processed information. Empirically, this is the case.

Not surprisingly, one relevant variable is actual exposure frequency. In a classic study of rumor transmission, Allport and Lepkin (1945) observed that the strongest predictor of belief in wartime rumors was simple repetition. Numerous subsequent studies demonstrated that a given statement is more likely to be judged "true" the more often it is repeated. This illusion of truth effect (Begg, Anas, & Farinacci, 1992) has been obtained with trivia statements or words from a foreign language (e.g., Hasher, Goldstein, & Toppino, 1977) as well as advertising materials (e.g., Hawkins & Hoch, 1992).

Illusions of truth are even observed when participants are explicitly told at the time of exposure that the information is *false*. Skurnik, Yoon, Park, and Schwarz (2005) exposed older and younger adults once or thrice to product statements such as, "Shark cartilage is good for your arthritis," and these statements were explicitly marked as "true" or "false." As may be expected, all participants were less likely to accept a statement as true the more often they were told that it was false—but only when they were tested immediately. After a 3-day delay, repeated warnings backfired for older adults: They were now more likely to assume that a statement was true, the more often they were explicitly told that it is false. This finding is consistent with the observation that explicit memory declines with age, whereas implicit memory remains largely intact (Park, 2000). Hence, after a 3-day delay, older adults could not recall whether the statement was originally marked as true or false, but they still experienced its content as highly familiar, leading them to accept it as true. Ironically, this mechanism turns warnings into recommendations, with important implications for public education campaigns (for a review, see Schwarz, Sanna, Skurnik, & Yoon, 2007).

Theoretically, any other variable that increases processing fluency should have the same effect as message repetition. Supporting this prediction, Reber and Schwarz (1999) found that participants were more likely to accept statements such as "Osorno is a city in Chile" as true when the statements were presented in colors that made them easy (e.g., dark blue) rather than difficult (e.g., light blue) to read against the background. Similarly, McGlone and Tofighbakhsh (2000) manipulated processing fluency by presenting substantively equivalent novel aphorisms in a rhyming (e.g., "woes unite foes") or nonrhyming form (e.g., "woes unite enemies"). As expected, participants judged substantively equivalent aphorisms as more true when they rhymed than when they did not.

In combination, these findings indicate that processing fluency serves as an experiential basis of truth judgments. In the absence of more diagnostic information, people draw on the apparent familiarity of the statement to infer its likely truth value. This inference is based on the (usually correct) assumption that widely shared opinions are both more likely to be familiar and to be correct than more idiosyncratic ones. Hence, if it seems like they have heard it before, there is probably something to it. By the same token, people should infer that apparently familiar information is likely to be false when they have reason to believe that false information is more common in the given context. Empirically, this is the case, and fluency can result in inferences of truth or falseness, depending on people's assumptions about the prevalence of truth and falseness in the relevant environment (e.g., Skurnik, Schwarz, & Winkielman, 2000; Unkelbach, 2007).

Fluency and Affect: Judgments of Preference and Beauty

The judgment effects reviewed so far can be plausibly traced to inferences based on the experience of fluent processing itself. However, a second factor contributes to the pervasive influence of processing fluency. High processing fluency is experienced as pleasant and elicits a positive affective reaction that can be captured with psychophysiological measures (Winkielman & Cacioppo, 2001). The positive affective reaction, in turn, can itself serve as a basis of judgment, providing an alternative pathway for fluency effects that is particularly relevant to judgments of preference (Winkielman et al., 2003). What is less clear is *why* processing fluency is experienced as affectively positive. Relevant proposals range from the adaptive value of a preference for familiar stimuli (Zajonc, 1968) to the adaptive value of fast stimulus identification (Winkielman, Schwarz, & Nowak, 2002), and their empirical evaluation awaits further research.

In his classic demonstration of the mere exposure effect, Zajonc (1968; for a review, see Bornstein, 1989) showed that repeated exposure to a stimulus results in more positive evaluations, and several researchers suggested that this observation is a function of increased processing fluency (e.g., Jacoby, Kelley, & Dywan, 1989; Seamon, Brody, & Kauff, 1983). If so, *any* variable that facilitates fluent processing should also facilitate positive evaluations, even with a single exposure. Numerous studies support this prediction. For example, Reber, Winkielman, and Schwarz (1998) presented participants with slightly degraded pictures of everyday objects and manipulated processing fluency through a visual priming procedure. Depending on conditions, the target picture was preceded by a subliminally presented, highly degraded contour of either the target picture or a different picture. As predicted, pictures preceded by matched contours were recognized faster, indicating higher fluency, and were liked more than pictures preceded by mismatched contours. Extending this work, Winkielman and Fazendeiro (reported in Winkielman et al., 2003) showed participants unambiguous pictures of common objects and manipulated processing fluency through semantic primes. In the high-fluency condition, the picture (e.g., of a lock) was preceded by a matching word (e.g., *lock*); in the moderate-fluency condition, by an associatively related word (e.g., *key*); and in the low-fluency condition by an unrelated word (e.g., *snow*). As predicted, pictures preceded by matching words were liked more than pictures preceded by related words, which, in turn, were liked more than pictures preceded by unrelated words. This positive effect of processing fluency was eliminated when participants attributed their positive affective response to music played in the background, as has previously been observed for the influence of moods (Schwarz & Clore, 1983).

Lee and Labroo (2004; see also Labroo, Dhar, & Schwarz, 2008) obtained similar findings in the consumer domain. They found, for example, that consumers reported more positive attitudes toward ketchup when they were previously exposed to a closely related product (mayonnaise) rather than an unrelated one. Presumably, the closely related product facilitated processing of the target product, much as related semantic primes facilitated processing of the target pictures in Winkielman and Fazendeiro's study.

Numerous other variables that affect processing fluency produce parallel effects, from figure–ground contrast and presentation duration (e.g., Reber et al., 1998) to the prototypicality of the stimulus (e.g., Halberstadt & Rhodes, 2000; Langlois & Roggman, 1990). Moreover, the influence of many variables addressed in the psychology of aesthetics (Arnheim, 1974), such as figural goodness, symmetry, and information density, can be traced to the mediating role of processing fluency: All of these variables facilitate stimulus identification and elicit more positive evaluations. Based on these and related findings, Reber, Schwarz, and Winkielman (2004) proposed a fluency theory of aesthetic pleasure that assigns a central role to the perceiver's processing dynamics: The more fluently perceivers can process a stimulus, the more positive their aesthetic response. This proposal provides an integrative account of diverse variables and traces their influence to the same underlying process. First, *image variables* that have long been known to influence aesthetic judgments, such as figural goodness, figure–ground contrast, symmetry, and prototypicality, exert their influence by facilitating or impairing fluent processing of the stimulus. Second, *perceiver variables*, such as a history of previous exposure or a motivational state to which the stimulus is relevant, similarly exert their influence through processing fluency. Third, *contextual variables*, such as visual or semantic priming, that play no role in traditional theories of aesthetics operate in the same fashion and also affect aesthetic appreciation through their influence on processing fluency.

Finally, it is worth noting that the relationship between perceived familiarity and affective response is bidirectional. As Monin (2003) demonstrated, stimuli that evoke a positive affective response are judged as more familiar, even when researchers control for fluency of processing. Similarly, Garcia-Marques and Mackie (2001) observed that participants in a good mood are more likely to perceive novel arguments as familiar, which may contribute to their acceptance of them as true.

Summary

In summary, processing fluency influences judgment through two related pathways. First, people attend to the dynamics of their own information processing and draw on the experience of fluent or disfluent processing as a source of information. What they conclude from their fluency experiences, however, depends on which of many potentially applicable naive theories of information processing is brought to mind by contextual variables, most notably, the task posed. Second, high fluency elicits spontaneous positive affective reactions, which provide further experiential information, paralleling the influence of moods and emotions. Neither source of experiential information exerts an influence when its informational value for the judgment at hand is called into question. This is the case when judges are aware that their fluency experience (for a review, see Kelley & Rhodes, 2002) or apparent affective reaction to the target (for a review, see Schwarz & Clore, 2007) is due to an irrelevant source.

Finally, some phenomena are likely to reflect the operation of both processes. For example, studying the role of processing fluency in consumer choice, Novemsky, Dhar, Schwarz, and Simonson (2007) presented participants with descriptions of two digital cameras. As expected, participants were less likely to defer choice when the print font of the description was easy (56% deferral) rather than difficult to read (71% deferral), unless their attention was explicitly drawn to the font (57% deferral). This result may reflect that the described cameras seemed less attractive under low-fluency conditions, or that the information seemed less familiar and credible, both of which could contribute to a higher rate of deferral.

THE EASE OF RECALL AND THOUGHT GENERATION: ACCESSIBILITY EXPERIENCES

The same conceptual logic applies to the ease or difficulty of recall and thought generation. Information can be easy or difficult to bring to mind for many different reasons, and what people conclude from these *accessibility experiences* depends on which of many naive theories of mental processes they bring to bear. Some naive theories link accessibility experiences to characteristics of the object of judgment, such as the frequency or temporal distance of events, whereas others link them to the state of one's own knowledge, such as one's expertise or interest, or to characteristics of the current situation, such as factors that may be distracting. Whenever the experience is attributed to a source that is irrelevant to the target judgment, its informational value is discredited, and people draw on other inputs, usually the declarative information they have brought to mind.

What Does the Experience Mean?

One widely applicable naive theory holds that the more exemplars that exist, the easier it is to bring some to mind. This correct belief is at the heart of Tversky and Kahneman's (1973) availability heuristic, and people infer higher frequency and probability from ease of recall. Because frequent exemplars are also more typical for their category, ease of recall further suggests high typicality. Accordingly, people infer that they use their bicycles more often after recalling few rather than many instances (Aarts & Dijksterhuis, 1999); rate themselves as more assertive after recalling few rather than many of their own assertive behaviors (Schwarz et al., 1991); like Tony Blair more after listing few rather than many favorable thoughts about him (Haddock, 2002); hold an attitude with more confidence after generating few rather than many supporting arguments (Haddock, Rothman, Reber, & Schwarz, 1999); consider an event more likely the more reasons they generate for why it might *not* have occurred (Sanna, Schwarz, & Stocker, 2002); and are more likely to defer choice after listing many rather than few reasons for making a choice (Novemsky et al., 2007).

When people apply this naive theory, their inferences are consistent with the implications of *what* comes to mind when recall or thought generation is easy, but opposite to these implications when it is difficult. Several lines of evidence indicate that these effects are due to metacognitive experiences rather than to differences in the quality of examples listed. First, external raters detect no quality difference between the first and last two examples listed (e.g., Schwarz et al., 1991). Second, yoked participants, who merely read the thoughts generated by another and are hence deprived of the generation experience, are more influenced when their partner lists many rather than few arguments, in contrast to the person who lists them (e.g., Wänke, Bless, & Biller, 1996). Third, and most important, the impact of a metacognitive experience is eliminated when the experience is misattributed to an external influence, such as music played in the background. In this case, participants draw on accessible content, and rate themselves as more assertive, the more examples of assertive behavior they list, thus reversing the otherwise observed pattern (Schwarz et al., 1991; for conceptual replications, see Haddock et al., 1999; Novemsky et al., 2007; Sanna, Schwarz, & Small, 2002).[1] Finally, the same effect can be observed when all participants list the same number of thoughts and their subjective experience of difficulty is manipulated through facial feedback in the form of *corrugator contraction*, an expression associated with mental effort (e.g., Sanna, Schwarz, & Small, 2002; Stepper & Strack, 1993).

Other naive theories of memory correctly hold, for example, that it is easier to recall events that are well rather than poorly represented in memory; that one found important when they occurred; or that happened in the recent rather than distant past. Accordingly, people infer higher childhood amnesia after successfully recalling 12 rather than four childhood events (Winkielman, Schwarz, & Belli, 1998) and consider past events less important, and date them as having occurred at a more distant time after recalling many rather than few details (Schwarz & Xu, 2009). People further assume that it is easier to recall material in their domain of interest, and that a lack of expertise renders recall and thought generation difficult. Hence, they infer, for example, that they are not very interested in politics when they find it difficult to answer political knowledge question—unless they can attribute the difficulty to an external source, such as a lack of media coverage (Schwarz & Schuman, 1997). Conversely, attributing any experienced difficulty to one's lack of knowledge renders it uninformative for judgments about states of the world (e.g., Sanna & Schwarz, 2003).

Determinants and Consequences of Theory Selection

Given that different naive theories are applicable to the same accessibility experience, it is important to understand the determinants of their use. As in the case of fluency experiences, a key determinant is the judgment task itself, which recruits an applicable inference rule that allows the perceiver to get from "here" (the available data) to "there" (the judgment of interest). For example, Schwarz and Xu (2009) asked students to list two or six "fine Italian restaurants" in town. If they were then asked how many fine Italian restaurants the city has, they inferred from the difficulty of listing six that there could not be many. This inference is consistent with Tversky and Kahneman's (1973) availability heuristic. However, if they were asked instead how much they knew about town, they inferred from the same difficulty that they were quite unfamiliar with their college town. Theoretically, each of these judgments entails an attribution of the recall experience to a specific source, either to the number of restaurants in town or to one's own expertise. Once this implicit attribution is made, the experience is "explained" and should become uninformative for judgments that require a different theory, making it likely that people turn to accessible thought content instead. Confirming this prediction, participants who first concluded that there were few fine Italian restaurants in town subsequently reported high expertise: After all, there aren't many such restaurants and they nevertheless could list quite a few, so they must know a lot about town. Conversely, those who first concluded that their difficulty reflects a lack of knowledge subsequently inferred that there are many fine Italian restaurants: After all, they had listed quite a few, and they did not even know much about town.

In a conceptual replication, Schwarz and Xu (2009) asked participants to recall details of the Oklahoma City bombing. When they were then asked to date the event, they inferred that it was more recent after recalling two rather than 10 details; but if they were asked instead how important the event was to them at the time, they inferred higher importance after recalling two rather than 10 details. Again, these judgments entail an attribution of the experience to a specific cause (here, recency or importance), rendering the experience uninformative for other judgments. Accordingly, participants who initially attributed the difficulty of recalling many details to the event's temporal distance subsequently reported that the event was quite important to them: After all, they had just recalled numerous details even though the event had apparently happened long ago. Conversely, participants who initially attributed difficulty of recall to low personal importance subsequently dated the event as closer in time: After all, they could still recall numerous details despite the event's low personal importance.

Summary

In summary, recall and thought generation can be experienced as easy or difficult. What people conclude from these accessibility experiences depends on which of many potentially applicable naive theories of memory and cognition is brought to mind by the present context. In most cases, applicable theories are recruited by the judgment task, and the same experience can result in different substantive conclusions, depending on the specific theory applied. Moreover, every theory-based judgment entails a causal attribution of the experience to the source specified in the naive theory. Accordingly, the first judgment can serve as a context that undermines the informational value of the experience for later judgments that require the application of a different theory, much as has been observed for other (mis)attribution manipulations (for a review, see Schwarz & Clore, 2007). Once the informational value of the experience is called into question, people turn to the content of their thoughts as an alternative source of information. Hence, subsequent judgments are content-based rather than experience-based, resulting in a reversal of the otherwise observed effects.

Although numerous studies converge on the conclusion that people rely only on their metacognitive experiences when their informational value is not called into question (Schwarz & Clore, 2007), less is known about the conditions that determine the relative impact of experiential and declarative information. On the one hand, some findings are compatible with a conceptualization of metacognitive experiences as heuristic cues that are more likely to dominate one's judgment when processing motivation (e.g., Rothman & Schwarz, 1998) or capacity (e.g., Greifeneder & Bless, 2008) is low. On the other hand, fluent processing usually increases people's confidence in the content of their thoughts (e.g., by suggesting high expertise or a large body of supportive evidence), which exerts more influence on judgment when processing motivation and capacity are high (for a review, see Petty, Briñol, Tormala, & Wegener, 2007). Hence, metacognitive experiences are likely to influence judgment under both heuristic/intuitive and systematic/analytic processing conditions. A systematic exploration of these contingencies promises further insight into the contextualized interplay of experiential and declarative information in human reasoning.

METACOGNITIVE EXPERIENCES AND THE CHOICE OF PROCESSING STRATEGIES

As already seen, people draw on their metacognitive experiences to assess their own knowledge and various task characteristics. These assessments also inform their choice of processing strategies. When asked to answer a question, for example, people may feel that they know the correct answer even though they are currently unable to bring it to mind. In many cases, this *feeling of knowing* is based on the ease with which partial information comes to mind (Koriat, 1993); in other cases, it is based on the apparent familiarity of the cues provided in the question (Reder & Ritter, 1992). In either case, the higher their feeling of knowing, the more likely people are to engage in detailed retrieval efforts (e.g., Costermans, Lories, & Ansay, 1992). On the other hand, easy retrieval of a plausible answer results in high *confidence* and truncates the search process, making more detailed scrutiny of the answer unlikely (for a discussion, see Petty et al., 2007).

While the above processing decisions are based on assessments of one's own knowledge, metacognitive experiences are likely to inform a wide range of strategy choices, a possibility that awaits systematic investigation. In general, people prefer processing strategies that have been characterized as analytic, systematic, bottom-up, and detail-oriented when they consider their current situation "problematic," but prefer strategies that have been characterized as intuitive, heuristic, and top-down when they consider their current situation as "benign" (Schwarz, 1990). Numerous variables, from task characteristics to incidental environmental cues, moods, and bodily approach or avoidance feedback, can convey this information and have been found to influence processing style (for reviews, see Schwarz, 2002; Schwarz & Clore, 2007). One of these variables is the fluency with which information can be processed. For example, when asked, "How many animals of each kind did Moses take on the ark?" most people answer "two" despite knowing that the biblical actor was Noah (Erickson & Mattson, 1981). Presenting this Moses question in a difficult-to-read print font dramatically reduces reliance on the first answer that comes to mind and increases the recognition that the question cannot be answered as asked; on the other hand, a difficult-to-read print font impairs performance when the first spontaneous association is correct (Song & Schwarz, 2008). Both observations presumably reflect the fact that familiar questions, and the associations they bring to mind, receive less scrutiny than unfamiliar ones. Similarly, Alter, Oppenheimer, Epley, and Norwick (2007) reported that manipulations that increased subjective processing difficulty improved participants' performance on reasoning tasks that benefit from a more analytic processing style.

Note, however, that the influence of metacognitive experiences on strategy choice is bound to be as malleable as their influence on judgment. Inferring that the task is unfamiliar, for example, may abort any attempt to engage in effortful analytic processing when the task seems to require background knowledge that one is likely to lack, given the task's low familiarity. Future research may fruitfully explore how contextual variables that shape the inferences drawn from a given metacognitive experience affect subsequent strategy choices.

CODA

After decades of pervasive "neglect of conscious experience" (Tulving, 1989, p. 4), it is now increasingly acknowledged that an understanding of human cognition requires attention to the subjective experiences that accompany cognitive processes. Consideration of these experiences adds new complexity to theorizing about the "mind in context," even if we limit the context to the immediate task environment and ignore the broader social and cultural context in which it is embedded. As numerous social cognition studies into the effects of knowledge accessibility demonstrate (for reviews, see Förster & Liberman, 2007; Higgins, 1996), contextual variables influence what comes to mind and which declarative information is used in forming a judgment. Knowing the accessible declarative inputs, however, is insufficient to predict the final judgment because the implications of the declarative information are qualified by accompanying subjective experiences (Schwarz & Clore, 2007), including the metacognitive experiences reviewed in this chapter. These metacognitive experiences, in turn, are themselves a function of contextual variables that influence how easily information can be retrieved from memory, thoughts can be generated, or novel material can be processed. Moreover, what people conclude from the experience of easy or difficult processing depends on which of many potentially applicable naive theories of mental processes they bring to bear, which, again, is a function of contextual variables, most notably, the tasks on their minds. Finally, application of a given theory to form an initial judgment entails an attribution of the experience to a specific source, which renders the experience uninformative for subsequent judgments that require the application of a different theory. Hence, the final judgment emerges from a systematic interplay of accessible declarative and experiential inputs, each of which is subject to multiple contextual influences—and a minor change in context, such as the order in which two questions are asked (Schwarz & Xu, 2009), may be sufficient to reverse the otherwise obtained outcome.

What are we to make of this contextual malleability of human judgment? Taking the reviewed experiments at face value, our perception of reality is subject to numerous haphazard influences, leaving us to wonder how we make it through the day. From a broader perspective, however, the observed contextual malleability is compatible with the assumption that thinking is for doing (James, 1890), which requires high sensitivity to the context in which things are to be done (see Smith & Collins, Chapter 7, this volume). Hence, information that is relevant in a given context should indeed be privileged at the expense of less relevant information, making context-dependent knowledge accessibility an adaptive feature. The accompanying metacognitive experience that the information comes to mind easily may further highlight its relevance, giving it an advantage over less accessible and presumably less relevant information. Similarly, the fluency with which new information can be processed indeed often reflects previous exposure, making it a valid indicator of familiarity. Moreover, the meaning we impose on a given metacognitive experience should indeed be the meaning that is most relevant to the task at hand, and the recruitment of task-relevant naive theories facilitates this. From this perspective, the basic processes identified in this chapter are adaptive rather than dysfunctional.

Unfortunately, however, this is only part of the story. Although we are very sensitive to our subjective experiences, we are utterly insensitive to their source. We mistake our preexisting moods as our reaction to the object of judgment (e.g., Schwarz & Clore, 1983), fail to recognize that recall is only difficult because we are asked to recall too large a number of examples (e.g., Schwarz et al., 1991), and misread the fluency resulting from easy- or difficult-to-read presentation formats (e.g., Reber & Schwarz, 1999) as indicative of the actual familiarity of the material. Throughout, we treat our thoughts and feelings as bearing on the specific task at hand and rarely consider the possible influence of incidental variables, unless our attention is explicitly drawn to them (Higgins, 1998; Schwarz, 1990). Although the resulting errors of judgment may be less common in the wild than in experiments with carefully managed incidental influences, the emergence of fluency (Alter & Oppenheimer, 2006) and mood (Hirshleifer & Shumway, 2003) effects on stock prices illustrates that they are certainly not restricted to laboratory studies with inconsequential tasks. Being blissfully unaware of incidental influences and alternative interpretations, we experience our judgments as a compelling reflection of reality, although a different question may result in the construction of a different reality from the same inputs—a naive realism that protects us from a continuous sense of uncertainty (for related discussions, see Dunham & Banaji, Chapter 10, this volume; Ross & Ward, 1996).

NOTE

1. These findings also bear on Tormala, Falces, Briñol, and Petty's (2007) observation that participants who attempt to list many thoughts may also have more unrequested thoughts; for example, those asked to list many favorable thoughts may also find a larger number of unfavorable thoughts coming to mind. Tormala and colleagues suggest that these unrequested thoughts, rather than the experience of difficulty per se, may drive the reviewed effects. If so, the pattern of participants' judgments should not reverse when the diagnostic value of the metacognitive experience is called into question:

Attributing one's difficulty to background music (Schwarz et al., 1991), for example, does nothing to discredit the substantive relevance of any unrequested thoughts one might have had. Although unrequested thoughts are probably part and parcel of the experience of difficulty, they do not provide a coherent account of the available findings.

REFERENCES

Aarts, H., & Dijksterhuis, A. (1999). How often did I do it?: Experienced ease of retrieval and frequency estimates of past behavior. *Acta Psychologica, 103*, 77–89.

Allport, F. H., & Lepkin, M. (1945). Wartime rumors of waste and special privilege: Why some people believe them. *Journal of Abnormal and Social Psychology, 40*, 3–36.

Alter, A. L., & Oppenheimer, D. M. (2006). Predicting short-term stock fluctuations by using processing fluency. *Proceedings of the National Academy of Sciences USA, 103*, 9369–9372.

Alter, A. A., Oppenheimer, D. M., Epley, N., & Norwick, R. (2007). *Overcoming intuition: Metacognitive difficulty activates analytic reasoning.* Unpublished manuscript, Princeton University.

Arnheim, R. (1974). *Art and visual perception: A psychology of the creative eye.* Berkeley: University of California Press.

Begg, I. M., Anas, A., & Farinacci, S. (1992). Dissociation of processes in belief: Source recollection, statement familiarity, and the illusion of truth. *Journal of Experimental Psychology: General, 121*, 446–458.

Bornstein, R. F. (1989). Exposure and affect: Overview and meta-analysis of research 1968–1987. *Psychological Bulletin, 106*, 265–289.

Costermans, J., Lories, G., & Ansay, C. (1992). Confidence level and feeling of knowing in question answering. *Journal of Experimental Psychology: Learning, Memory, and Cognition, 18*, 142–150.

Erickson, T. A., & Mattson, M. E. (1981). From words to meaning: A semantic illusion. *Journal of Verbal Learning and Verbal Behavior, 20*, 540–552.

Festinger, L. (1954). A theory of social comparison processes. *Human Relations, 7*, 123–146.

Förster, J., & Liberman, N. (2007). Knowledge activation. In A. Kruglanski & E. T. Higgins (Eds.), *Social psychology: Handbook of basic principles* (2nd ed., pp. 201–231). New York: Guilford Press.

Garcia-Marques, T., & Mackie, D. M. (2001). The feeling of familiarity as a regulator of persuasive processing. *Social Cognition, 19*, 9–34.

Greifeneder, R., & Bless, H. (2007). Relying on accessible content vs. accessibility experiences: The case of processing capacity. *Social Cognition, 25*, 853–881.

Haddock, G. (2002). It's easy to like or dislike Tony Blair: Accessibility experiences and the favorability of attitude judgments. *British Journal of Social Psychology, 93*, 257–267.

Haddock, G., Rothman, A.J., Reber, R., & Schwarz, N. (1999). Forming judgments of attitude certainty, importance, and intensity: The role of subjective experiences. *Personality and Social Psychology Bulletin, 25*, 771–782.

Halberstadt, J., & Rhodes, G. (2000). The attractiveness of nonface average: Implications for an evolutionary explanation of the attractiveness of average faces. *Psychological Science, 11*, 285–289.

Hasher, L., Goldstein, D., & Toppino, T. (1977). Frequency and the conference of referential validity. *Journal of Verbal Learning and Verbal Behavior, 16*, 107–112.

Hawkins, S. A., & Hoch, S. J. (1992). Low-involvement learning: Memory without evaluation. *Journal of Consumer Research, 19*, 212–225.

Higgins, E. T. (1996). Knowledge activation: Accessibility, applicability, and salience. In E. T. Higgins & A. W. Kruglanski (Eds.), *Social psychology: Handbook of basic principles* (pp. 133–168). New York: Guilford Press.

Higgins, E. T. (1998). The aboutness principle: A pervasive influence on human inference. *Social Cognition, 16*, 173–198.

Hirshleifer, D., & Shumway, T. (2003). Good day sunshine: Stock returns and the weather. *Journal of Finance, 58*, 1009–1032.

Jacoby, L. L., Kelley, C. M., & Dywan, J. (1989). Memory attributions. In H. L. Roediger & F. I. M. Craik (Eds.), *Varieties of memory and consciousness: Essays in honour of Endel Tulving* (pp. 391–422). Hillsdale, NJ: Erlbaum.

James, W. (1890). *The principles of psychology* (Vol. 2). New York: Henry Holt.

Johnson, E., & Tversky, A. (1983). Affect, generalization, and the perception of risk. *Journal of Personality and Social Psychology, 45*, 20–31.

Kelley, C. M., & Rhodes, M. G. (2002). Making sense and nonsense of experience: Attributions in memory and judgment. *Psychology of Learning and Motivation, 41*, 293–320.

Koriat, A. (1993). How do we know that we know?: The accessibility model of the feeling of knowing. *Psychological Review, 100*, 609–639.

Labroo, A. A., Dhar, R., & Schwarz, N. (2008). Of frog wines and smiling watches: Semantic priming of perceptual features and brand evaluation. *Journal of Consumer Research, 34*, 819–831.

Langlois, J. H., & Roggman, L. A. (1990). Attractive faces are only average. *Psychological Science, 1*, 115–121.

Lee, A. Y., & Labroo, A. A. (2004). The effect of conceptual and perceptual fluency on brand evaluation. *Journal of Marketing Research, 41*, 151–165.

Masson, M. E. J., & Caldwell, J. I. (1998). Conceptually driven encoding episodes create perceptual misattributions. *Acta Psychologica, 98*, 183–210.

McGlone, M. S., & Tofighbakhsh, J. (2000). Birds of a feather flock conjointly (?): Rhyme as reason in aphorisms. *Psychological Science, 11*, 424–428.

Monin, B. (2003). The warm glow heuristic: When liking leads to familiarity. *Journal of Personality and Social Psychology, 85*, 1035–1048.

Novemsky, N., Dhar, R., Schwarz, N., & Simonson, I. (2007). Preference fluency in choice. *Journal of Marketing Research, 44*, 347–356.

Park, D.C. (2000). The basic mechanisms accounting for age-related decline in cognitive function. In D. C. Park & N. Schwarz (Eds.), *Cognitive aging: A primer* (pp. 3–22). Philadelphia: Psychology Press.

Petty, R. E., Briñol, P., Tormala, Z. L., & Wegener, D. T. (2007). The role of metacognition in social judgment. In A. Kruglanski & E. T. Higgins (Eds.), *Social psychology: Handbook of basic principles* (2nd ed., pp. 254–284). New York: Guilford Press.

Reber, R., & Schwarz, N. (1999). Effects of perceptual fluency on judgments of truth. *Consciousness and Cognition*, *8*, 338–342.

Reber, R., Schwarz, N., & Winkielman, P. (2004). Processing fluency and aesthetic pleasure: Is beauty in the perceiver's processing experience? *Personality and Social Psychology Review*, *8*, 364–382.

Reber, R., Winkielman, P., & Schwarz, N. (1998). Effects of perceptual fluency on affective judgments. *Psychological Science*, *9*, 45–48.

Reder, L. M., & Ritter, F. E. (1992). What determines initial feelings of knowing?: Familiarity with question terms, not with answers. *Journal of Experimental Psychology: Learning, Memory, and Cognition*, *18*, 435–451.

Ross, L., & Ward, A. (1996). Naive realism in everyday life: Implications for social conflict and misunderstanding. In E. S. Reed, E. Turiel, & T. Brown (Eds.), *Values and knowledge* (pp. 103–135). Hillsdale, NJ: Erlbaum.

Rothman, A. J., & Schwarz, N. (1998). Constructing perceptions of vulnerability: Personal relevance and the use of experiential information in health judgments. *Personality and Social Psychology Bulletin*, *24*, 1053–1064.

Sanna, L. J., & Schwarz, N. (2003). Debiasing hindsight: The role of accessibility experiences and attributions. *Journal of Experimental Social Psychology*, *39*, 287–295.

Sanna, L. J., Schwarz, N., & Small, E. (2002). Accessibility experiences and the hindsight bias: I-knew-it-all-along versus It-could-never-have-happened. *Memory and Cognition*, *30*, 1288–1296.

Sanna, L. J., Schwarz, N., & Stocker, S. L. (2002). When debiasing backfires: Accessible content and accessibility experiences in debiasing hindsight. *Journal of Experimental Psychology: Learning, Memory, and Cognition*, *28*, 497–502.

Schwarz, N. (1990). Feelings as information: Informational and motivational functions of affective states. In E. T. Higgins & R. M. Sorrentino (Eds.), *Handbook of motivation and cognition: Vol. 2. Foundations of social behavior* (pp. 527–561). New York: Guilford Press.

Schwarz, N. (2002). Situated cognition and the wisdom of feelings: Cognitive tuning. In L. Feldman Barrett & P. Salovey (Eds.), *The wisdom in feelings: Psychological processes in emotional intelligence* (pp. 144–166). New York: Guilford Press.

Schwarz, N. (2007). Attitude construction: Evaluation in context. *Social Cognition*, *25*, 638–656.

Schwarz, N., Bless, H., Strack, F., Klumpp, G., Rittenauer-Schatka, H., & Simons, A. (1991). Ease of retrieval as information: Another look at the availability heuristic. *Journal of Personality and Social Psychology*, *61*, 195–202.

Schwarz, N., & Clore, G. L. (1983). Mood, misattribution, and judgments of well-being: Informative and directive functions of affective states. *Journal of Personality and Social Psychology*, *45*, 513–523.

Schwarz, N., & Clore, G. L. (2007). Feelings and phenomenal experiences. In A. Kruglanski & E. T. Higgins (Eds.), *Social psychology: Handbook of basic principles* (2nd ed., pp. 385–407). New York: Guilford Press.

Schwarz, N., Sanna, L., Skurnik, I., & Yoon, C. (2007). Metacognitive experiences and the intricacies of setting people straight: Implications for debiasing and public information campaigns. *Advances in Experimental Social Psychology, 39*, 127–161.

Schwarz, N., & Schuman, H. (1997). Political knowledge, attribution, and inferred political interest: The operation of buffer items. *International Journal of Public Opinion Research, 9*, 191–195.

Schwarz, N., & Xu, J. (2009). *Constructing heuristics on the spot: Divergent inferences from ease of recall.* Unpublished manuscript, University of Michigan.

Seamon, J. G., Brody, N., & Kauff, D. M. (1983). Affective discrimination of stimuli that are not recognized: Effects of shadowing, masking, and central laterality. *Journal of Experimental Psychology: Learning, Memory, and Cognition, 9*, 544–555.

Skurnik, I., Schwarz, N., & Winkielman, P. (2000). Drawing inferences from feelings: The role of naive beliefs. In H. Bless & J. Forgas (Eds.), *The message within: The role of subjective experience in social cognition and behavior* (pp. 162–175). Philadelphia: Psychology Press.

Skurnik, I., Yoon, C., Park, D. C., & Schwarz, N. (2005). How warnings about false claims become recommendations. *Journal of Consumer Research, 31*, 713–724.

Song, H., & Schwarz, N. (2008). Fluency and the detection of distortions: Low processing fluency attenuates the Moses illusion. *Social Cognition, 26*, 791–799.

Song, H., & Schwarz, N. (2009). If it's difficult-to-pronounce, it must be risky: Processing fluency and risk perception. *Psychological Science, 20*, 135–138.

Stepper, S., & Strack, F. (1993). Proprioceptive determinants of emotional and nonemotional feelings. *Journal of Personality and Social Psychology, 64*, 211–220.

Tormala, Z. L., Falces, C., Briñol, P., & Petty, R. E. (2007). Ease of retrieval effects in social judgment: The role of unrequested cognitions. *Journal of Personality and Social Psychology, 93*, 143–157.

Tulving, E. (1989). Memory: Performance, knowledge, and experience. *European Journal of Cognitive Psychology, 1*, 3–26.

Tversky, A., & Kahneman, D. (1973). Availability: A heuristic for judging frequency and probability. *Cognitive Psychology, 5*, 207–232.

Unkelbach, C. (2007). Reversing the truth effect: Learning the interpretation of processing fluency in judgments of truth. *Journal of Experimental Psychology: Learning, Memory, and Cognition, 33*, 219–230.

Wänke, M., Bless, H., & Biller, B. (1996). Subjective experience versus content of information in the construction of attitude judgments. *Personality and Social Psychology Bulletin, 22*, 1105–1113.

Weaver, K., Garcia, S. M., Schwarz, N., & Miller, D. T. (2007). Inferring the popularity of an opinion from its familiarity: A repetitive voice can sound like a chorus. *Journal of Personality and Social Psychology, 92*, 821–833.

Whittlesea, B. W. A. (1993). Illusions of familiarity. *Journal of Experimental Psychology: Learning, Memory, and Cognition, 19*, 1235–1253.

Whittlesea, B. W. A., Jacoby, L. L., & Girard, K. (1990). Illusions of immediate memory: Evidence of an attributional basis for feelings of familiarity and perceptual quality. *Journal of Memory and Language, 29*, 716–732.

Winkielman, P., & Cacioppo, J. T. (2001). Mind at ease puts a smile on the face: Psychophysiological evidence that processing facilitation leads to positive affect. *Journal of Personality and Social Psychology, 81*, 989–1000.

Winkielman, P., Schwarz, N., & Belli, R.F. (1998). The role of ease of retrieval and attribution in memory judgments: Judging your memory as worse despite recalling more events. *Psychological Science, 9*, 124–126.

Winkielman, P., Schwarz, N., Fazendeiro, T., & Reber, R. (2003). The hedonic marking of processing fluency: Implications for evaluative judgment. In J. Musch & K. C. Klauer (Eds.), *The psychology of evaluation: Affective processes in cognition and emotion* (pp. 189–217). Mahwah, NJ: Erlbaum.

Winkielman, P., Schwarz, N., & Nowak, A. (2002). Affect and processing dynamics. In S. Moore & M. Oaksford (Eds.), *Emotional cognition: From brain to behavior* (pp. 111–138). Amsterdam: Benjamins.

Witherspoon, D., & Allan, L. G. (1985). The effects of a prior presentation on temporal judgments in a perceptual identification task. *Memory and Cognition, 13*, 103–111.

Zajonc, R. B. (1968). Attitudinal effects of mere exposure. *Journal of Personality and Social Psychology: Monograph Supplement, 9*, 1–27.

7

Situated Cognition

ELIOT R. SMITH
ELIZABETH C. COLLINS

What does it mean to say that *mind*—including all the processes that underlie our thoughts, feelings, and behavior—emerges from interactions among and between individual persons and their contexts? Can it be meaningful to suggest that cognition is not implemented solely within the brain but is somehow extended by aspects of a person's physical and social context, including other people? This chapter seeks to answer these questions, with a special focus on the *social* (rather than physical) context of cognition. Human cognition is fundamentally shaped by people's immediate social and communicative goals, personal relationships, and group memberships. Our social worlds not only frequently make up the *content* of our thoughts and feelings, but they also shape the *processes* underlying our cognition and behavior (Smith & Conrey, 2009). The viewpoint taken in this chapter owes much to the broader situated cognition perspective in the social and cognitive sciences, which we first introduce.

THE SITUATED COGNITION PERSPECTIVE

A conceptual focus on the interaction between the individual and the context is characteristic of a recently emerging intellectual movement termed *situated cognition* (Clancey, 2009; Clark, 1997; Robbins & Aydede, 2009). The core themes of situated cognition have attained significant influence in many fields beyond psychology, from anthropology to education to robotics and artificial intelligence. Among the themes with the most direct relevance to this book are the following:

1. *A broad critique of models postulating abstract, amodal, autonomous inner representations and processes.* Situated cognition can be a label for a grab bag of widely diverse (even inconsistent) ideas and principles. A core common thread among these ideas is what they oppose (Clancey, 2009; Wilson & Clark, 2009): the image of cognition as implemented by abstract computational processes, isolated from the real world—an image that has largely dominated psychology since the 1950s and 1960s (Fodor, 1975; Newell, 1980; Pylyshyn, 1984). Situated cognition replaces *computation* with *biology* as the fundamental guiding metaphor for understanding mind. As Clark (1997, p. 1) writes: "We imagined mind as a kind of logical reasoning device coupled with a store of explicit data—a kind of combination logic machine and filing cabinet. In so doing, we ignored the fact that minds evolved to make things happen. We ignored the fact that the biological mind is, first and foremost, an organ for controlling the biological body."

2. *Cognition and adaptive behavior depend on detailed, moment-by-moment, sensorimotor interaction with the environment.* Agre (1997) likened living in the world to canoeing down a white-water stream. Formulating a detailed plan or behavioral "script" in advance and then reading it out from memory to follow it will not suffice; instead, one must make continual adjustments in the canoe's position and path as unexpected waves and currents buffet the boat. The situated perspective sees the mind not as primarily in the business of constructing, storing, and retrieving inner representations, but rather as a controller for behavior, continually transforming incoming information into specifications of what to do *right now*.

3. *Organisms rely on perception of the environment over inner representations when possible.* Brooks (1991) perhaps pushed this principle the farthest with his insistence that the world is its own best representation. Previously, theorists assumed that an organism had to construct, update, and rely on an internal representation of the world—for example, theories of social cognition assumed that social perceivers form inner representations of other persons, social groups, and so forth, on which they draw to make judgments and plan behaviors. Brooks argued that this approach is inefficient. An inner representation of the world would be cognitively costly, necessarily inaccurate, insufficiently detailed, and unable to track ongoing dynamic changes in the real world. Clark (1989, p. 64) proposed as a general principle that "evolved creatures will neither store nor process information in costly ways when they

can use the structure of the environment and their operations upon it as a convenient stand-in for the information-processing operations concerned." Indeed, research on "change blindness" (Simons & Ambinder, 2005) demonstrates that our intuitive feeling that we continually maintain a relatively complete inner representation of our visual surroundings is actually illusory. Instead, we use our perceptual systems to access the world when needed.

4. *Environmental supports are crucial scaffolds for cognition (the extended mind thesis).* Hutchins (1995), in the article "How the Cockpit Remembers Its Speeds," describes how an airliner *cockpit*—a cognitive system encompassing two pilots and a great deal of specialized hardware—remembers crucial items of information that apply to the current flight. Much of the information is stored not in the brains of the pilots (because that type of memory is fragile, fallible, and slow) but in the form of indicators, penciled or taped marks, and so forth, on the instrument panel. A more everyday example (Wilson & Clark, 2009) is that few of us would have an easy time multiplying two three-digit numbers in our heads, but the task becomes trivial when we are given pencil and paper. External memory reduces the task to a series of perception–action cycles, such as recognizing which column to process next and accessing a few well-learned multiplication and addition facts. The *extended mind thesis* (Clark & Chalmers, 1998) is the idea that such performances are best described by considering the whole mind plus environment as a cognitive system rather than maintaining a basically arbitrary dividing line to consider the environment only as "input" to a cognitive system that is rigorously kept inside the head. This thesis "very explicitly identifies cognitive systems themselves as reaching beyond individuals into their physical and social environments" (Wilson & Clark, 2009, p. 58). Illustrating the impact of situated cognition in education (Lave, 1997), some experts advocate not teaching children facts (i.e., stocking their minds with inner representations), but teaching reasoning skills and information about how to gather facts together—in essence, teaching how to use the environment as an extension of the mind.

5. *Social supports are crucial scaffolds for cognition (the socially extended mind thesis).* Not only the physical environment but other people, and—more broadly—sociocultural systems, also participate in cognition. Thus, committees integrate, store, and retrieve information to make decisions; transactive memory systems let each of us offload memory storage to others, and larger cultural systems serve as a repository of information that can be transmitted to new generations (Hutchins, 1995; Nijstad & Stroebe, 2006; Wegner, 1986). Again, as we discuss later, it seems less than fruitful to insist that other people only provide

"input," while all cognition or information processing takes place within the mind of the individual. Rather, a group discussion can be insightfully analyzed as an integrated, multiagent cognitive system, implementing informational processes such as memory, scrutiny and integration of information, and decision making (Mason, Conrey, & Smith, 2007; Stasser, 1988).

The interdependence of the mind with its context in the generation of cognition and adaptive behavior is perhaps the core idea of situated cognition, as expressed by Clancey (2009):

> Can we summarize the meaning of situated cognition itself[?] ... The one essential theoretical move is contextualization (perhaps stated as "anti-localization," in terms of what must be rooted out): We cannot locate meaning in the text, life in the cell, the person in the body, knowledge in the brain, a memory in a neuron. Rather, these are all active, dynamic processes, existing only in interactive behaviors of cultural, social, biological, and physical environment systems. (p. 28)

We focus especially on the social rather than physical (nonsocial) context. Although nonsocial contexts have been more often investigated in the situated cognition literature (e.g., Kirsh, 1995), we believe that cognition is fundamentally social: Social contexts, motives, and identities constrain and constitute our thoughts and behavior whether or not we are physically in the presence of other people (Smith & Semin, 2004). We flesh out this idea in discussions of three main topics: the interdependence of cognition and behavior with (1) immediate situational contexts, (2) communicative concepts and relationships, and (3) the socially defined self. We must leave aside the issue of embodiment (Pfeifer & Bongard, 2007). Embodiment is closely related to the general principles of situated cognition, for the body is the most immediate physical context for mind. Recent thinking (e.g., Barsalou, 1999) emphasizes the importance of the body and sensorimotor systems in all cognition, even abstract conceptual thought, but space precludes our going into these important matters.

IMMEDIATE SITUATIONAL CONTEXTS

As we have noted, a core principle of the situated cognition approach is that human judgments, decisions, and adaptive behaviors are generally constructed from locally available resources and situational cues. This means that communications, self-reports of attitudes or other judgments, and decisions about how to act are not simply "readouts" of stable, abstract inner knowledge representations. We first address this point generally, then discuss the interdependence of cognition with contextual resources, under the headings of the extended mind and the socially extended mind.

Cognition and Behavior Depend on the Immediate Situation

Barsalou's (1999) perceptual symbol systems model holds that conceptual knowledge is reconstructed as a "situated simulation" that differs in every relevant context rather than being retrieved in static form. Many types of knowledge about an object (e.g., a car: wheels, engine, visual appearance, sound) are represented in memory, and subsets of that information are recombined to yield a context-appropriate representation (say, an old Volvo station wagon or a flashy sports car). Schwarz (1999) and Wilson and Hodges (1992) have argued generally that social knowledge is contextually reconstructed. And Garcia-Marques, Santos, and Mackie (2006) provide recent evidence that social group stereotypes, despite their reputation as stable and difficult to change, actually show as much variability as nonsocial conceptual representations within individuals across time (Barsalou, 1987; Yeh & Barsalou, 2006).

Judgments or evaluations of objects depend on not only situation-specific representations of the object itself but also implicit comparison standards, which Kahneman and Miller (1986) termed *norms*. Norms arise from not only preexisting expectations about a situation but also situationally salient counterfactuals. Thus, an object encountered in a specific situation elicits the online construction of its own norm, against which it is compared and evaluated, and similar objects may be perceived very differently if they trigger divergent norms. For example, Greenberg and Pyszczynski (1985) found that if participants overheard an ethnic slur about an African American target who had just lost a debate, then they evaluated the target's skill more negatively than did participants who did not hear the ethnic slur. When the African American target won the debate, participants who had heard the ethnic slur actually gave a more positive evaluation of the target than those who had not. Evidently judgment of the debate performance was based on information that was momentarily accessible, including negative constructs activated by the slur (but only if they were applicable).

The "shifting standards" model of judgments (Biernat & Manis, 1994) describes how one element of the situation, stereotype-relevant group membership, can influence social judgments. Because stereotypes imply expectations, standards and meanings shift when members of different groups are judged in a domain that is stereotype relevant. As a result, evaluative judgments are usually made in comparison to the group; that is, subjective language ("good" or "bad") is typically used and understood with reference to the category of the person being described. This can lead to seemingly paradoxical effects. For example, in one study (Biernat & Manis, 1994, Study 1) participants rated articles on feminine topics (healthy cooking tips and eye makeup trends) subjectively better when they were said to be written by a man rather than a woman, although they thought that the male author should be paid less than the female (and the opposite for masculine topics). Their subjective evaluation, in effect, was "It's pretty good—*for a man*." Thus, the context of the object being judged (specifically, the gender of the author) alters the standards used for judgment.

Power, whether originating in relatively permanent organizational roles or in situation-specific interdependence relationships, is another crucial aspect of a person's social context that has consequences for cognition. Research has examined how power influences stereotype use, with contradictory results. Some studies find that highly powerful people use stereotypes more (Fiske, 1993), whereas others find that the powerful use them less (Overbeck & Park, 2001). In a recent review Guinote (2007) proposed that the reason for this discrepancy is that power affects cognition at a more basic level than does stereotyping. She posits that an increase in a person's power increases selective information-processing abilities and attunement to the important elements in the situation. Thus, people with low power are likely to use a consistent strategy to deal with the situation, whereas people with high power are more flexible, individuating the people they need information about, and stereotyping the people they do not. As a consequence, high power leads to different strategies and behaviors depending on the needs of the situation, whereas low power leads to relatively consistent behavior across situations.

There is other evidence that behavioral decisions are constructed online from momentarily available information as well—rather than being read out from stable inner representations. Shafir (2007) reviews numerous lines of evidence that even highly abstracted, stripped-down decisions (e.g., choices between monetary gambles) are constructed based on locally salient information instead of the perceiver's stable, general preferences and beliefs about the world. As a result, it is easy to produce examples that lead people to violate fundamental principles of rationality, such as framing effects, in which logically irrelevant details can reverse people's preferences between a pair of options; intransitive preferences, in which *A* is preferred to *B*, and *B* to C, but C is preferred to *A*; or anchoring effects, in which a clearly irrelevant number can influence people's numerical estimates.

Situational construction means that in many cases not only our judgments but also our overt behaviors are strongly influenced by minor details of situations (see also Mischel & Shoda, Chapter 8, this volume). Bargh, Chen, and Burrows (1996) have illustrated how situational primes can subtly activate behavioral representations, such as the concept of "politeness," and actually cause people to behave in a more polite fashion. Similarly, primes activating concepts about older adults cause people to walk slowly, consistent with the stereotype of that group. Do these kinds of situational effects influence only nondeliberative behaviors, such as how fast to walk down a corridor? Fascinating research by Morwitz, Johnson, and Schmittlein (1993) shows that even major, presumably well-considered decisions, such as purchasing a new automobile, can be influenced by seemingly trivial situational events. Some consumers answered a question about the likelihood that they would buy a new car in the next 6 months in the context of a multipage marketing survey. Regardless of the answers they gave, they were 35% more likely actually to buy a car during that period compared to those who did not respond to the intent question. Similar results are obtained when people answer other behavioral intent questions (Levav & Fitzsimons, 2006).

All these effects are examples of how we construct our judgments and behaviors using whatever cues the current situation and context makes available or seemingly attractive, rather than being driven solely by our stable, long-term preferences, values, and inner representations of the world.

The Extended Mind

The situated cognition perspective focuses attention on how people offload cognitive work onto the environment by using *cognitive artifacts* (most obviously, computers and calculators but also calendars, pencil and paper, etc.) in ways that meaningfully extend their cognitive abilities. Importantly, even language is a shared sociocultural resource that extends cognition. Wilson and Clark (2009) discuss the key question arising from this perspective: Why should we talk about an "extended mind" rather than making the more conventional assumption that the environment simply provides inputs to the mind (viewed as implemented solely by the brain)? What differentiates a true "extension" of the mind from a simple input? Wilson and Clark discuss a radio as an analogy. The radio's purpose is to receive and decode sounds carried on radio waves, so anything that makes the radio better able to perform that function (e.g., a modification or addition of an electronic circuit) is best regarded as an augmentation or extension rather than a simple input. By analogy, cognitive augmentation or extension can be said to occur when "new resources help accomplish a recognizable cognitive task in an intuitively appropriate manner, e.g., by enabling the faster or more reliable processing of information"—when the resources operate "together with the rest of some cognitive system that serves the kinds of purposes that that cognitive system has served: to perceive, to decide, to remember, to behave" (p. 63).

Viewed in this light, earlier examples, such as the taped marks indicating critical speeds in an airport cockpit, or the pencil and paper that augment our calculating abilities, qualify as true cognitive extensions: They participate in tasks (memory, computation) that are intrinsically cognitive in nature and that we would perform less well without such external aids. The case would be even clearer for cognitive extensions that are durable and reliable, according to Wilson and Clark (2009), an argument that makes language or a hypothetical implanted memory chip a better candidate for being a true extension of mind compared to a Post-it note or a calculator.

The Socially Extended Mind

People extend their cognition with not only technological and sociocultural resources from the environment but also other people. Transactive memory (Wegner, 1986) is a prime example. Sometimes people do not store an item of information in their own memory, but instead store a "pointer" (in the computer science sense) to another person who knows the information and can report it. Two or more people can specialize and divide cognitive labor in this way, resulting in a social, supraindividual memory system with greater capacity than that of any one individual. Not only memory but also other types of information construal, integration, and decision processes are often implemented by groups, and not just by isolated individuals (Gigone & Hastie, 1997; Hutchins, 1991; Levine & Moreland, 1998). For example, in a group discussion, people may contribute items of information relevant to the decision being made. Stasser's (1988) model of this process includes both within-individual cognitive processes (e.g., being reminded of an item of information by something that another group member has said) and supraindividual social processes (e.g., social influence from others' opinions, or the way individual contributions become part of the group's "common ground" in the discussion). As these multilevel processes operate over time, they may have nonobvious effects, such as a group's tendency to focus on information that is widely shared among group members. No individual group member may have this focus as a goal, or even be aware of it, but it nevertheless emerges as a result of the cognitive and social processes within the group.

It is even possible to think of collective cognition as primary over individual cognition rather than the other way around. It has been argued that many features of the human cognitive system evolved specifically to participate in socially shared or collective cognition at several different levels, from the dyad to the small work group, to the larger "deme" or linguistic community (Caporael, 1997). In fact, recognizing the special characteristics of group information processing, cognitive scientists, as well as social psychologists, are now beginning to study collective cognition or *swarm intelligence* (Goldstone & Janssen, 2005; Kennedy, Eberhart, & Shi, 2001; Mason et al., 2007; Nijstad & Stroebe, 2006). Along similar lines, it is clear that individual cognition is fundamentally shaped and enabled by language, which itself is a socially shared and socially learned system. Developmentally, it has been argued that individual thought follows from and builds on the prior accomplishment of interpersonal communication (Vygotsky, 1962/1986). In other words, thinking is like holding a conversation with oneself, an ability that obviously owes nearly everything to one's ability to hold a conversation with another person.

COMMUNICATIVE CONTEXTS

A basic principle of the situated cognition perspective is that cognition is for action (Smith & Semin, 2004). Because communication is a frequent and important type of action, communicative goals and relationships (e.g., whether one is speaking or listening to another) shape and constrain cognition and behavior. As communication is shaped by contexts including dyads, communities, and cultures, not only do biases appear in what is transmitted from one person to another, but also changes are introduced in the individual speaker's own cognition and behavior. Human communication is not merely the translation and output of preexisting cognitions but involves online construction of cognitions, attitudes, and actions in response to all elements of the situation.

One significant aspect of communication in a group is that group members tend to discuss information that is shared by many in preference to information that is unique to specific group members (Stasser & Titus, 1985). Similarly, stereotype-consistent information is communicated in preference to stereotype-inconsistent information, even when equal amounts of each type of information are available to the speaker (see Ruscher, 1998, for a review). These effects may be related; stereotype-consistent information may be favored because participants regard it as culturally shared knowledge. Interestingly, even when members of a dyad spend equal amounts of time discussing stereotype-consistent and -inconsistent information about a target, both members still tend to end up with a stereotype-consistent impression of the target (Ruscher, Hammer, & Hammer, 1996).

In *serial reproduction* research an initial communicator is exposed to information and must pass it on to another, who then communicates to a third individual, and so on. Kashima (2000; Lyons & Kashima, 2003) found that, over time, stereotype-*consistent* information was retained more than stereotype-*inconsistent* information. However, when participants believed they were writing the story as a memory rather than storytelling task, stereotype-consistent information was not favored (Lyons & Kashima, 2003). This finding illustrates that not some purely intraindividual "schematic" interpretive or memory process but the fact of having an audience causes participants to focus on stereotype-consistent information. These results are clearly related to the processes that cause people to discuss shared and stereotype-consistent information more in groups.

Grice's (1975) *principle of relevance* states that people will provide information that is relevant to the conversation. Thus, cues to an audience's interests can shape what others communicate. Norenzayan and Schwarz (1999) found that participants gave more situational explanations for behavior on a questionnaire whose letterhead read "Institute for Social Research" rather than "Institute for Personality Research." Presumably the title served as a subtle cue about what the researcher was interested in, thereby biasing participants' responses.

Communicative roles and contexts can go beyond shaping what is overtly communicated; they can also shape the private thoughts and attitudes of the individuals involved. Zajonc (1960) examined how communicative roles influence the way individuals encode information. He found that people prepare mentally in different ways depending on whether they expect to play the role of communicator or listener in an upcoming interaction, leading to differences in the ways they organize and judge information.

The tendency for a speaker to "socially tune" to an audience's attitudes or expectations can influence not only the overt content of the communication but also the speaker's own beliefs and attitudes (Higgins & Rholes, 1978). If a speaker knows that an audience likes a target person, the speaker's communication about that target is likely to be skewed in a positive direction. Furthermore, if the speaker sees the audience as similar to him- or herself, or as positive in other ways, the speaker's resulting long-term impression and memory of the target become biased in the same direction as well (Echterhoff, Higgins, & Groll, 2005). People even take on stereotypical characteristics and endorse stereotypes more when they know that a liked audience endorses those stereotypes (Sinclair, Huntsinger, Skorinko, & Hardin, 2005; Sinclair, Lowery, Hardin, & Colangelo, 2005). This effect is found even when the audience is not physically present when the participant completes the measures. Control conditions in these studies show that the cognitive process of simply formulating a biased message is insufficient to produce these results. Instead, the communication context and the speaker's relationship to the audience are a necessary part of the process that causes the change in attitude within the speaker.

Expectations regarding the target of communication (not just the audience) also influence communication choices. One example is *linguistic intergroup bias* (LIB) (Maass, 1999), the tendency for people to describe negative outgroup and positive ingroup behaviors using abstract language (implying that they are stable and general characteristics), and to describe positive outgroup and negative ingroup behaviors more concretely (framing them as specific acts). For example, if John is an ingroup member, then a prosocial behavior might be described as "John is kind," but an outgroup member doing the same thing might elicit "John comforted the hurt child" (cf. Semin & Fiedler, 1988). As with social tuning, the LIB does not seem to occur automatically or unconditionally as a result of autonomous, inner cognitive processes. Rather, it occurs when the descriptions serve communicative goals, but not otherwise (Semin, de Montes, & Valencia, 2003).

The research described here illustrates how cognition is socially situated within communication contexts, by showing some of the ways that both meaning and choice of language are influenced by salient communicative roles and relationships. Some of this research demonstrates effects of communication on the communicator's own thoughts, as well as on recipients, opening the door for future research on the results of interactions over time among multiple individuals who mutually influence each other as they communicate (Mason et al., 2007).

THE SELF AND IDENTITY AS CONTEXT

The psychological self has been accorded increasing importance in social-psychological theory in recent years (Baumeister, 1998). The self not only serves as a repository of information about "who I am" (e.g., one's traits, abilities, roles, and other personal characteristics) but also plays a crucial role in regulating responses to situations and generating behavior. For example, self-relevance is the underlying appraisal that makes a situation important, and the self is widely assumed to include *self-standards*, or guides for behavior (e.g., Higgins, 1987). Recognizing the centrality of the self, Clancey (1997, p. 366) writes from a situated cognition perspective that the "overarching content of thought is not ... [descriptions or symbolic representations of states of the world], but coordination of an identity" in a social context. These considerations mean that effects of the social context on the self will have important consequences for cognition and behavior.

Context Sensitivity of the Self

An influential theoretical tradition including social identity theory and self-categorization theory (Turner, Hogg, Oakes, Reicher, & Wetherell, 1987) places much emphasis on the flexibility and context-specificity of the social self, especially those aspects of the self that derive from important social group memberships. Each of us has an identity as a man or woman, as well as national, ethnic, religious, professional, and many other group memberships. Which identity is salient depends on the current context; for example, being the only woman in a room full of men at a meeting makes gender identity highly salient, whereas a different social context might cue a different identity. In fact, the characteristics that people mention in describing themselves tend to be those that are unusual in their social context (home, school, etc.) (McGuire & Padawer-Singer, 1978). Based on such evidence, the current self cannot be seen as a static representation, but as one whose construction is based on the salience of group memberships in the current situation. "The concept of the self as a separate mental structure does not seem necessary, because we can assume that any and all cognitive resources—long-term knowledge, implicit theories, ... and so forth—are recruited, used, and deployed when necessary" (Turner, Oakes, Haslam, & McGarty, 1994, p. 459).

Thinking of oneself as a member of one or another group (e.g., by age or gender or nationality) in turn is highly consequential. It makes a difference in not only the ways one thinks about or describes the self, but also in the ways one thinks about and acts toward other people. This is because a shift in self-categorization changes some other people from being ingroup members (who are generally evaluated favorably, treated with fairness and altruism, and seen as being similar to the self) to being outgroup members (who generally are not favored in these ways), and vice versa (Mullen, Brown, & Smith, 1992; Turner et al., 1987). We are more easily persuaded by ingroup than by outgroup members (Mackie, Worth, & Asuncion, 1990), share emotions and attitudes with them (Norton, Monin, Cooper, & Hogg, 2003; Smith, Seger, & Mackie, 2007), and see ourselves as similar to them (Robbins & Krueger, 2005). The salience of different group memberships affects whether stereotypes seem relevant to the self or not (Ambady, Shih, Kim, & Pittinsky, 2001), with resulting effects on behavior via stereotype threat (Steele & Aronson, 1995).

Aspects of the self influence cognition and judgment in other ways as well, through motivational pressures aimed at self-enhancement. When we judge other people on common trait dimensions (e.g., *smart*, *honest*, or *conscientious*), our definitions of such traits are not fixed and objective, but depend on our own perceived standing on those traits (Dunning & Cohen, 1992). And consider the case of a person who is ambiguous, in that both positive and negative stereotypes might potentially apply to him or her. If the person praises the perceiver, the positive stereotype is likely to be applied; in contrast, criticism triggers application of the negative stereotype. Our self-enhancing motives to believe praise and discount criticism, in other words, alter the information we use in judging other people (Sinclair & Kunda, 1999).

Shifting Norms for Behavior

A situation-specific self influences not only the way a person thinks about him- or herself and treats other ingroup or outgroup members but also all types of behavior. This is because group memberships are associated with *norms*, or group-based standards for correct and appropriate beliefs, opinions, and behaviors (Turner et al., 1987). People regularly follow the norms of their groups because they have internalized them—they believe them to be proper guides for behavior—and not simply because they think that other group members will enforce them. Norms govern a wide range of our behaviors, from the way we stand facing the door of an elevator even when we are alone, to the types of groups against which we experience and report prejudice (Crandall, Eshleman, & O'Brien, 2002). As a result, when a group membership becomes salient because of the context, people tend to conform to the norms of that group, even if no other group members are physically present. To illustrate this point, Baldwin, Carrell, and Lopez (1990) found that the attitudes of Roman Catholic students were more consistent with their religious teachings when they were tested in a room with a photo of the Pope visible on the wall.

In all these ways, the social context influences cognition and behavior "from the inside out." It influences the psychological self and therefore influences the ways people think about themselves and others, and shapes behavior in accordance with relevant norms. Because it operates even when we are alone, this type of influence is even more basic and fundamental than effects of context that operate "from the outside in," such as when other people monitor and reward or punish an individual's behavior, or make information salient in the immediate environment.

CONCLUSIONS

The idea of situated cognition and related concepts, such as embodiment, invite us to move beyond mind–body dualism and reliance on computation as the guiding metaphor for understanding mind. The view of mind as an isolated, autonomous processor of abstract information is not as fruitful as the view of mind as inextricably intertwined with its social context (see also Mischel & Shoda, Chapter 8, this volume). Effects of social context on cognition and behavior are both powerful and pervasive. The actions of others and social situations cue behaviors directly (Chartrand & Bargh, 1999); our relationships and communications with others shape our own attitudes and beliefs (Higgins, 1992); and socially constructed group memberships and identities affect many of our thoughts, feelings, and actions. Instead of being a "logic machine and filing cabinet" (Clark, 1997, p. 1), the mind is built for action—almost always, action in a social context. Hence, social motives and relationships not only influence but also constitute cognition and behavior.

Considering cognition as an abstract computational process does have advantages: It simplifies the picture substantially, and understanding of human cognition did advance greatly in the decades during which this was the standard assumption. However, we have come to the point where further leaps in understanding require that we must grapple with the complexity introduced by the interdependence of cognition with the situation (as well as the body, an issue on which we have been unable to follow up in this chapter). Conceptual progress will be maximized when we ask not how people translate their stable, abstract inner representations, goals, and so on, into judgments and behavioral decisions, but rather how people interact with and exploit the social and physical environment to navigate their lives, moment by moment.

Given the research discussed in this book, it even seems appropriate to ask whether there are any instances when cognition is *not* situated. In one sense, the answer is clearly affirmative. There is some discussion in the situated cognition literature (e.g., Clark, 1997, pp. 166–175) of types of cognition that are nonsituated and hence must rely more heavily on inner representational resources, such as thinking about things that are not currently present (in fictional worlds, counterfactuals, future plans, daydreams). But even these forms of cognition do not completely evade situational constraints. First, we conceptualize counterfactual worlds or future plans in major part by flexibly recombining elements of the world we have concretely experienced (Barsalou, 1993; Glenberg, 1997), for our representational abilities remain grounded in sensorimotor systems. Second, even when reminiscence, planning, or storytelling free our cognition from the constraints of the immediate situation, cognition is still shaped by elements of our social context: our personal self-identities (gender, occupation, nationality, etc.), the nature of our bodies, and our socially constrained life experiences and personal relationships.

ACKNOWLEDGMENT

Preparation of this chapter was supported by National Science Foundation Grant No. BCS0527249.

REFERENCES

Agre, P. E. (1997). *Computation and human experience*. New York: Cambridge University Press.

Ambady, N., Shih, M., Kim, A., & Pittinsky, T. L. (2001). Stereotype susceptibility in children: Effects of identity activation on quantitative performance. *Psychological Science*, *12*, 385–390.

Baldwin, M. W., Carrell, S. E., & Lopez, D. F. (1990). Priming relationship schemas: My advisor and the Pope are watching me from the back of my mind. *Journal of Experimental Social Psychology*, *26*, 435–454.

Bargh, J. A., Chen, M., & Burrows, L. (1996). Automaticity of social behavior: Direct effects of trait construct and stereotype activation on action. *Journal of Personality and Social Psychology*, *71*, 230–244.

Barsalou, L. W. (1987). The instability of graded structure: Implications for the nature of concepts. In U. Neisser (Ed.), *Concepts and conceptual development: Ecological and intellectual factors in categorization* (pp. 101–140). New York: Cambridge University Press.

Barsalou, L. W. (1993). Flexibility, structure, and linguistic vagary in concepts: Manifestations of a compositional system of perceptual symbols. In A. F. Collins, S. E. Gathercole, M. A. Conway, & P. E. Morris (Eds.), *Theories of memory* (pp. 29–101). Hillsdale, NJ: Erlbaum.

Barsalou, L. W. (1999). Perceptual symbol systems. *Behavioral and Brain Science, 22*, 577–660.

Baumeister, R. F. (1998). The self. In D. T. Gilbert & S. T. Fiske (Eds.), *The handbook of social psychology* (4th ed., Vol. 2, pp. 680–740). New York: McGraw-Hill.

Biernat, M., & Manis, M. (1994). Shifting standards and stereotype-based judgments. *Journal of Personality and Social Psychology, 66*, 5–20.

Brooks, R. A. (1991). New approaches to robotics. *Science, 253*, 1227–1232.

Caporael, L. R. (1997). The evolution of truly social cognition: The core configurations model. *Personality and Social Psychology Review, 1*, 276–298.

Chartrand, T. L., & Bargh, J. A. (1999). The chameleon effect: The perception–behavior link and social interaction. *Journal of Personality and Social Psychology, 76*, 893–910.

Clancey, W. J. (1997). *Situated cognition: On human knowledge and computer representations.* New York: Cambridge University Press.

Clancey, W. J. (2009). Scientific antecedents of situated cognition. In P. Robbins & M. Aydede (Eds.), *Cambridge handbook of situated cognition* (pp. 11–34). New York: Cambridge University Press.

Clark, A. (1989). *Microcognition.* Cambridge, MA: MIT Press.

Clark, A. (1997). *Being there.* Cambridge, MA: MIT Press.

Clark, A., & Chalmers, D. (1998). The extended mind. *Analysis, 58*, 7–19.

Crandall, C. S., Eshleman, A., & O'Brien, L. (2002). Social norms and the expression and suppression of prejudice: The struggle for internalization. *Journal of Personality and Social Psychology, 82*, 359–378.

Dunning, D., & Cohen, G. L. (1992). Egocentric definitions of traits and abilities in social judgment. *Journal of Personality and Social Psychology, 63*, 341–355.

Echterhoff, G., Higgins, E. T., & Groll, S. (2005). Audience-tuning effects on memory: The role of shared reality. *Journal of Personality and Social Psychology, 89*, 257–276.

Fiske, S. T. (1993). Controlling other people: The impact of power on stereotyping. *American Psychologist, 48*, 621–628.

Fodor, J. A. (1975). *The language of thought.* Cambridge, MA: Harvard University Press.

Garcia-Marques, L., Santos, A. S. C., & Mackie, D. M. (2006). Stereotypes: Static abstractions or dynamic knowledge structures? *Journal of Personality and Social Psychology, 91*, 814–831.

Gigone, D., & Hastie, R. (1997). The impact of information on small group choice. *Journal of Personality and Social Psychology, 72*, 132–140.

Glenberg, A. M. (1997). What memory is for. *Behavioral and Brain Sciences, 20*, 1–55.

Goldstone, R. L., & Janssen, M. A. (2005). Computational models of collective behavior. *Trends in Cognitive Sciences, 9*, 424–430.

Greenberg, J., & Pyszczynski, T. (1985). The effect of an overheard ethnic slur on evaluations of the target: How to spread a social disease. *Journal of Experimental Social Psychology, 21*, 195–211.

Grice, H. P. (1975). Logic and conversation. In P. Cole & J. L. Morgan (Eds.), *Syntax and semantics 3: Speech acts* (pp. 41–58). New York: Academic Press.

Guinote, A. (2007). Behaviour variability and the situated focus theory of power. *European Review of Social Psychology, 18*, 256–295.

Higgins, E. T. (1987). Self-discrepancy: A theory relating self and affect. *Psychological Review, 94*, 319–340.

Higgins, E. T. (1992). Achieving "shared reality" in the communication game: A social action that creates meaning. *Journal of Language and Social Psychology, 11*, 107–131.

Higgins, E. T., & Rholes, W. S. (1978). "Saying is believing": Effects of message modification on memory and liking for the person described. *Journal of Experimental Social Psychology, 14*, 363–378.

Hutchins, E. (1991). The social organization of distributed cognition. In L. B. Resnick & J. M. Levine (Eds.), *Perspectives on socially shared cognition* (pp. 283–307). Washington, DC: American Psychological Association.

Hutchins, E. (1995). How a cockpit remembers its speeds. *Cognitive Science, 19*(3), 265–288.

Kahneman, D., & Miller, D. T. (1986). Norm theory: Comparing reality to its alternatives. *Psychological Review, 93*, 136–153.

Kashima, Y. (2000). Maintaining cultural stereotypes in the serial reproduction of narratives. *Personality and Social Psychology Bulletin, 26*, 594–604.

Kennedy, J., Eberhart, R. C., & Shi, Y. (2001). *Swarm intelligence.* San Francisco: Kaufmann.

Kirsh, D. (1995). The intelligent use of space. *Artificial Intelligence, 73*, 31–68.

Lave, J. (1997). The culture of acquisition and the practice of understanding. In D. I. Kirshner & J. A. Whitson (Eds.), *Situated cognition: Social, semiotic, and psychological perspectives* (pp. 17–35). Mahwah, NJ: Erlbaum.

Levav, J., & Fitzsimons, G. J. (2006). When questions change behavior: The role of ease of representation. *Psychological Science, 17*, 207–213.

Levine, J. M., & Moreland, R. L. (1998). Small groups. In D. T. Gilbert & S. T. Fiske (Eds.), *The handbook of social psychology* (Vol. 2, 4th ed., pp. 415–469). New York: McGraw-Hill.

Lyons, A., & Kashima, Y. (2003). How are stereotypes maintained through communication?: The influence of stereotype sharedness. *Journal of Personality and Social Psychology, 85*, 989–1005.

Maass, A. (1999). Linguistic intergroup bias: Stereotype perpetuation through language. In M. P. Zanna (Ed.), *Advances in experimental social psychology* (Vol. 31, pp. 79–121). San Diego, CA: Elsevier.

Mackie, D. M., Worth, L. T., & Asuncion, A. G. (1990). Processing of persuasive in-group messages. *Journal of Personality and Social Psychology, 58*, 812–822.

Mason, W. A., Conrey, F. R., & Smith, E. R. (2007). Situating social influence processes: Dynamic, multidirectional flows of influence within social networks. *Personality and Social Psychology Review, 11*, 279–300.

McGuire, W. J., & Padawer-Singer, A. (1978). Trait salience in the spontaneous self-concept. *Journal of Personality and Social Psychology, 33*, 743–754.

Morwitz, V. G., Johnson, E. J., & Schmittlein, D. (1993). Does measuring intent change behavior? *Journal of Consumer Research, 20*, 46–61.

Mullen, B., Brown, R., & Smith, C. (1992). Ingroup bias as a function of salience, relevance, and status: An integration. *European Journal of Social Psychology, 22*, 103–122.

Newell, A. (1980). Physical symbol systems. *Cognitive Science: A Multidisciplinary Journal, 42*, 135–183.

Nijstad, B. A., & Stroebe, W. (2006). How the group affects the mind: A cognitive model of idea generation in groups. *Personality and Social Psychology Review, 10*, 186–213.

Norenzayan, A., & Schwarz, N. (1999). Telling what they want to know: Participants tailor causal attributions to researchers' interests. *European Journal of Social Psychology, 29*, 1011–1020.

Norton, M. I., Monin, B., Cooper, J., & Hogg, M. A. (2003). Vicarious dissonance: Attitude change from the inconsistency of others. *Journal of Personality and Social Psychology, 85*, 47–62.

Overbeck, J. R., & Park, B. (2001). When power does not corrupt: Superior individuation processes among powerful perceivers. *Journal of Personality and Social Psychology, 81*, 549–565.

Pfeifer, R., & Bongard, J. (2007). *How the body shapes the way we think*. Cambridge, MA: MIT Press.

Pylyshyn, Z. (1984). *Computation and cognition*. Cambridge, MA: MIT Press.

Robbins, J. M., & Krueger, J. I. (2005). Social projection to ingroups and outgroups: A review and meta-analysis. *Personality and Social Psychology Review, 9*, 32–47.

Robbins, P., & Aydede, M. (Eds.). (2009). *Cambridge handbook of situated cognition*. New York: Cambridge University Press.

Ruscher, J., Hammer, E. Y., & Hammer, E. D. (1996). Forming sharing impressions through conversation: An adaptation of the continuum model. *Personality and Social Psychology Bulletin, 22*, 705–720.

Ruscher, J. B. (1998). Prejudice and stereotyping in everyday communication. In M. P. Zanna (Ed.), *Advances in experimental social psychology* (Vol. 30, pp. 241–307). San Diego, CA: Elsevier.

Schwarz, N. (1999). Self-reports: How the questions shape the answers. *American Psychologist, 54*, 93–105.

Semin, G. R., de Montes, G. L., & Valencia, J. F. (2003). Communication constraints on the linguistic intergroup bias. *Journal of Experimental Social Psychology, 39*, 142–148.

Semin, G. R., & Fiedler, K. (1988). The cognitive functions of linguistic categories in describing persons: Social cognition and language. *Journal of Personality and Social Psychology, 54*, 558–568.

Shafir, E. (2007). Decisions constructed locally: Some fundamental principles of the psychology of decision making. In A. W. Kruglanski & E. T. Hig-

gins (Eds.), *Social psychology: Handbook of basic principles* (2nd ed., pp. 334–352). New York: Guilford Press.
Simons, D. J., & Ambinder, M. S. (2005). Change blindness: Theory and consequences. *Current Directions in Psychological Science*, *14*, 44–48.
Sinclair, L., & Kunda, Z. (1999). Reactions to a black professional: Motivated inhibition and activation of conflicting stereotypes. *Journal of Personality and Social Psychology*, *77*, 885–904.
Sinclair, S., Huntsinger, J., Skorinko, J., & Hardin, C. D. (2005). Social tuning of the self: Consequences for the self-evaluations of stereotype targets. *Journal of Personality and Social Psychology*, *89*, 160–175.
Sinclair, S., Lowery, B. S., Hardin, C. D., & Colangelo, A. (2005). Social tuning of automatic racial attitudes: The role of affiliative motivation. *Journal of Personality and Social Psychology*, *89*, 583–592.
Smith, E. R., & Conrey, F. R. (2009). The social context of cognition. In P. Robbins & M. Aydede (Eds.), *Cambridge handbook of situated cognition* (pp. 454–466). New York: Cambridge University Press.
Smith, E. R., Seger, C. R., & Mackie, D. M. (2007). Can emotions be truly group level?: Evidence regarding four conceptual criteria. *Journal of Personality and Social Psychology*, *93*, 431–446.
Smith, E. R., & Semin, G. R. (2004). Socially situated cognition: Cognition in its social context. *Advances in Experimental Social Psychology*, *36*, 53–117.
Stasser, G. (1988). Computer simulation as a research tool: The DISCUSS model of group decision making. *Journal of Experimental Social Psychology*, *24*(5), 393–422.
Stasser, G., & Titus, W. (1985). Pooling unshared information in group decision making: Biased information sampling during discussion. *Journal of Personality and Social Psychology*, *48*, 1467–1478.
Steele, C. M., & Aronson, J. (1995). Stereotype threat and the intellectual test performance of African Americans. *Journal of Personality and Social Psychology*, *69*, 797–811.
Turner, J. C., Hogg, M. A., Oakes, P. J., Reicher, S. D., & Wetherell, M. S. (1987). *Rediscovering the social group: A self-categorization theory*. Cambridge, MA: Blackwell.
Turner, J. C., Oakes, P. J., Haslam, S., & McGarty, C. (1994). Self and collective: Cognition and social context. *Personality and Social Psychology Bulletin*, *20*, 454–463.
Vygotsky, L. (1986). *Language and thought*. Cambridge, MA: MIT Press. (Original work published 1962)
Wegner, D. M. (1986). Transactive memory: A contemporary analysis of the group mind. In B. Mullen & G. R. Goethals (Eds.), *Theories of group behavior* (pp. 185–208) New York: Springer-Verlag.
Wilson, R. A., & Clark, A. (2009). How to situate cognition: Letting nature take its course. In P. Robbins & M. Aydede (Eds.), *Cambridge handbook of situated cognition* (pp. 55–77). New York: Cambridge University Press.

Wilson, T. D., & Hodges, S. D. (1992). Attitudes as temporary constructions. In L. L. Martin & A. Tesser (Eds.), *The construction of social judgments* (pp. 37–65). Hillsdale, NJ: Erlbaum.

Yeh, W., & Barsalou, L. W. (2006). The situated nature of concepts. *American Journal of Psychology, 119*, 349–384.

Zajonc, R. (1960). The process of cognitive tuning in communication. *Journal of Abnormal and Social Psychology, 61*, 159–167.

PART III

THE PERSON

8

The Situated Person

WALTER MISCHEL
YUICHI SHODA

The view of mind, and of other psychological constructs (e.g., personality traits, attitudes, cognitions), as Platonic situation–free entities, impervious to contexts, and reflected consistently in cognition, affect, and social behavior across diverse situations, has dominated not just personality but much of psychology since its inception, as discussed throughout this volume, for example, in the varieties and consequences of "Platonic blindness" (Dunham & Banaji, Chapter 10, this volume). In social psychology the decontextualized entity view has cast a long shadow, motivating the protest movement toward "situated cognition" (Smith & Collins, Chapter 7, this volume). The fact that the intellectual shifts reflected in the core themes of the present book now extend across our subdisciplines is seen in the strikingly close parallels between *situated cognition* and the *situated person* perspective.

As early advocates of a situated view of the person in interaction with contexts (Mischel, 1968, 1973; Mischel & Shoda, 1995), it is gratifying to see this convergence across diverse areas of psychological science. We hope the present volume, and this chapter, will help us all more clearly see the common themes and parallel developments, and build a more cumulative, less discipline-driven and discipline-insulated psychological science. The parallel findings and remarkably similar reconceptualizations that seem to be emerging across many of our subfields suggest we may indeed be living within a paradigm shift, and invite us to extract its essential ingredients to our mutual benefit.

MIND AND PERSON IN CONTEXT

The *situated person* view was rooted in the recognition that the classic Western assumptions about mental entities isolated from contexts, and their expected expressions in consistent social behavior across diverse situations, were clearly contradicted by the empirical evidence available even 40 years ago (Mischel, 1968). Most important, the traditional entity conceptions were untenable if one examines how the mind works as people attempt to adapt to diverse situations (Mischel, 1973). As noted then, because such adaptability and the ability to discriminate even among subtly different situations is essential for survival, humans could not have evolved to behave consistently across situations that vary in the challenges they pose and the solutions they require.

Humans are not unique in this regard. But what sets them (and other species with complex central nervous systems) apart is their vast capacity for learning. They learn not only to associate old stimuli to new outcomes, but also learn to selectively tune into certain aspects of stimuli and form new functional equivalence classes with increasingly find distinctions. People make meaning out of the situations they encounter and use this to adapt their behavior (what they think, feel, and do) accordingly to each situation. And not all individuals give the same meaning to a situation because of their individual learning history, their culture, and perhaps their unique genetic makeup. They behave in ways that are consistent with the meanings that particular situations have for them: Individual differences arise from the distinctive ways that the person processes and understands situations or contexts, which in turn reflects the individual's psychosocial and biological history (Mischel, 1973). In short, as an alternative to the classic personality model, a constructivist, dynamic, contextualized view needs to account for the situated person as a meaning-maker (Mischel, 2004; Mischel & Shoda, 1995).

Furthermore, instead of broad traits, the contextualized, situated person view proposed, as basic units for a conceptualization of personality and individual differences, the cognitive–affective processes and cognitive–affective mental representations through which individuals interpret situations and experiences, and that guide their social behavior adaptively across different situations (Cervone & Shoda, 1999; Mischel, 1973, 2004; Mischel & Shoda, 1995; Van Mechelen, 2009; Vansteelandt & Van Mechelen, 1998, 2006). The focus is on how the person's encoding or construal and interpretations of the situation, and the expectations, goals, and affects activated by those interpretations, generate the contextualized, conditionally hedged patterns of variability observed in behavior.

Emerging theory and research on the situated person indicate that

1. Situational features (e.g., rejection cues) activate cognitive–affective units or mental representations (e.g., construals, expectations, goals, affects) in the individual's social information-processing system based on the person's prior experience with those features.
2. The individual's system is sensitized to particular features of situations.
3. The psychological features of the situation (stimuli-as-encoded) are the active ingredients of situations to which the system reacts.
4. Individuals are characterized by distinctive and stable *if* ... *then* ... or situation–behavior signatures (e.g., she is warm and friendly *if* ... but cold and hostile *if*. ...
5. Psychological individual differences also can be characterized by stable situational profiles (i.e., the sets of interpersonal situations the person characteristically experiences in the psychological life space). These "belong" neither to the person nor to the situation.
6. Individual experiences within a relationship are an emergent property of each interpersonal system (rather than a simple combination of personalities of the individuals that constitute the relationship).

A reader who compares this situated person conception with the situated cognition perspective (Smith & Collins, Chapter 7, this volume) will quickly note their commonalities. To reduce parallel play and move toward becoming a more cumulative psychological science, we need at least to be aware of, and benefit from each others' contributions, even when they come from different subdisciplines dealing with the same basic issues, which makes this book a particularly welcome and timely development.

In this chapter we discuss these points and their implications for the contextualized view of person at the psychological level of analysis. We also summarize key features of the Cognitive–Affective Processing System (CAPS) model that we designed, intended as a metatheory for studying the mind in context within diverse domains and subfields of psychological science (Mischel & Shoda, 1995, 1998). Our goal then, and our hope now, is that such a broad meta-level framework, applicable across diverse content domains (e.g., attitudes, cognitions, memory representations, including representations of the self) (Mischel & Morf, 2004), will help to enhance and integrate diverse lines of work dealing with the multiple expressions of the "mind in context."

THE SITUATED PERSON VIEW VERSUS TRADITIONAL PERSONALITY TRAIT PSYCHOLOGY

In ancient Greece, for Hippocrates the essential psychological trait entities consisted of the Big Four humors (blood, bile, cholera, phlegm). In current traditional models of personality, traits as situation-free entities are still alive, as seen in the Big Five—Open-mindedness, Conscientiousness, Extraversion, Neuroticism, and Sociability (e.g., McCrae & Costa, 1999)—as global traits, with little attention to situations and even less to the interactions of persons and situations. Flying in the face of traditional entity trait assumptions, and directly contradicting them, Mischel (1968, 1973) showed that rigorous study after study failed to support those assumptions, and pointed instead to the crucial importance of context and the specific meaning of the situation. The findings revealed that, for example, the aggressive child at home may be less aggressive than most when in school; the man who is exceptionally hostile when rejected in love may be unusually tolerant about criticism of his work; the one who always shakes with anxiety in the doctor's office may be a calm mountain climber; the high-risk business entrepreneur may take few social risks; the model of morality and self-control in public life may show an opposite side in private life. The conception of the situated person stirred a paradigm crisis, and in the 40 years that followed an increasingly detailed contextualized view of the situated person was developed, with supporting evidence (e.g., Cervone & Shoda, 1999; Fleeson, 2001; Fournier, Moskowitz, & Zuroff, 2008; Mischel, 2004; Mischel & Mischel, 1973; Mischel & Shoda, 1995, 1998; Shoda, 2003; Shoda, Mischel, & Wright, 1989, 1994).

The contextualized view of personality and individual differences shocked the field when it was first proposed. Reacting against it, researchers made diverse attempts to find evidence to support the consistency of social behavior and personality indicators across diverse situations. In spite of decades of such efforts (reviewed elsewhere; e.g., Cervone & Shoda, 1999; Mischel, 2004; Mischel, Shoda, & Ayduk, 2008), most studies found that such consistency, while not zero, is only slightly above chance, rarely accounting for more than a small percent of the variance when behavior is directly observed, consistent with the original observations made in *Personality and Assessment* (Mischel, 1968, 1973; Mischel & Peake, 1982a; Peterson, 1968; Shoda et al., 1994; Vernon, 1964).

Eliminating Context by Aggregation across Situations

In the traditional uncontextualized view of traits, the findings on the role of situations reflect the noise and error of measurement. This interpretation acknowledges the importance of situations and the low correlations found in the individual's behavior from situation to situation (Epstein, 1979), but after lip service to context, it still aggregates the individual's behavior on a given dimension (e.g., "conscientiousness," "sociability") over many different situations to estimate an overall "true score" (as discussed in Epstein 1979, 1980; Mischel, 2004; Mischel & Peake 1982b; Pervin, 1994). Getting rid of the situation by aggregation follows the core assumption of classic trait theory, which makes "personality" independent of, and unconnected with, situations, and attributes causal powers either to the person *or* to the situation, while ignoring their psychological interconnection. In that view, one then tries to take out the variability introduced by different situations rather than focusing on it. In contrast, in the contextualized view, the analysis of the person's variability across situations provides the route to understanding the underlying stable organization of the mind (Mischel & Shoda, 1995).

Historically, the zero-sum conception of the relationship between personality and situation, in which to the degree that the person was important in causal explanations of behavior, the situation was not, and vice versa, generated a heated and misguided "person *versus* situation" debate. It raged for many years of intense controversy from the 1970s into the 1980s, with arguments about which one accounts for the bigger variance, whose aftereffects still linger. Most personality psychologists continued the search for consistencies in the situation-free person, and on the other side social psychologists kept demonstrating the power of the situation (Nisbett & Ross, 1980; Ross & Nisbett, 1991). The encouraging shift is seen in the increasing attention to the nature of person–context interactions and their implications for understanding the individual's mind in context, as the present volume documents. In the area of personality, after decades of futile debates about the power of the "person versus the situation," it seems to be a growing trend (e.g., Cervone & Orom, 2009; Fleeson, 2001; Magnusson & Endler, 1977; Moskowitz, 1982, 1994; Van Mechelen, 2009; Vansteelandt & Van Mechelen, 1998).

The glaring discrepancies between the high levels of consistency expected by decontexualized theories and intuition, and what was actually observed made the challenge clear: If the classic theories could not accurately predict the observed behavior, a new understanding was needed. This reconceptualization began with the idea that the field was searching for consistency in the wrong places: It was looking for the "personality as it is," apart from situations, treating contexts as the noise or "error of measurement" that needed to be stripped out. Instead, the field needed to turn the standard view and practice upside down: By including the situation or context as it is perceived by the person, and by analyzing behavior in this encoded situational context, the consistencies that characterize the person, far from disappearing as had been assumed, would be found (Mischel, 1973; Mischel & Shoda, 1995). But these individual differences would not be expressed in consistent cross-situational behavior; instead consistency would be found in distinctive but stable patterns of if ... then ... situation–behavior relations that form contextualized, psychologically meaningful personality signatures (e.g., "she does *A* when *X*, but *B* when *Y*").

To go from theoretical conceptualization to supporting evidence required two types of empirical demonstrations: (1) evidence for the existence and meaningfulness of the hypothesized stable *if ... then ...* situation–behavior signatures of personality and (2) compelling demonstrations of the person's ability to mediate the impact of situations by creating their meaning through cognitive reappraisal. Evidence on the first point supports the idea that the consistency and stability that distinctively characterizes an individual is found in the stable patterns of variability: When the perceived situation or "if" changes, so does the behavior, but the *if ... then ...* pattern itself is stable and distinctively characterizes each individual. Evidence on the second point supports the view, now widely accepted, that the impact of contexts or stimuli depends on their meaning and mental representation; when the meaning changes, so does the behavior. Both findings are considered next.

Evidence for the Situated Person Perspective: Distinctive, Stable *If ... Then ...* ***Behavioral Signatures***

On the first point, evidence for the *if ... then ... situation–behavior signatures of personality*, such evidence came initially from the Carlton College study (Mischel & Peake, 1982a), and then in a massive fine-grained observational study at the Wediko Summer Camp (Shoda, Mischel, & Wright, 1989, 1993a, 1993b, 1994). The latter provided arguably the "thickest" data archive to date for the analysis of social behavior across multiple repeated situations over time (Mischel & Shoda, 1995). Contradicting the classic assumptions, the data showed that individuals who were similar in average levels of behavior, for example, in their aggression, nevertheless differed predictably and dramatically in the types of situations in which they aggressed. As expected (Mischel, 1973), they were characterized by highly psychologically informative *if ... then ...* behavioral signatures. Consider, for example, two children who showed similar mean amounts of physical and verbal aggression, observed closely over the course of the 6-week summer in the residential camp setting. One was characterized by being exceptionally aggressive whenever approached by adults, but was much less aggressive than most when interacting with peers, whereas the other child was characterized by the opposite pattern: highly aggressive with peers, exceptionally docile with adults. Although both were similar in overall aggression, their distinctively different behavioral *if ... then ...* patterns suggested quite different processing dynamics and motivations (Mischel & Shoda, 1995; Shoda et al., 1994).

The basic findings on these stable, contexualized patterns of variability have been supported in diverse studies and populations (e.g., Borkenau, Riemann, Spinath, & Angleitner, 2006; Fournier et al., 2008; Moskowitz, Suh, & Desaulniers, 1994). These stable and distinctive *if ... then ...* situation–behavior patterns form *behavioral signatures of personality* (Shoda et al., 1994), and suggest the existence of a higher order consistency on which the intuitive belief in personality may be based (Shoda & Mischel, 1993). To understand these intraindividual patterns of variability requires a theory and research paradigm that goes beyond the traditional investigation of personality and social situations. The findings yield both new answers and new questions about the nature of personality and the interactions of persons and situations within particular contexts.

Our conceptualization of the "situated person," as noted earlier, requires not only demonstrating the existence and meaningfulness of stable *if ... then ...* situation–behavior signatures but also evidence to show that the impact of the "ifs" or situations depends on their meaning and mental representation by the individual. Beginning in the late 1960s and early 1970s, studies of the young child's willingness and ability to delay immediate gratification showed that it was not the objective temptations faced in the situation, as earlier theories had suggested, but how the rewards were subjectively represented (e.g., Mischel, 1974a, 1974b; Mischel, Shoda, & Rodriguez, 1989). Contradicting the behaviorists' emphasis on "stimulus control," these experiments showed that delay behavior and self-control could be changed readily and radically by altering how the stimuli were cognitively appraised or encoded (Mischel, 1974a, 1974b; Mischel et al., 1989; Mischel & Ayduk, 2004). The preschool child could wait for otherwise unbearable delay periods for tempting treats, such as a marshmallow, by focusing on its nonconsummatory "cool" qualities (e.g., its shape). On the other hand, the same child would yield immediately to the temptation by focusing on its consummatory "hot" or arousing features (e.g., its yummy, sweet, chewy taste).

Thus, by reappraising the situation, or by focusing attention on selected mental representations, individuals can exert some control over their own cognitions and affects, and transform the impact of the stimulus. They can select, structure, influence, and reinterpret or cognitively and emotionally transform situations to which they are exposed, and are not merely passive victims of the situations or stimuli that they encounter (e.g., Eigsti et al., 2006; Kross, Ayduk, & Mischel, 2005; Mischel, 1996; Mischel, Cantor, & Feldman, 1996). They also can enhance their control over the context and situational pressures through *if ... then ...* implementation planning strategies for achieving even highly difficult and distal goals, as elaborated in the work of Gollwitzer and colleagues (e.g., Gollwitzer, 1996; Gollwitzer & Bargh, 1996).

A COGNITIVE–AFFECTIVE PROCESSING SYSTEM FOR THE MIND IN CONTEXT

CAPS was intended as a metatheory that incorporates situations or contexts into the conception of the person (Bandura, 1986; Mischel, 1968, 1973; Ross & Nisbett, 1991; Shoda et al., 1993a; Wright & Mischel, 1987). The concept of the situation, however, is not like the simple stimulus in early behaviorism that mechanically pulls responses from an organism's repertoire. Features of situations activate a set of internal reactions—not just cognitive but also affective—based on the individual's prior experience with those features (Mischel, 1973). These features of situations are encountered in the external environment, but they also are generated in thought, planning, fantasy, and imagination (e.g., Antrobus, 1991; Gollwitzer, 1999; Mischel et al., 1989). And they encompass not just social and interpersonal situations (as when lovers "reject" or peers "tease and provoke") but also intrapsychic situations, as in mood states (e.g., Isen, Niedenthal, & Cantor, 1992; Schwarz, 1990), as well as in the everyday stream of experience and feeling (e.g., Bolger & Eckenrode, 1991; Cantor & Blanton, 1996; Emmons, 1991; Smith & Lazarus, 1990; Wright & Mischel, 1988).

Nominal and Psychological Situations

Most important, CAPS theory (Shoda et al., 1994) distinguishes between "nominal situations" (e.g., meeting in the dean's office) and the "active ingredients" or "psychological features" of situations (e.g., having your ideas rejected). *Nominal situations* refer to the particular places and activities in the particular setting, for example, woodworking activities in a summer camp, or arithmetic tests and dining halls, or playgrounds in a school setting (e.g., Hartshorne & May, 1928; Newcomb, 1929). Individual differences in relation to such specific nominal situations, even if highly stable, would be of limited generalizability. These are valid and reliable definitions, but they don't tell us what aspects of each situation are responsible for the observed pattern of behavior variation. If Mary is usually relaxed in the nominal situation "meeting with Jane" but often tense in the situation "having lunch with Joe," will she be anxious when picking up a job candidate at the airport? It is this lack of generalizability that made demonstrations of situation specificity a threat to the fundamental goal of personality psychology. It is therefore important to try to characterize "situations" in terms of their common psychological features (Shoda & LeeTiernan, 2002). Once the feature of the situation to which the individual is responding is identified (e.g., having one's ideas rejected by an authority), prediction to other situations that contain known features becomes possible, even if they are nominally quite different.

Identifying the Psychological Features (Active Ingredients) of Situations

Identifying the psychological features of situations is a key challenge not just for CAPS theory or personality psychology but more generally for models of the mind in context, all of which need a language to understand the meaning of various social situations or contexts for the individuals who experience them. This challenge is analogous to one faced by an allergy specialist. Suppose a patient has reliably identified that he has an allergic reaction every time he eats breakfast cereal brands *A* and *E*, but he can eat brands *B*, *C*, and *D* without problems. Note that the "situations," the brands of cereal, are defined nominally. The pattern of variation in the patient's reactions across the situations (brands of cereal) is reliable and reflects some stable characteristics of his immune system. But to go beyond it and to predict whether or not he can safely eat brand *X*, a new brand he has not tried before, it would first be necessary to identify just what it is about brands *A* and *E* that cause the allergic reaction.

Equally important, the features of situations that activate the person's processing dynamics are not just triggered by external situations encountered in the social world. They also are generated internally within the personality system through thought, planning, fantasy, and imagination (e.g., Antrobus, 1991; Gollwitzer, 1996; Klinger, 1996; Mischel et al., 1989; Nolen-Hoeksema, Parker, & Larson, 1994). And they encompass not just social and interpersonal (as when lovers are perceived as "rejecting") but also mood states (e.g., Isen, Niedenthal, & Cantor, 1992; Schwarz, 1990), as well as the everyday stream of experience and feeling (e.g., Bolger & Eckenrode, 1991; Emmons, 1991; Smith & Lazarus, 1990; Wright & Mischel, 1988). Whether externally or internally produced, they activate the individual's processing dynamics, generating characteristic cognitive–affective–behavioral reaction patterns (e.g., Shoda & Mischel, 1998).

Two Basic Assumptions

The CAPS model of the situated person makes only two basic assumptions. First, people differ in the *chronic accessibility*, that is, the ease with which particular cognitive and affective mental representations or units, CAUs for short, become activated. These CAUs refer to the cognitions and affects or feelings that are available to the person (Mischel, 1973; Mischel & Shoda, 1995). Such mediating units become activated or triggered by the specific psychological features of situations, and seem similar to the concept of "situated cognitions" (Smith & Collins, Chapter 7, this volume). However, we named them CAUs to make explicit that they include more than "cool" cognitions but also "hot" affective reactions (Mischel & Shoda, 1995).

Second, CAUs (e.g., encodings or construals, efficacy and outcome expectancies, beliefs, goals and values, affects and feeling states, as well as competencies and self-regulatory plans and strategies), are not conceptualized as isolated, static, components. They are organized, for example, into subjective equivalence classes, as illustrated in theory and research on encoding, person prototypes and personal constructs, (e.g., Cantor & Mischel, 1977, 1979; Cantor, Mischel, & Schwartz, 1982; Forgas, 1983a, 1983b; Higgins, King, & Mavin, 1982; Kelly, 1955; Linville & Clark, 1989; Vallacher & Wegner, 1987). Some aspects of the organization of relations among the cognitions and affects, such as evaluative-affective associations, and inter-concept relations (e.g., Cantor & Kihlstrom, 1987; Mendoza-Denton & Mischel, 2007; Murphy & Medin, 1985) are common among members of a culture, whereas others may be unique for an individual (e.g., Rosenberg & Jones, 1972). But whether common or unique, cognitive-affective representations are not unconnected discrete units that are simply elicited as discrete "responses" in isolation: rather, these cognitive representations and affective states interact dynamically and influence each other reciprocally within an essentially connectionist model loosely analogous to neural networks models of the brain in biology. It is the relatively stable organization of the relationships among the CAUs that forms the core of the structure, and that guides and constrains their effects.

Individual Differences in the Stable Organization of Interconnections among Cognitive–Affective Units

Thus the CAPS model makes a second assumption: individual differences reflect not only the accessibility of particular cognitions and affects but also the distinctive *organization of relationships* among them (see Figure 8.1, which shows a schematic, greatly simplified CAPS system). This organization (conceptualized as a connectionist network analogous to neural networks in the brain), characterizes the basic stable *nature of the processing system*. It is this organization that guides and constrains the activation of the particular cognitions and affects that are available within the system and that are expressed in behavior in the contextualized *if* ... *then* ... signatures that distinctively characterize individuals.

As Figure 8.1 illustrates, when the individual perceives certain features of a situation, a characteristic pattern of cognitions and affects

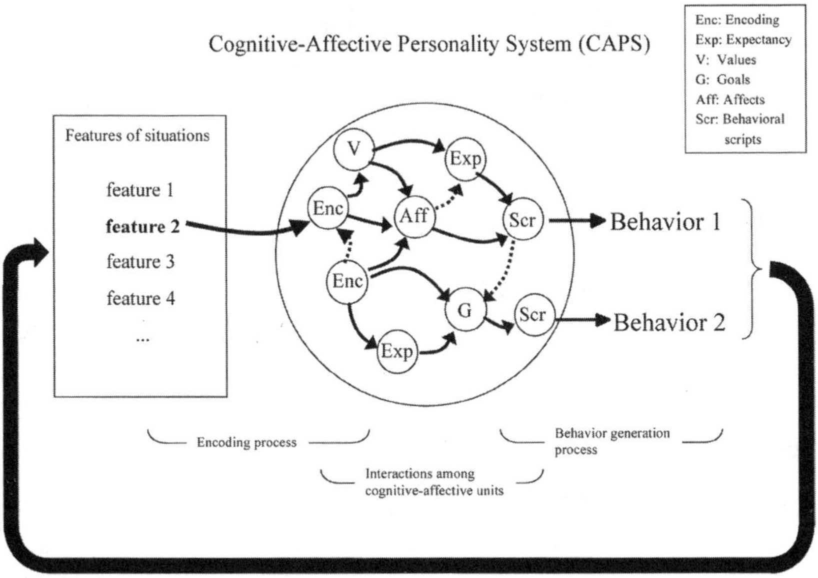

FIGURE 8.1. The Cognitive–Affective Personality System (CAPS). Situational features activate a given mediating unit, which activates specific subsets of other mediating units through a stable network of relations that characterize an individual, generating a characteristic pattern of behavior in response to different situations. The relation may be positive (solid line), which increases the activation, or negative (dashed line), which decreases the activation. From Mischel and Shoda (1995, p. 254). Copyright 1995 by the American Psychological Association. Adapted with permission.

(shown schematically as circles) becomes activated through this distinctive network of connections. Mediating units in the system become activated in relation to some situation features (positive connections) but are deactivated or inhibited in relation to others (negative connections, shown as broken lines), which decreases the activation, and not affected by the rest. The CAPS system interacts continuously and dynamically with the social world in which it is contextualized. The interactions with the external word involve a two-way reciprocal interaction: The behaviors that the personality system generates influence the interpersonal situations the person subsequently faces and that, in turn, influence the person.

An Example: Rejection Sensitivity Signature and Processing Dynamics

To illustrate, consider the behavioral signature and processing dynamics that have been identified for the high "rejection-sensitivity type" (Ayduk & Gyurak, 2008; Downey, Feldman, & Ayduk, 2000; Feldman & Downey, 1994). These individuals have highly accessible intense anxieties about interpersonal rejection and abandonment that become activated *if* they encounter in their close relationships what could be perceived as uncaring behavior (e.g., partner is attentive to someone else). They tend to scan interpersonal situations looking for cues about rejection, appraise them in terms of their potential rejection threats, anxiously expect them, and are vigilantly alert to finding them. When they do, they become easily concerned and ruminate about whether or not they are loved, or might become abandoned, which may in turn trigger a cascade of anger, resentment, and rage. This readily activates coercive and overcontrolling behaviors that then are readily blamed on the partner's behavior. A self-fulfilling prophecy plays out in which fears of abandonment become validated by the rejections that highly rejection-sensitive individuals in part create for themselves. But for the present discussion, it is notable that if all their behavior is aggregated, regardless of context, they may not be more aggressive on the whole than others or more likely to express anger, disapproval, and coercive behaviors. Indeed, under some conditions they can be remarkably caring, loving, and thoughtful to their partners.

SIGNATURES OF THE INDIVIDUAL'S PSYCHOLOGICAL ENVIRONMENT: DIAGNOSTIC CONTEXTUALIZED PROFILES

The individuals' behaviors influence the environments or situations that they subsequently experience and select, an observation for which there is wide agreement among researchers (e.g., Bolger, DeLongis, Kessler, & Schilling, 1989; Bolger & Schilling, 1991; Buss, 1987; Ross & Nisbett, 1991; Smith & Rhodewalt, 1986; Snyder, 1983; Snyder & Gangestad, 1982) ranging from behavior geneticists (e.g., Plomin, DeFries, McClearn, & Rutter, 1997) to social-cognitive interactionists (e.g., Bandura, 1986; Mischel & Shoda, 1995). Ultimately this results in a degree of stability or equilibrium in the situations the person characteristically experiences in the psychological life space. Such stability "belongs" neither to the person nor to the situation in isolation. Rather, it is a reflection of the enduring pattern of reciprocal interactions between the individual and his or her distinctive interpersonal world as they dynamically influence each other, each impacting on the other.

Illustrative Situational Profiles Characterizing the Individual's Social World (Life Space)

To illustrate, Figures 8.2, 8.3, and 8.4 show the frequency (in *z* scores) with which each of these three children from the Wediko Summer Camp (Shoda, 1990) experienced the five types of situations measured repeatedly over the course of 6 weeks. For Child #6, everything happened often; he was positively approached by peers, teased by them, praised by adults, and also warned and given time-outs by them. In stark contrast, for Child #20 we see an empty summer, with much less experience, either positive or negative, than the average camper. It is a portrait of an isolated child, avoided or ignored by the social world around him.

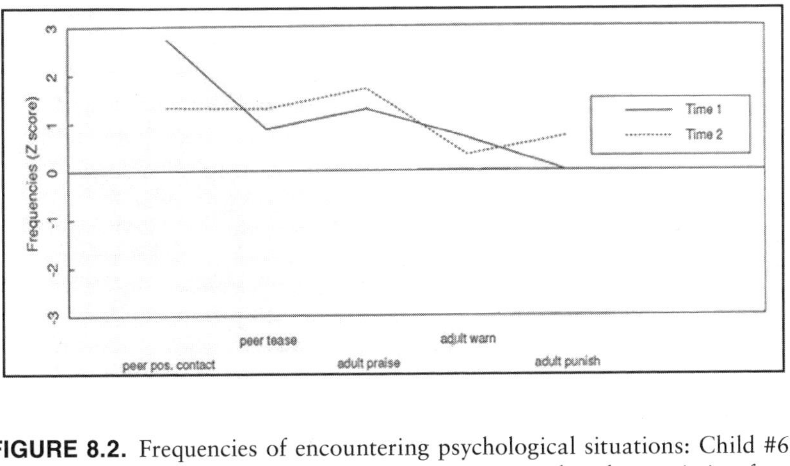

FIGURE 8.2. Frequencies of encountering psychological situations: Child #6, profile stability: $r = .53$. From Shoda (1990). Reprinted with permission from the author.

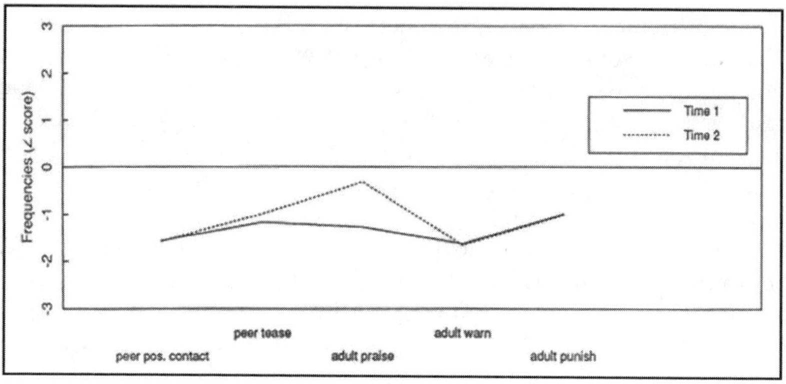

FIGURE 8.3. Frequencies of encountering psychological situations: Child #20, profile stability: $r = .63$. From Shoda (1990). Reprinted with permission from the author.

Child #78 experienced a world in which the outstanding feature was the exceptional amount of teasing (and threatening/provoking) he endured from peers. If such different patterns of interpersonal encounters are characteristic and stable for each individual across different activities and contexts—and they often are—they constitute an aspect of behavioral coherence that needs to be incorporated into the conception and assessment of personality consistency (Mischel & Shoda, 1995).

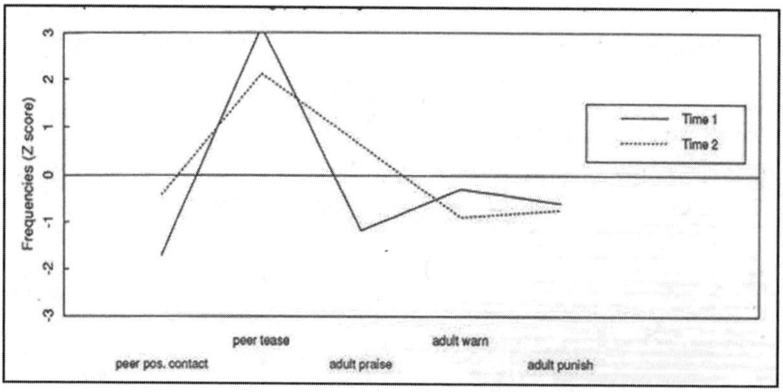

FIGURE 8.4. Frequencies of encountering psychological situations: Child #78, profile stability: $r = .77$. From Shoda (1990). Reprinted with permission from the author.

Beyond predicting that individuals are characterized by a distinct set of social situations to which they are exposed, the CAPS theory makes it possible to analyze the process that underlies the emergence of such individual differences. This is possible because, for human social behaviors, a key component of the "environment" consists of other people. Thus, a model of people that explicitly relates the situational input to behavioral output, such as the CAPS model, can simultaneously also function as a model of the environment (e.g., Shoda, LeeTiernan, & Mischel, 2002). For example, in a close relationship, one person's behavioral output becomes the other person's situational input, and vice versa, forming a dyadic system (Zayas, Shoda, & Ayduk, 2002). Then, to the extent that each partner's personality is characterized by a stable "*if . . . then . . .* " behavioral signature, it becomes possible to model the interactions between them, and predict the "personality" of the interpersonal system they form, with its own distinctive relationship "signature" with characteristic dynamics.

Computer simulations using a parallel constraint satisfaction network confirmed this prediction, showing how each interpersonal system formed by a combination of two individuals has predictable and distinctive behaviors and patterns of interactions (Shoda et al., 2002). Most interestingly, the model and the computer simulation predict that sometimes the cognitive and affective states that an individual experiences often, in a given relationship, are different from those the same individual experiences in other relationships, or in isolation; that is, they are an emergent property of each interpersonal system rather than a simple combination of the personalities of the individuals that constitute the system.

Intuitively and theoretically, it has long been observed that every interpersonal relationship has its own personality. Qualities of an interpersonal relationship are not simply an average of the personalities of the individuals that form it. For example, the marriage of two generally agreeable individuals may turn out to be full of discord and unhappiness, whereas the opposite can also occur, in which two generally disagreeable individuals form a happy and invigorating, if not quiet, partnership. Past efforts to answer these questions were hampered by a conceptualization of personality that did not provide for ways to take effects of situations into account. The CAPS theory illustrates that by incorporating situations into the conception of the person, and more specifically, by characterizing each individual by a stable and distinct set of *if . . . then . . .* pattern or *behavioral signature*, where "if" is the psychological features present in a situation, and "then" is the cognitions and affects that become activated by them, it becomes possible to model explicitly the process by which the "personality" of a relationship emerges out of the interactions among individuals (see Shoda et al., 2002).

CONTROLLING THE "TEMPERATURE" THROUGH COGNITIVE REAPPRAISAL

To take account of the affective or "hot" aspects of social information processing, the CAPS model was extended to encompass two interacting subsystems: a cool, cognitive, reflective "know" system and a hot, reflexive, impulsive, automatic, emotional "go" system (Metcalfe & Mischel, 1999; Mischel & Ayduk, 2004). The interactions between these systems allow prediction of long-term developmental outcomes of not only goal-directed delay of gratification but also cognitive and emotional self-regulation in contexts that range from drug addiction and impulse disorders to economic decision making, to conflict in interpersonal relationships (Mischel, 2004; Mischel, Ayduk, & Mendoza-Denton, 2003).

Hot and Cool System Characteristics and Interactions

The effects of the context on behavior, the *if* ... *then* ... relations that characterize the CAPS system, are sometimes simple and reflexive, and sometimes more complex and highly mediated, requiring self-regulation, for example, when prepotent impulsive reactions are inhibited in light of anticipated future consequences (e.g., Mischel & Ayduk, 2004). To account for such differences in *self*-regulation, Metcalfe and Mischel (1999) proposed a theory in which self-regulation reflects the interaction between the *hot* system and *cool* system. The *hot system* is specialized for quick emotional processing and responding based on unconditional or conditional trigger features, as when rejection sensitive people become abusive to their partners as automatic reactions to perceived rejection cues. It is conceptualized as the basis of emotionality, fears as well as passions—impulsive and reflexive—initially controlled by innate releasing stimuli (thus, literally under "stimulus control"); it is fundamental for emotional (classical) conditioning and undermines efforts at self-control, reflective thought, and planfulness (Metcalfe & Mischel, 1999). In contrast, the *cool cognitive system* is specialized for complex spatiotemporal and episodic representation and thought. It is cognitive, emotionally neutral, contemplative, flexible, integrated, coherent, spatiotemporal, slow, episodic, and strategic—the seat of self-regulation and self-control.

The hot and cool systems interact continuously: As one becomes more activated, the other becomes less activated, and the balance between them is determined by stress, developmental level, and the individual's self-regulatory dynamics. Whereas stress—both chronic and situational—enhances the hot system and attenuates the cool system, with increasing development and maturation, the cool system becomes more developed and active, and the impact of the hot system becomes attenuated. The interactions between these systems allow prediction and explanation of findings on diverse phenomena involving the interplay of emotion and cognition, including goal-directed delay of gratification and the operation of "willpower" and self-directed change. Thus, strategic interventions may be used to influence the interaction of the hot and cool systems to overcome the power of stimulus control as people attempt purposefully to prevent powerful situations and hot trigger stimuli from eliciting their impulsive immediate responses and dispositional vulnerabilities in potentially maladaptive ways.

Working Through Negative Emotional Experiences: Getting the Temperature Right

Research also shows how mental operations can be harnessed as effective interventions to deal with intense negative feelings and experiences. An example of such intervention possibilities comes from research examining the common belief that in order to "get over" intense negative emotional experiences such as rejection by significant others, one needs to work through and understand those negative feelings. However, people's attempts to do this are often counterproductive, leading to rumination that increases distress (Nolen-Hoeksema, 1991; Teasdale, 1988). Kross and colleagues (2005), guided by CAPS and the hot–cool system model, facilitated "emotional cooling" by instructing participants to adopt a *psychologically distanced* perspective (i.e., to take a step back and watch the conflict happening to them from a distance) immediately after cueing them to recall an intense anger-arousing experience. Such distancing helped people to rerepresent their experiences cognitively and the emotions they elicited in relatively cool, cognitive terms, making sense of them and working through them without becoming overwhelmed by them, or becoming engulfed in rumination and depression. The overall findings are beginning to explain when people's attempts to understand their negative feelings are likely to be adaptive and when they are likely instead to trigger rumination. Kross and colleagues' work suggests a moderate level of activation in both the hot and cool system seems ideal: When the "temperature" gets too hot, extreme negative affect becomes reactivated; when the cool system dominates, rationalization and intellectualization, rather than working through and getting over it, become more likely. The continuing challenge will be to specify with increasing precision the mental operations for getting the right thermostat settings for coping with different types of emotional dilemmas.

CONTEXTUALIZED, SITUATED PERSONS: RECOGNIZING THE WITHIN-PERSON VARIABILITY

In conclusion, in the traditional decontextualized view of human traits and behavior, the inconsistencies and variability that characterize people are perplexing; in a contextualized view, they are expected. The emerging contextualized view of human nature and the situated person now has been buttressed by solid data, and conceptualized in a CAPS framework that allows us to make some sense of human complexity and plasticity—for good or ill—and at least not to be shocked by it.

Notable examples are commonplace in the characters that have always inhabited serious fiction and literature, and are regularly found in daily life. In recent history, recall ex-President Bill Clinton's impeachment experience: He was a model of self-control when dealing with foreign policy with heads of state in the Rose Garden but not when with young interns in the Oval Office. Or the fall of the honorable Sol Wachtler from his role as Chief Judge of the State of New York and the Court of Appeals, and a model of jurisprudent wisdom, to incarceration in a federal prison. Respected for laws to make marital rape a punishable crime, the judge nevertheless spent 13 months writing obscene letters, making lewd phone calls, and threatening to kidnap the daughter of the mistress who had left him for another man. For more in the same vein, the headline stories in 2008 depicted in detail the quick descent of Eliot Spitzer from Governor of New York State, and its previous widely feared Attorney General, for apparently violating federal laws whose enforcement he had himself helped to strengthen.

Traditional analyses of such "inconsistencies" in personality lead to the questions: "Which one of these two people is the real one? What is simply the effect of the situation?" Such questions may be reminiscent of the history of other sciences. Before the birth of modern chemistry, debates such as "Which is the true nature of this substance—combustible, or not combustible?" could have arisen in light of the fact that certain substances are extremely reactive in some contexts but not in others. Chemistry solves this problem by transitioning from conceptualizing the "nature" of a substance by its "behavior," such as being more combustible, to understanding the interaction between substances. The reaction between substances in turn is now understood with regard to the electrons that occupy the outer quantum orbital of the atoms that make them up, not by their "combustibility." Similarly, modern physics does not view color as a property of an object. It depends on the nature of light shining on the object, the visual system of the perceiving organism (humans, dogs, bees), as well as the nature of the object. The nature of the object is not conceptualized by its "color." Instead it is conceptualized by the quantum mechanical structure of the atom (in this case, electrons in any of the atomic orbitals, not just the outermost one). Color is an emergent phenomenon that arises out of the interactions of an object and its context (i.e., the light shining on it, and the visual system of the perceiving organism). Seen this way, it is not puzzling that the same object may appear to have different colors in different contexts.

Similarly, CAPS theory allows the same person to have contradictory facets that are equally genuine. The surface contradictions become comprehensible when one analyzes the network of relations among cognitions and affects, and how they interact with situations. The research problem becomes to understand when and why different cognitions and affects become activated predictably in relation to different features of situations, external and internal. In the situated person view, the individual's distinctive patterns of variability in different contexts are not necessarily internal contradictions; they may be potentially predictable expressions of a stable underlying system that itself may remain relatively unchanged in its organization. It raises such questions as: Are the caring and uncaring behaviors seen within the same person two scripts in the service of the same goal? If so, how are they connected to, and guided by, the person's self-conceptions and belief system in relation to the psychological features of situations that activate them? The challenge is to discriminate, understand, and predict when each aspect will be activated, and the dynamics that underlie the pattern, with increasing detail and precision, at diverse levels of analysis. And that promises to open an agenda in which we psychological scientists accord to our "subjects" the same complexity, plasticity, and depth that we assume characterizes us.

ACKNOWLEDGMENTS

The preparation of this chapter was supported by a grant from the National Institute of Mental Health (MH39349). Both authors contributed equally in the preparation of this chapter.

REFERENCES

Antrobus, J. (1991). Dreaming: Cognitive processes during critical activation and high afferent thresholds. *Psychology Review*, *98*, 96–121.

Ayduk, O., & Gyurak, A. (2008). Applying the Cognitive-Affective Processing Systems approach to conceptualizing rejection sensitivity. *Social and Personality Psychology Compass*, 2, 2016–2033.

Bandura, A. (1986). *Social foundations of thought and action: A social cognitive theory*. Englewood Cliffs, NJ: Prentice-Hall.

Bargh, J. A., & Gollwitzer, P. M. (Eds.). (1996). *The psychology of action: Linking cognition and motivation to behavior.* New York: Guilford Press.

Bolger, N., DeLongis, A., Kessler, R. C., & Schilling, E. A. (1989). Effects of daily stress on negative mood. *Journal of Personality and Social Psychology, 57,* 808–818.

Bolger, N., & Eckenrode, J. (1991). Social relationships, personality, and anxiety during a major stressful event. *Journal of Personality and Social Psychology, 61,* 440–449.

Bolger, N., & Schilling, E. A. (1991). Personality and the problems of everyday life: The role of neuroticism in exposure and reactivity to daily stressors. *Journal of Personality, 59,* 355–386.

Borkenau, P., Riemann, R., Spinath, F. M., & Angleitner, A. (2006). Genetic and environmental influences on person *X* situation profiles. *Journal of Personality, 74,* 1451–1479.

Buss, D. M. (1987). Selection, evocation, and manipulation. *Journal of Personality and Social Psychology, 53,* 1214–1221.

Cantor, N., & Blanton, H. (1996). Effortful pursuit of personal goals in daily life. In P. M. Gollwitzer & J. A. Bargh (Eds.), *The psychology of action: Linking cognition and motivation to behavior* (pp. 338–359). New York: Guilford Press.

Cantor, N., & Kihlstrom, J. F. (1987). *Personality and social intelligence.* Englewood Cliffs, NJ: Prentice-Hall.

Cantor, N., & Mischel, W. (1977). Traits as prototypes: Effects on recognition memory. *Journal of Personality and Social Psychology, 35,* 38–48.

Cantor, N., & Mischel, W. (1979). Prototypicality and personality: Effects on free recall and personality impressions. *Journal of Research in Personality, 13,* 187–205.

Cantor, N., Mischel, W., & Schwartz, J. C. (1982). A prototype analysis of psychological situations. *Cognitive Psychology, 14,* 45–77.

Cervone, D., & Orom, H. (2009). Identifying cross-situational coherence by assessing personality architecture. *Journal of Research in Personality, 43,* 228–240.

Cervone, D., & Shoda, Y. (1999). Social-cognitive theories and the coherence of personality. In D. Cervone & Y. Shoda (Eds.), *The coherence of personality: Social-cognitive bases of consistency, variability, and organization* (pp. 3–33). New York: Guilford Press.

Downey, G., Feldman, S., & Ayduk, O. (2000). Rejection sensitivity and male violence in romantic relationships. *Personal Relationships, 7,* 45–61.

Eigsti, I., Zayas, V., Mischel, W., Shoda, Y., Ayduk, O., Dadlani, M. B., et al. (2006). Predicting cognitive control from preschool to late adolescence and young adulthood. *Psychological Science, 17,* 478–484.

Emmons, R. A. (1991). Personal strivings, daily life events, and psychological and physical well-being. *Journal of Personality, 59,* 453–472.

Epstein, S. (1979). The stability of behavior: I. On predicting most of the people much of the time. *Journal of Personality and Social Psychology, 37,* 1097–1126.

Epstein, S. (1980). The stability of behavior: II. Implications for psychological research. *American Psychologist, 35*, 790–806.

Feldman, S., & Downey, G. (1994). Rejection sensitivity as a mediator of the impact of childhood exposure to family violence on adult attachment behavior. *Development and Psychopathology, 6*, 231–247.

Fleeson, W. (2001). Toward a structure- and process-integrated view of personality: Traits as density distributions of states. *Journal of Personality and Social Psychology, 80*, 1011–1027.

Forgas, J. P. (1983a). Episode cognition and personality: A multidimensional analysis. *Journal of Personality, 51*, 34–48.

Forgas, J. P. (1983b). Social skills and the perception of interaction episodes. *British Journal of Clinical Psychology, 22*, 195–207.

Fournier, M. A., Moskowitz, D. S., & Zuroff, D. C. (2008). Integrating dispositions, signatures, and the interpersonal domain. *Journal of Personality and Social Psychology, 90*, 283–289.

Gollwitzer, P. M. (1996). The volitional benefits of planning. In J. A. Bargh & P. M. Gollwitzer(Eds.), *The psychology of action: Linking cognition and motivation to behavior* (pp. 297–312). New York: Guilford Press.

Gollwitzer, P. M. (1999). Implementation intentions: Strong effects of simple plans. *American Psychologist, 54*, 493–503.

Hartshorne, H., & May, M. A. (1928). *Studies in the nature of character: Vol. 1. Studies in deceit.* New York: Macmillan.

Higgins, E. T., King, G. A., & Mavin, G. H. (1982). Individual construct accessibility and subjective impressions and recall. *Journal of Personality and Social Psychology, 43*, 35–47.

Isen, A. M., Niedenthal, P. M., & Cantor, N. (1992). An influence of positive affect on social categorization. *Motivation and Emotion, 16*, 65–78.

Kelly, G. (1955). *The psychology of personal constructs.* New York: Basic Books.

Klinger, E. (1996). Emotional influences on cognitive processing, with implications for theories of both. In J. A. Bargh & P. M. Gollwitzer (Eds.), *The psychology of action: Linking cognition and motivation to action* (pp. 168–189). New York: Guilford Press.

Kross, E., Ayduk, O., & Mischel, W. (2005). When asking "*why*" doesn't hurt: Distinguishing rumination from reflective processing of negative emotions. *Psychological Science, 16*, 709–715.

Linville, P. W., & Clark, L. F. (1989). Can production systems cope with coping? *Social Cognition, 7*, 195–236.

Magnusson, D., & Endler, N. S. (1977). Interactional psychology: Present status and future prospects. In *Personality at the crossroads: Current issues in interactional psychology* (pp. 3–31). Hillsdale, NJ: Erlbaum.

McCrae, R. R., & Costa, P. T., Jr. (1999). A five-factor theory of personality. In L. A. Pervin & O. P. John (Eds.), *Handbook of personality: Theory and research* (2nd ed., pp. 139–153). New York: Guilford Press.

Mendoza-Denton, R., & Mischel, W. (2007). Integrating system approaches to culture and personality: The Cultural Cognitive–Affective Processing System. In S. Kitayama & D. Cohen (Eds.), *Handbook of cultural psychology* (pp. 175–195). New York: Guilford Press.

Metcalfe, J., & Mischel, W. (1999). A hot/cool system analysis of delay of gratification: Dynamics of willpower. *Psychological Review, 106*, 3–19.

Mischel, H. N., & Mischel, W. (1973). *Readings in personality.* New York: Holt, Rinehart & Winston.

Mischel, W. (1968). *Personality and assessment.* Hillsdale, NJ: Erlbaum.

Mischel, W. (1973). Toward a cognitive social learning reconceptualization of personality. *Psychological Review, 80*, 252–283.

Mischel, W. (1974a). Cognitive appraisals and transformations in self-control. In B. Weiner (Ed.), *Cognitive views of human motivation* (pp. 33–49). New York: Academic Press.

Mischel, W. (1974b). Processes in delay of gratification. In L. Berkowitz (Ed.), *Advances in experimental social psychology* (Vol. 7, pp. 249–292). New York: Academic Press.

Mischel, W. (1996). From good intentions to willpower. In J. A. Bargh & P. M. Gollwitzer (Eds.), *The psychology of action: Linking cognition and motivation to action* (pp. 197–218). New York: Guilford Press.

Mischel, W. (2004). Toward an integrative science of the person [Prefatory chapter]. *Annual Review of Psychology, 55*, 1–22.

Mischel, W., & Ayduk, O. (2004). Willpower in a Cognitive–Affective Processing System: The dynamics of delay of gratification. In R. F. Baumeister & K. D. Vohs (Eds.), *Handbook of self-regulation: Research, theory, and applications* (pp. 99–129). New York: Guilford Press.

Mischel, W., Ayduk, O., & Mendoza-Denton, R. (2003). Sustaining delay of gratification over time: A hot/cool systems perspective. In G. Loewenstein, D. Read, & R. Baumeister (Eds.), *Time and decision: Economic and psychological perspectives on intertemporal choice* (pp. 175–200). New York: Russell Sage Foundation.

Mischel, W., Cantor, N., & Feldman, S. (1996). Principles of self-regulation: The nature of willpower and self-control. In E. T. Higgins & A. W. Kruglanski (Eds.), *Social psychology: Handbook of basic principles* (pp. 329–360). New York: Guilford Press.

Mischel, W., & Morf, C. (2003). The self as a psycho-social dynamic processing system: A meta-perspective on a century of the self in psychology. In M. R. Leary & J. P. Tangney (Eds.), *Handbook of self and identity* (pp. 15–43). New York: Guilford Press.

Mischel, W., & Peake, P. K. (1982a). Beyond déjà vu in the search for cross-situational consistency. *Psychological Review, 89*, 730–755.

Mischel, W., & Peake, P. (1982b). In search of consistency: Measure for measure. In M. P. Zanna, E. T. Higgins, & C. P. Herman (Eds.), *Consistency in social behavior: The Ontario Symposium* (Vol. 2, pp. 187–207). Hillsdale, NJ: Erlbaum.

Mischel, W., & Shoda, Y. (1995). A cognitive–affective system theory of personality: Reconceptualizing situations, dispositions, dynamics, and invariance in personality structure. *Psychological Review, 102*, 246–268.

Mischel, W., & Shoda, Y. (1998). Reconciling processing dynamics and personality dispositions. *Annual Review of Psychology, 49*, 229–258.
Mischel, W., Shoda, Y., & Ayduk, O. (2008). *Introduction to personality: Toward an integrative science of the person* (8th ed.). New York: Wiley.
Mischel, W., Shoda, Y., & Rodriguez, M. L. (1989, May). Delay of gratification in children. *Science, 244*, 933–938.
Moskowitz, D. S. (1982). Coherence and cross-situational generality in personality: A new analysis of old problems. *Journal of Personality and Social Psychology, 43*, 754–768.
Moskowitz, D. S. (1994). Cross-situational generality and the interpersonal circumplex. *Journal of Personality and Social Psychology, 66*, 921–933.
Moskowitz, D. S., Suh, E. J., & Desaulniers, J. (1994). Situational influences on gender differences in agency and communion. *Journal of Personality and Social Psychology, 66*, 753–761.
Murphy, G. L., & Medin, D. L. (1985). The role of theories in conceptual coherence. *Psychological Review, 92*, 289–316.
Newcomb, T. M. (1929). *Consistency of certain extrovert–introvert behavior patterns in 51 problem boys.* New York: Columbia University, Teachers College, Bureau of Publications.
Nisbett, R. E., & Ross, L. D. (1980). *Human interference: Strategies and shortcomings of social judgment.* Englewood Cliffs, NJ: Prentice-Hall.
Nolen-Hoeksema, S. (1991). Responses to depression and their effects on the duration of depressive episodes. *Journal of Abnormal Psychology, 100*, 569–582.
Nolen-Hoeksema, S., Parker, L. E., & Larson, J. (1994). Ruminative coping with depressed mood following loss. *Journal of Personality and Social Psychology, 67*, 92–104.
Pervin, L. A. (1994). A critical analysis of trait theory. *Psychological Inquiry, 5*, 103–113.
Peterson, D. R. (1968). *The clinical study of social behavior.* New York: Appleton–Century–Crofts.
Plomin, R., DeFries, J. C., McClearn, G. E., & Rutter, M. (1997). *Behavioral genetics* (3rd ed.). New York: Freeman.
Rosenberg, S., & Jones, R. (1972). A method for investigating and representing a person's implicit theory of personality. *Journal of Personality and Social Psychology, 22*, 372–386.
Ross, L., & Nisbett, R. E. (1991). *The person and the situation: Perspectives of social psychology.* New York: McGraw-Hill.
Schwarz, N. (1990). Feelings and information: Informational and motivational functions of affective states. In E. T. Higgins & R. M. Sorrentino (Eds.), *Handbook of motivation and cognition: Vol. 2.Foundations of social behavior* (pp. 527–561). New York: Guilford Press.
Shoda, Y. (1990). *Conditional analyses of personality coherence and dispositions.* Unpublished doctoral dissertation, Columbia University.
Shoda, Y. (2003). Individual differences in social psychology: Understanding situations to understand people, understanding people to understand situ-

ations. In C. Sansone, C. Morf, & A. Panter (Eds.), *Handbook of methods in social psychology* (pp. 117–141). Thousand Oaks, CA: Sage.

Shoda, Y., & LeeTiernan, S. (2002). What remains invariant?: Finding order within a person's thoughts, feelings, and behaviors across situations. In D. Cervone & W. Mischel (Eds.), *Advances in personality science* (pp. 241–270). New York: Guilford Press.

Shoda, Y., LeeTiernan, S., & Mischel, W. (2002). Personality as a dynamical system: Emergence of stability and consistency from intra- and inter-personal interactions. *Personality and Social Psychology Review*, 6, 316–325.

Shoda, Y., & Mischel, W. (1993). Cognitive social approach to dispositional inferences: What if the perceiver is a cognitive-social theorist? *Personality and Social Psychology Bulletin*, *19*, 574–585.

Shoda, Y., & Mischel, W. (1998). Personality as a stable cognitive–affective activation network: Characteristic patterns of behavior variation emerge from a stable personality structure. In S. Read & L. C. Miller (Eds.), *Connectionist models of social reasoning and social behavior* (pp. 175–208). Mahwah, NJ: Erlbaum.

Shoda, Y., Mischel, W., & Wright, J. C. (1989). Intuitive interactionism in person perception: Effects of situation–behavior relations on dispositional judgments. *Journal of Personality and Social Psychology*, *56*, 41–59.

Shoda, Y., Mischel, W., & Wright, J. C. (1993a). Links between personality judgments and contextualized behavior patterns: Situation–behavior profiles of personality prototypes. *Social Cognition*, *4*, 399–429.

Shoda, Y., Mischel, W., & Wright, J. C. (1993b). The role of situational demands and cognitive competencies in behavior organization and personality coherence. *Journal of Personality and Social Psychology*, *65*, 1023–1035.

Shoda, Y., Mischel, W., & Wright, J. C. (1994). Intra-individual stability in the organization and patterning of behavior: Incorporating psychological situations into the idiographic analysis of personality. *Journal of Personality and Social Psychology*, *67*, 674–687.

Smith, C. A., & Lazarus, R. S. (1990). Emotion and adaptation. In L. A. Pervin (Ed.), *Handbook of personality: Theory and research* (pp. 609–637). New York: Guilford Press.

Smith, T. W., & Rhodewalt, F. (1986). On states, traits, and processes: A transactional alternative to the individual difference assumptions in Type A behavior and physiological reactivity. *Journal of Research in Personality*, *20*, 229–251.

Snyder, M. (1983). The influence of individuals on situations: Implications for understanding the links between personality and social behavior. *Journal of Personality*, *51*, 497–516.

Snyder, M., & Gangestad, S. (1982). Choosing social situations: Two investigations of self-monitoring processes. *Journal of Personality and Social Psychology*, *43*, 123–135.

Teasdale, J. D. (1988). Cognitive vulnerability to persistent depression. *Cognition and Emotion*, 2, 247–274.

Vallacher, R. R., & Wegner, D. M. (1987). What do people think they're doing?:

Action identification and human behavior. *Psychological Review*, *94*, 3–15.

Van Mechelen, I. (2009). A royal road to understanding the mechanisms underlying person-in-context behavior. *Journal of Research in Personality*, *43*, 179–186.

Vansteelandt, K., & Van Mechelen, I. (1998). Individual differences in situation–behavior profiles: A triple typology model. *Journal of Personality and Social Psychology*, *75*, 751–765.

Vansteelandt, K., & Van Mechelen, I. (2006). Individual differences in anger and sadness: Pursuit of active situational features and psychological processes. *Journal of Personality*, *74*, 871–909.

Vernon, P. E. (1964). *Personality assessment: A critical survey*. New York: Wiley.

Wright, J. C., & Mischel, W. (1987). A conditional analysis of dispositional constructs: The local predictability of social behavior. *Journal of Personality and Social Psychology*, *53*, 1159–1177.

Wright, J. C., & Mischel, W. (1988). Conditional hedges and the intuitive psychology of traits. *Journal of Personality and Social Psychology*, *3*, 454–469.

Zayas, V., Shoda, Y., & Ayduk, O. N. (2002). Personality in context: An interpersonal systems perspective. *Journal of Personality*, *70*, 851–898.

9

Implicit Independence and Interdependence

A Cultural Task Analysis

SHINOBU KITAYAMA
TOSHIE IMADA

Over the last few decades, cultural-psychological work has made significant progress. Focusing primarily on East Asians and North Americans, researchers have provided convincing evidence for cultural variations in a variety of psychological tendencies. Thus, we now know that relative to East Asians, North Americans are more likely to be focused in attention (e.g., Kitayama, Duffy, Kawamura, & Larsen, 2003; Masuda & Nisbett, 2001), to draw dispositional (as opposed to situational) inferences (e.g., Miyamoto & Kitayama, 2002; Morris & Peng, 1994), to show self-enhancing or self-serving biases (Heine, Kitayama, & Hamamura, 2007; Rose, Endo, Windschitl, & Suls, 2008), to experience disengaging (rather than engaging) emotions (e.g., Kitayama, Mesquita, & Karasawa, 2006), to enjoy personal (vs. social) happiness (e.g., Kitayama et al., 2006; Oishi & Diener, 2003; Uchida, Kitayama, Mesquita, Reyes, & Morling, 2008), to seek uniqueness of the self (Kim & Sherman, 2007), and to be motivated by private (rather than public) choices (e.g., Iyengar & Lepper, 1999; Kitayama & Imada, in press; Na & Kitayama, 2008). Conversely, East Asians are highly holistic in attention; less prone to dispositional bias in social inference and less likely to show self-enhancing or self-serving biases; and more likely to experience engaging rather than disengaging emotions, to enjoy social rather than personal happiness, to seek to remain conventional, and to be motivated by public rather than private choices (see, e.g., Kitayama, Duffy, & Uchida, 2007, for a recent review).

One overarching pair of constructs used to account for this diverse array of cross-cultural variation is independence and interdependence (Kitayama et al., 2007; Markus & Kitayama, 1991, 2004). The effects indicate that North Americans are operating on the assumption that the self is independent, that is, separate from context, internally motivated, and distinct and unique. In contrast, the effects suggest that East Asians are operating on the assumption that the self is interdependent, that is, connected to context, externally motivated, and similar to others and embedded.

This chapter presents a cultural task analysis of the influences of independence and interdependence on the array of psychological tendencies. The central premise of the cultural task analysis is that the notion of "cultural context" must be taken seriously. We argue that cultural context comprises myriad cultural tasks of independence and interdependence (organized sets of goals and procedures to accomplish them). These tasks are created, accumulated, and passed across generations in any given culture. The cultural context matters because individuals participate in these cultural tasks to realize their culture's mandate of the self as either independent in many Western cultural contexts or interdependent in many Eastern cultural contexts. Through this engagement with the cultural tasks of independence or interdependence, individuals may be expected to acquire and eventually internalize psychological tendencies that are required by the pertinent cultural tasks. In what follows, we elaborate on the cultural task analysis, present evidence for it, and draw additional implications of the analysis. We then discuss some historical antecedent conditions of independence and interdependence.

CULTURAL TASK ANALYSIS

Independent Model of Self

Along with a number of colleagues, we have argued that cultures vary in the extent to which either independence or interdependence is sanctioned (Kitayama et al., 2007; Markus & Kitayama, 1991; Shweder & Bourne, 1982; Triandis, 1989). Western cultural contexts have emphasized a view of the self as independent, defined primarily by internal attributes, such as preferences, desires, and traits. It would be a mistake to assume that this view has always been hegemonic throughout the long history of Western civilization. Nevertheless, it is also true that such a view was evident in the ancient Greek civilization, where logic was invented as a practical means of differentiating good arguments from bad ones, and rhetoric was developed as a tool for debate (Morris, 1991; Nisbett, 2003). Although dormant to a large extent throughout the Dark Age and confined largely to monasteries throughout Europe, the view of the self as independent was rediscovered and extensively elaborated in Western Europe during the Reformation and Renaissance eras. The birth of Protestantism in the 14th and 15th centuries was one of the most crucial events. Some novel conceptions, such as calling and predestination, underscored the idea that each person has his or her inherent merit; moreover, he or she is in direct communication with God (Weber, 1958). Soon a number of prominent thinkers in the era of Enlightenment reinforced similar themes. All these forces converged to yield a general conception of self as independent, autonomous, and separate, or socially disengaged. Within this framework, social relations are conceived as voluntary and thus optional (Morris, 1991).

Interdependent Model of Self

In contrast, in Eastern civilizations, a contrasting view of the self as interdependent, interpersonally connected, and socially embedded has been elaborated. This general view of the self can be found in the ontology of Buddhism (which emphasizes a unity of the universe, including all creatures, both past and present), Confucian ethics (which is grounded in the central significance given to hierarchical relationships at both societal and personal levels), and a variety of indigenous, holistic beliefs, such as Bushido and Taoism. Of course, the relational, interdependent view of the self acknowledges one's internal attributes, such as desires, intentions, and attitudes. However, these attributes are not considered as primary. Instead, they are seen as coexisting with, contingent on, and often subordinated to the social order.

Cultural Tasks of Independence and Interdependence

We have argued that the two cultural views of the self as independent and interdependent are used to organize social practices and institutions; as a consequence, they provide a number of cultural tasks that people perform to participate in their social lives (Fiske, Kitayama, Markus, & Nisbett, 1998; Kitayama & Markus, 1994, 1999; Markus & Kitayama, 2004; see also Cantor, 1994; Greenwald, 1982).

The independent view is associated with cultural tasks such as "expressing unique self," "being a strong leader," "taking an initiative to achieve a personal success," and "being in charge and under control." These tasks are likely to be present in many, if not all, cultures and historical times. However, they are also likely to be highly sanctioned in

Western cultures. By habitually and repeatedly engaging in these tasks individuals are likely to acquire the various psychological tendencies required by them. Because independent tasks require people to focus on personal self as separate from both other such selves and context, they foster psychological tendencies that distinguish the self from its surroundings. Moreover, many of the independent tasks require one's action to be internally motivated and guided. As a consequence, the independent tasks tend to encourage both a focus of attention on goal-relevant objects, and decontextualized decisions and judgments.

The interdependent view is typically associated with a contrasting set of cultural tasks, such as "conforming and being obedient," "being similar to others," and "following social norms and fitting-in" and "achieving social harmony." Again, although these tasks are likely present in many, if not all, cultures and historical times, they are strongly sanctioned in Asian cultures. Like the independent tasks, the interdependent cultural tasks afford a number of psychological tendencies, but the tendencies fostered by the interdependent tasks are bound to be diametrically opposite to those fostered by the independent tasks. Most importantly, interdependent tasks require people to attend broadly to social context. Thus, these tasks may foster psychological tendencies that connect the self to the context, and experience it as part of that context. Furthermore, many of the interdependent tasks require the self to be closely attuned to expectations and norms of the surrounding situation and, accordingly, may require both a broad allocation of attention to social context and decisions, and judgments that are context-dependent and situation-sensitive.

To explore the nature of independent and interdependent tasks in both the United States and Japan, we recently asked both American and Japanese participants to describe freely real-life episodes in which they felt either "separate and independent" or "connected and interdependent" (Imada & Kitayama, 2006). These episodes were then content-coded. Fifteen distinct categories were identified for independence. They included "financial and professional autonomy," "separation from others," "difference from others," "personal achievement," "responsibility," "being respected," and "freedom." Likewise, 13 distinct categories were identified for interdependence. They included "collective activity," "similarities with others," "help and support," "group affiliation," and "being appreciated."

Notably, virtually all of these categories were present in both the United States and Japan. However, in support of the idea that American culture provides a wide array of independence tasks, American independent episodes were more equally distributed across the 15 categories. It is evident that American culture provides its people with a wide variety of ways in which to become independent. We suggest that individuals engaging in the American culture selectively adopt some subset of the independent cultural tasks in their effort to be independent. For example, some people may try to be independent by taking on an important societal responsibility, whereas others may try to do so by achieving financial and professional success. Although these individuals are likely to be highly unique in their selection of cultural tasks, they are similar in their pursuit of the cultural imperative of independence. In contrast, more than half of Japanese independent episodes were accounted for by only two categories ("being different from others" and "social exclusion"), indicating that Japanese culture provides its people with a relatively small number of ways to be independent. It is clear, then, that even when Japanese try to be independent, their options are bound to be limited because the culture offers relatively few resources to do so.

We also expected Japanese culture to provide an equally wide array of tasks to achieve interdependence. This in fact was the case. Thus, Japanese episodes were distributed across the 13 categories quite evenly. Clearly, Japanese culture offers a large number of ways to be interdependent. We suggest that people engaging in this cultural context seek to accomplish the cultural imperative of interdependence in their own unique ways. Thus, some people may try to be interdependent by affiliating themselves with important groups, such as companies, schools, or the country itself. But other people may try to do so by being similar and inconspicuous in attitudes, mannerisms, their clothing, and the like. In contrast, nearly 70% of American interdependent episodes were accounted for by three categories alone ("collective activity," "personal relationship," and "communication"). Clearly, interdependence exists in the American cultural context, but this culture offers relatively few resources, even if people seek to accomplish this value in their personal lives.

Cultural Tasks and Implicit Psychological Tendencies

One important implication of the cultural task analysis is that many psychological tendencies, such as focused versus holistic attention, activation of different emotions, and promotion- or prevention-focus, are gradually fostered, acquired, and internalized through repeated engagement in and performance of pertinent cultural tasks. This perspective, then, strongly suggests that, for most adults of any given cultural group, the pertinent psychological tendencies will be habitual, automatic, and largely non-self-reflective.

These tendencies may be called "implicit" and distinguished from "explicit" beliefs about the self as independent or interdependent. Roughly speaking, by *implicit* tendencies, we refer to how people habitually think, feel, and act, whereas by *explicit* beliefs, we refer to what people believe themselves to be. We have roughly classified these implicit tendencies into cognition, emotion, and motivation (Markus & Kitayama, 1991). These implicit psychological tendencies may or may not be aligned closely to explicit personal beliefs about the self as independent or interdependent (Kitayama, 2002; Kitayama & Markus, 1999).

We suggest that in adapting to their own cultural context, people are motivated to be independent or interdependent in accordance with the overarching imperative of the culture. Furthermore, they do so by performing various relevant cultural tasks. It is very unlikely, however, that any single person wholeheartedly takes up and performs all pertinent tasks available in his or her culture. For example, in the aforementioned study by Imada and Kitayama (2006), there were a number of ways in which to be independent in the American context. Even though these options are available for everyone in this culture, it is highly unlikely that everyone seriously pursues all of them because they can be independent by adopting only a small number of such options and performing them well. In other words, the available cultural tasks represent alternative ways for one to attain his or her culture's mandate of the self as independent or interdependent. The person may therefore become independent or interdependent in his or her own way. As noted earlier, specific psychological features that define independence or interdependence may be expected to vary from one individual to the next within any given cultural group.

Acculturation and Individual Development

Needless to say, which tasks people choose for the sake of realizing or living up to their own culture's mandate or imperative (i.e., independence or interdependence) is likely to depend on myriad factors. For example, early socialization may play an important role. Likewise, contemporary social contexts may also have an important impact on the selection of cultural tasks (Cantor, 1994). Furthermore, all these factors are embedded in macro-, societal-, or collective-level contexts such as social class, ecology, and economy, among others (e.g., Berry, 1976; Inglehart & Baker, 2000; Kitayama & Markus, 1999; Oyserman & Lee, 2007). Configurations of these various factors are likely to be highly idiosyncratic. This explains why individuals are so diverse and unique. At the same time, individuals in a given sociocultural context are bound to be quite similar at a higher level of analysis, to the extent that the available diverse cultural tasks are similar to one another in terms of the cultural imperative they are designed to address. Accordingly, the cultural task analysis explicitly acknowledges that people in different cultures are systematically different, yet people within any given culture are similar in terms of broad cultural themes or ideas to which they are committed, such as independence and interdependence.

An analogy may help. Think about a sports gym. People who come regularly to a gym are all committed to health. As a consequence, if they are compared with people who do not come to the gym, there will be massive "cultural" differences on some relevant dimensions, especially those related to health orientations. At the same time, however, gym goers also differ from one another. Some swim, others do weights, and still others jog; moreover, many others mix activities in different combinations. As a consequence, gym goers are similar and, simultaneously, different from one another. They are similar in a very general theme of health consciousness and general physical fitness, yet very different in terms of specific means by which to realize this theme.

The cultural task analysis maintains that the ways people participate in a local gym apply equally well to their engagement in and acquisition of culture in general. Thus, all European Americans tend to share a certain degree of commitment to cultural ideas and ideals having to do with independence, such as self-esteem, self-initiative, promotion, and personal success. Yet they are very different from one another in the specific ways to realize these ideas and ideals. Likewise, all Asians tend to share a certain degree of commitment to the cultural ideas and ideals having to do with interdependence, such as filial piety, conformity and docility, adjustment and flexibility and the like. However, they are very different from each other in ways to realize such ideas and ideals.

IMPLICIT INDEPENDENCE AND INTERDEPENDENCE: A BRIEF REVIEW

One straightforward implication of the cultural task analysis is that there are a number of differences in implicit psychological tendencies implicated in the cultural tasks of independence and interdependence. Here we provide a brief review of the evidence demonstrating this point.

Self-Definition

When we describe who we are, we define ourselves in culturally specific ways, so independent or interdependent forms of the self gain tangible forms that become readily accessible in our minds. In fact, culturally variant descriptions of the self can be demonstrated by the 20-Statements

Test (TST), in which individuals are asked to describe themselves in 20 different ways. With this method, Cousins (1989) found that Americans listed more personal traits (e.g., "I am friendly") than did Japanese, whereas Japanese listed more social categories (e.g., "I am a college student") than did Americans. When Japanese listed traits, they did so only in a contextualized format (e.g., "I am diligent in school"). The prevalence of personal traits in Western independent cultural contexts and the prevalence of social categories in Asian interdependent contexts were also observed by other researchers (Rhee, Uleman, Lee, & Roman, 1995; Trafimow, Triandis, & Goto, 1991; Uchida, Park, & Kitayama, 2009). By defining the self with purely internal aspects, such as personal traits, individuals extract the absolute constituents of the self that are unique to them. Also, by doing so, individuals can fortify the self as independent and separate from the environment. In contrast, by defining the self in terms of social roles and situational contexts, individuals can form the interdependent self. Because of its socially flexible and boundless nature, it is difficult for the interdependent self to maintain itself without the social structures of which it is a part.

Positive Self-Images

Despite the culturally variable definitions of the self, people across cultures seem to be concerned about their self-images. However, the nature of the self-images about which individuals care the most seems to differ cross-culturally. For example, European Americans are typically motivated to hold positive views of the self. This strong tendency is demonstrated in their pursuit of high self-esteem and self-efficacy (Taylor & Brown, 1988). In contrast, Asians typically show a strong concern with their public self-image—how others think about them. This tendency is demonstrated in their strong concern with honor and saving face (e.g., Cohen, Hoshino-Browne, & Leung, 2007; Kitayama, Snibbe, Markus, & Suzuki, 2004). To attain a positive view of the self, European Americans tend to take credit for success and blame external circumstances for failure (Miller & Ross, 1975). However, such self-enhancing efforts are virtually absent among Asians (for reviews, see Heine, Lehman, Markus, & Kitayama, 1999; Kitayama & Markus, 1999). This may be because one's positive evaluation of the self does not affect but possibly hurts one's public self-image (e.g., being conceited) in Asian cultural contexts. Thus, quite to the contrary, Asians show a tendency toward self-criticism or self-effacement (Kitayama, Markus, Matsumoto, & Norasakkunkit, 1997). Perhaps, in this way Asians can generate others' sympathy or approval and, most importantly, improve their public self-image as humble, hard-working persons.

Several studies provide additional evidence for the notion that one's internally held positive self-image is important to European Americans, but positive appraisals of the self by others are much more important to Asians. For example, European Americans work harder when they choose a task to work on, but Asians work harder when meaningful others choose a task for them (Iyengar, & Lepper, 1999) or when they choose a task in the presence of public scrutiny (Na & Kitayama, 2008). Similarly, European Americans tend to show a personal dissonance effect; that is, they justify their choice that was made privately (thus, self-expressive), protecting their personal positive self-image as good decision makers. In contrast, Asians tend to show an interpersonal dissonance effect; that is, they justify their choice if it is made for friends (Hoshino-Browne et al., 2005) or under public scrutiny (Imada & Kitayama, 2007; Kitayama et al., 2004), so that they protect their public self-images.

Emotions

Kitayama and colleagues have proposed that some emotions are related to the success or failure of independence whereas others are more pertinent to success or failure of interdependence (e.g., Kitayama & Park, 2007). Emotions such as pride in self and feelings of self-confidence result from success in achieving one's independence, but emotions such as anger and frustration stem from a failure to do so, and from an effort to restore much-needed independence. The researchers refer to these emotions as *socially disengaging*. In contrast, emotions such as feelings of connectedness and communal feelings result from success in maintaining harmonious interdependence, whereas emotions such as guilt and shame stem from a failure to do so, and a subsequent effort to restore a much-valued state of interdependence. These emotions are called *socially engaging*. One straightforward prediction is that people who chronically engage in independent tasks should experience more disengaging emotions (e.g., pride and anger), and those who chronically engage in interdependent tasks should experience more engaging emotions (e.g., friendly feelings and shame).

This in fact is the case in recent studies that compared Americans and Japanese in mainland Japan. Kitayama, Mesquita, and colleagues (2006) asked American and Japanese participants to keep an "emotion diary" every day for a 2-week period. At the end of each day, participants remembered the "most emotional event of the day" and reported how strongly they experienced each different emotion. The emotions differed in both pleasantness and social orientation (i.e., engaging vs.

disengaging). As predicted, overall, across the two weeks, Americans reportedly experienced more disengaging emotions (e.g., pride in self, feelings of self-confidence, anger, and frustration) than engaging emotions (e.g., friendly feelings, respect, shame, and guilt). In contrast, Japanese in mainland Japan reportedly experienced more engaging emotions than disengaging emotions.

Sensitivity to Vocal Tone

Because vocal tone is one of the most potent relational cues in daily communication, sensitivity to it can serve as an important index of the interdependence (as opposed to independence) orientation. To measure this vocal sensitivity, Kitayama, Ishii, and colleagues devised a vocal Stroop paradigm (Ishii, Reyes, & Kitayama, 2003; Kitayama & Ishii, 2002). Within this paradigm, words that are either positive or negative in meaning (*wedding*, *funeral*) are spoken either in an emotionally positive or an emotionally negative tone. Thus, the word–tone pairings are either congruent or incongruent. Participants are explicitly instructed to ignore the attendant vocal tone in making judgments of the affective meaning of the words. Interference by the to-be-ignored tone on the meaning judgment is the key dependent variable.

Cumulative evidence suggests that the vocal sensitivity measured in this paradigm is highly valid as an index of interdependence or strong relational orientation. Within the United States, vocal sensitivity as indexed by the vocal interference effect is greater for more relational Catholics compared to more independent Protestants, especially when the latter are in "business" mode (Sanchez-Burks, 2002). More importantly, Americans become more sensitive to vocal tone when they are primed to be more social or interdependent (Gray, Ambady, Ishii, & Kitayama, 2006; Pickett, Gardner, & Knowles, 2004). Likewise, Ishii, Kobayashi, and Kitayama (in press) found that surreptitious exposure to schematic human faces (presented as illustrations of a rating scale for the vocal Stroop task) was sufficient to produce a significant increase in sensitivity to vocal cues.

Kitayama, Ishii, and colleagues have tested both Asians (Japanese and Filipinos) and North Americans (Ishii et al., 2003; Kitayama & Ishii, 2002). Stimuli were created in such a way that evaluative extremity of word meanings and of vocal tone were roughly equivalent across the languages. The data provided strong support for the hypothesis that Asians are more sensitive to vocal tone and more interdependent than North Americans; that is, Asians were more strongly influenced than Americans by competing vocal tone.

Attribution

Whereas virtually all independent cultural tasks (e.g., self-initiatives, personal goal pursuit, being unique) are based on an assumption that individuals act on the basis of their own attitudes and preferences, virtually all interdependent cultural tasks (e.g., conformity and obedience, social harmony, being similar) are based on a belief that people act in reference to norms and expectations. These contrasting beliefs are likely to bias social inferences. Those chronically engaged in independent tasks should be more likely than those chronically engaged in interdependent tasks to infer that another person's behavior is caused internally by the person's dispositional characteristics, such as attitudes and preferences, while ignoring potentially important external or situational determinants of the behavior.

Cross-cultural evidence for this prediction is strong. Numerous studies have shown that the dispositional bias in social explanation is more pronounced among North Americans than among Asians (e.g., Kitayama, Mesquita, et al., 2006; Miller, 1984; Morris & Peng, 1994). For example, in a recent study Kitayama, Ishii, and colleagues presented Japanese in mainland Japan and Americans with a series of vignettes that described a target person who committed either a socially desirable or a socially undesirable behavior. The participants were then asked to indicate the degree to which they felt that internal factors, such as the target's attitude and temperament, and external factors, such as social norms and social atmospheres, were implicated in the behavior. As predicted, Americans were more likely to endorse the internal factors than the external factors as a significant cause of the behavior. In contrast, no such difference or bias was evident among mainland Japanese participants.

Attention

Cultural tasks may also result in attention differences. Independent tasks often require personal goals and, as a consequence, people engaging in these tasks may focus their attention on goal-relevant objects, while ignoring other contextual cues. In contrast, interdependent tasks often require broad attention to the social surroundings, resulting in more holistic attentional tendencies.

Evidence shows that such attention differences exist in North America (where independence is highlighted) and Asia (where interdependence is highlighted). Masuda and Nisbett (2001) found that when asked to describe what is happening in a video vignette of an underwater scene,

North Americans begin their story by pointing to focal (i.e., big and centrally located) fish and describing features of the fish. Only later do they mention features in the background. In contrast, Japanese begin their story by referring to the background, describing the entire scene first, then moving on to mention the fish that is moving therein. The researchers also used a recognition memory task to show that whereas Americans tend to encode the focal fish separately from its background, Asians tend to encode the fish and its background as inherently connected. Conceptually equivalent findings have subsequently been obtained with diverse measures, including behavioral performance (Kitayama et al., 2003; Masuda & Nisbett, 2001), eye movement (Chua, Boland, & Nisbett, 2005), and neural measures such as electroencephalography (Lewis, Goto, Kong, & Lowenberg, 2008) and functional magnetic resonance imaging (Hedden, Ketay, Aron, Markus, & Gabrieli, 2008).

FURTHER IMPLICATIONS OF THE CULTURAL TASK ANALYSIS

Explicit Self-Beliefs on Independence and Interdependence

The cultural task analysis of independence and interdependence maintains that cultures vary in terms of the repertoires of cultural tasks created and accumulated therein over the course of history (Kitayama, 2002; Kitayama & Markus, 1999). Moreover, these cultural tasks require, and thus foster, a variety of implicit psychological tendencies. In general, independent tasks are much more likely than interdependent tasks to yield implicit psychological tendencies that separate and disengage the self, such as focused attention, dispositional bias, disengaging emotion, and personal happiness. For those who repeatedly engage in the pertinent cultural tasks, the corresponding psychological tendencies will be well rehearsed, become automatized, and thus implicit. This analysis has received substantial support from the bulk of research summarized above.

In many cross-cultural studies, however, independence and interdependence have frequently been studied as beliefs people have about themselves. One typical measure was invented by Singelis (1994). Self-beliefs about independence are measured by items such as "I am comfortable with being singled out for praise or rewards." Likewise, self-beliefs about interdependence are measured by items such as "It is important for me to maintain harmony within my group." When measured in this way, independence and interdependence are mostly orthogonal.

Does cultural task analysis apply equally to the self-beliefs of independent and interdependent individuals? There is reason to suspect that explicit beliefs of the self may rarely be involved in either the acquisition or the operation of implicit psychological tendencies. These beliefs are likely to be formed only after basic implicit personal and interpersonal inclinations are inculcated through early socialization, much before adolescence (Keller, 2007). Moreover, these tendencies are not required to perform many cultural tasks, such as being unique or similar to others, being a strong leader or a good follower, and being creative or conventional, for these psychological tendencies are habitual, automatic, and non-self-reflective. Accordingly, the explicit beliefs may be quite independent of the implicit psychological tendencies and may have formed under the influence of a number of haphazard factors. For example, many young people in contemporary Japan may be wedded to a "Western" idea of individualism (Matsumoto, 1999; Oyserman, Coon, & Kemmelmeier, 2002), yet this explicit belief about the self and its values may be acquired during adolescence or even later, quite independent of the earlier socialization that makes people think, feel, and act in a highly interdependent fashion. If this is the case, we may expect that cross-cultural variation in explicit beliefs about the self's independence and interdependence may prove to be less systematic and more unpredictable than the corresponding variation in implicit psychological tendencies of independence and interdependence.

In a recent review, Oyserman and colleagues (2002) examined numerous studies that used the explicit scale measures of independence and interdependence and observed that Americans are, in general, more independent and less interdependent than many other cultural groups of the world. The researchers also warned, however, that this generalization could not be taken too far because one can find a number of exceptions to the generalization. This skepticism on the notions of independence and interdependence is also echoed in recent writings by Matsumoto (1999) and Takano and Osaka (1999), who also refuted a characterization of independent Americans and interdependent Asians as no more than faulty cultural stereotyping. It is important to keep in mind, however, that these researchers also relied nearly exclusively on existing evidence regarding explicit self-beliefs on independence and interdependence.

If, as Matsumoto (1999), Takano and Osaka (1999), and others imply, the characterization of American and Asian cultures as independent and interdependent is no more than an incorrect stereotyping, then this should also apply to more implicit measures of independence and interdependence. If, however, our cultural task analysis is correct, it is entirely reasonable to expect that explicit beliefs are a crude and rather misleading index of cultural ethos. For example, some Japanese may strongly believe that they are independent, but they may form, express, and communicate this personal belief in an entirely interdependent fashion. It is possible, for example, that they try to be independent because it is shameful not to be independent. Notice, however, that the emotion of shame is highly interdependent and relationally bound. It is also possible that they try to be independent because their peers also try to be so. Yet this strong reference to peer group is also a signature of interdependence. The cultural task analysis suggests that the implicit manner in which they think, feel, and act—that is, how they form the concept of the self as independent or interdependent, maintain it, and express it—is a far more important marker of independence or interdependence. In comparison, the explicit belief of the self may be less significant. If this analysis is correct, there should be a contrasting systematic cultural variation once implicit measures are used.

This specific implication of the usefulness of the cultural task analysis has received strong evidence in the last two decades of research in cultural psychology. We already reviewed this literature in an earlier section. To make the point more clearly, it is worth describing a recent study by Kitayama, Park, Servincer, Karasawa, and Uskul (2009). These researchers used several implicit indicators of independence and interdependence, and found that compared to the Japanese, both West Europeans (British and Germans) and North Americans are more focused in attention and more prone to dispositional bias, to experiencing disengaging rather than engaging emotions, to experiencing personal rather than social happiness, and to a strong, symbolic ego-inflation. Simultaneously, the researchers administered one explicit self-belief measure of independence and interdependence (the Singelis scale of independent and interdependence self-construals).

The results were highly instructive. Replicating earlier findings, the implicit measures showed a highly systematic cross-cultural variation. In contrast, the explicit self-belief measure yielded results that were neither systematic nor readily interpretable. When the researchers looked at a difference between each person's explicit independence score and interdependence score as a rough approximation, Germans were much more independent than either Americans or British. Even more puzzlingly, Japanese were more independent than Americans and British, although they were still less independent than Germans. Thus, this work simultaneously demonstrated within a single study both a highly systematic cross-cultural variation in implicit independence and interdependence, and a completely anomalous pattern obtained with an explicit measure of independence and interdependence.

Relations among Different Facets of Implicit Independence and Interdependence

There is yet another important implication of the cultural task analysis. This analysis assumes that people strive for the cultural mandate of either independence or interdependence in their own idiosyncratic ways by choosing cultural tasks in which they purposefully and repeatedly engage. Even though any given culture provides numerous cultural tasks of either independence or interdependence, any given individual in the culture will participate in a relatively small number of them. Because different cultural tasks require very different kinds of cognitive, emotional, and motivational psychological tendencies, which of these tendencies are nurtured and reinforced will depend very much on the specific set of cultural tasks in which each individual chooses to engage on a regular, habitual basis. This implies that although people in a given cultural group, when taken as a whole, tend to show psychological features that are characteristic of the group, they may not show any coherent patterns; that is, just because one is quite independent or interdependent in one psychological feature (e.g., attention), one may or may not be so in another feature (e.g., emotion).

Support comes from some recent studies. In the aforementioned study by Kitayama and colleagues (2009), the researchers observed that compared to Japanese, both West Europeans (Britons and Germans) and North Americans are more focused in attention and more prone to dispositional bias in attribution, to experiencing disengaging rather than engaging emotions and personal rather than social happiness, and to showing a strong symbolic ego-inflation. As predicted by the foregoing analysis, however, the average correlation among the five implicit tendencies measured here was virtually zero in all four of the cultures tested.

In another recent study, Uchida and colleagues (2008) focused on the self. They used four implicit measures and one explicit measure. The implicit measure was the Implicit Association Test, designed to assess the ease of associating personal versus social acts with positive or negative valence. Americans more readily associated "personal" with "positive" than with "negative," showing that they have more positive implicit attitudes toward "personal" than toward "social." This effect was substantially weaker for Japanese. Another implicit measure was the TST. Americans were more likely than Japanese to produce personal pronouns. The remaining two measures related to emotions. As in the previous work by Kitayama, Mesquita, and colleagues (2006) reviewed earlier, Uchida and colleagues (2008) showed that Americans were more likely than Japanese to experience disengaging (vs. engaging) emotions.

Moreover, Americans were also more likely than Japanese to experience personal happiness than social happiness. These implicit measures showed a highly systematic and predicted pattern. As also predicted, however, the average correlation among the four implicit measures was again nearly zero within each of the two countries.

According to the criterion of psychometrics (Allen & Yen, 2002), the null correlations among the pertinent measures demonstrate that the concepts of independence and interdependence are not "real." In contrast, explicit measures of independence and interdependence, such as the scale by Singelis, are highly reliable. So the same concepts appear "real" when assessed explicitly, but not so when assessed implicitly.

Although paradoxical at first glance, this is precisely what one ought to predict on the basis of the cultural task analysis. This analysis implies that there will be little or no association among different features of independence or interdependence within a given culture, even when the culture varies systematically, on aggregate, at the collective level, on the very dimensions defined by these psychological features. Even when apparently invalid in one criterion (i.e., psychometrics), culturally significant constructs such as independence and interdependence can still be valid both psychologically and culturally because their influences are mediated by collective, societal, and historical processes. What is required is a more elaborate process model connecting culture to psychology, and vice versa. The cultural task analysis is the first step in this direction.

HISTORICAL ORIGINS OF INDEPENDENCE AND INTERDEPENDENCE

So far, we have assumed that Western cultures are organized in terms of the view of the self as independent. That is to say, many varieties of cultural tasks are rooted in the notion of independence. Even social relations are sometimes constructed as means to achieve personal, independent goals. For example, Miller and colleagues have shown that people in North American culture are more likely to engage in prosocial, altruistic behaviors (donation) when the behaviors can be seen as serving their own self-interest. In contrast, Eastern cultures are organized in terms of the view of the self as interdependent. That is to say, many varieties of cultural tasks are based on the notion of interdependence. Actions that are self-endorsed and thus experienced as fully personal are often constructed in service of certain communal interests, such as group harmony or conformity to social expectations. For example, Chirkov, Ryan,

Kim, and Kaplan (2003) have shown that Asians are much more likely than North Americans to self-endorse collectivistic or interdependent goals.

What are the origins of these cross-cultural variations in the composition of dominant cultural tasks? This question is historical in nature because cultural tasks are accumulated over generations in a given cultural group's history. In all likelihood an assortment of factors is involved. For example, according to Triandis (1995), a variety of ecological and economic factors, such as wealth, low-population density, social mobility, and herding, is likely to encourage an independent cultural ethos and the ideology of individualism. Conversely, a contrasting set of factors, such as poverty, high-population density, sedentary form of living, and agriculture, is likely to contribute to an interdependent ethos and the social ideology of collectivism. Although it is impossible to examine whether these factors were truly involved in the historical development of the contemporary cultural ethos of either Western or Eastern cultures, it is possible to test some implications of some hypotheses related to these historical considerations. Four such hypotheses appear promising.

Pathogen Prevalence

In their unique ecobiological thesis, Fincher, Thornhill, Murray, and Schaller (2008) have pointed out that societies vary considerably, both today and in the past, in their susceptibility to a variety of pathogens (e.g., malaria, leprosy, and tuberculosis), and proposed that susceptible societies would likely develop certain mechanisms that defend them against the pathogens. In particular, the researchers proposed that the susceptible societies are likely to develop strong ingroup orientations (or *ethnocentrism*) and conformity to group norms. A society could defend itself against pathogens if interactions are limited largely to ingroup members and, moreover, if the members' behaviors are tightly regulated. Notice that both of these features are commonly associated with interdependence and collectivism. In contrast, two features of a cultural group—relative absence of ethnocentrism and preference for innovation and uniqueness—are typically associated with independence and individualism. Although these features can entail very different benefits for the society, such as cosmopolitanism and technological innovations, they are also likely to expose the society to a variety of potential pathogens. Notice that some of the factors mentioned by Triandis and others, including population density, sedentary living or low mobility, and poverty, may increase pathogen prevalence. So the pathogen susceptibility hypothesis of cultural collectivism may potentially account for the hypothesized effects of these factors.

To test their hypothesis, Fincher and colleagues (2008) first estimated pathogen prevalence for 93 regions of the world from old atlases of infectious diseases and other historical epidemiological information. The estimate's validity was strongly supported by its high correlation with contemporary data based on the current scientific database. As a measure of individualism and collectivism, Fincher and colleagues used four different measures that are available in the literature. All these indices of cultural ethos were strongly related to pathogen prevalence, such that collectivism was in fact closely linked to pathogen prevalence in the past.

Mode of Subsistence

Farming typically requires a settled form of living. It further requires close cooperation and coordination of community activities. Moreover, some forms of fishing also appear to require similar social coordination. In contrast, herding is far more individualistic. It requires a far greater degree of individual initiative, yet it depends far less on the community and its cohesion. It is also possible that settled forms of living lend themselves to pathogen prevalence, at least historically (Diamond, 1997). Accordingly, farming and fishing may be expected to lead to a greater degree of interdependent, collectivistic ethos than does herding.

In support of these considerations, Edgerton (1965) found that East African farmers consulted each other more frequently and acted less individually than did East African herders. Likewise, Barry, Child, and Bacon (1959) have shown that child socialization practices in agricultural societies emphasize compliance, conscientiousness, and conservatism. In contrast, hunting and gathering societies emphasize individualism, assertiveness, and venturesomeness. Furthermore, in a large cross-national comparison, Berry (1967, 1979) found that agricultural societies are associated with greater degrees of conformity, whereas hunting and gathering societies are associated with greater degrees of independent decision making.

More recently, Uskul, Kitayama, and Nisbett (2008) examined whether cognitive styles also vary as a function of the mode of subsistence. On the basis of the evidence we have discussed, farmers and fishermen may be expected to have a more holistic cognitive style than do herders. To exclude all potential confounding variables, such as global national culture, climate, language, and ethnicity, Uskul and colleagues tested people in the three economies in Turkey's eastern Black Sea region and provided support for the prediction. For example, using a cognitive task designed to assess holistic attention, Uskul and colleagues found that both farmers and fishermen were more holistic in attention than herders.

Social Mobility

Although social mobility is inherent to the mode of subsistence, it can have effects above and beyond those attributed to traditional forms of subsistence. Specifically, more stable forms of living may foster greater attachment and identification with place, whereas more mobile styles of living may encourage a form of identity that is relatively separate from the place of living. In a series of studies conducted within the United States, Oishi and colleagues have amassed evidence for this hypothesis (Oishi, Lun, & Sherman, 2007; Oishi, Rothman, et al., 2007). For example, with a self-description task, Oishi, Lun, and colleagues (2007) found that personal self is more salient for frequent movers, but the collective self is more salient for nonmovers. Moreover, using an experience sampling method, they have found evidence for the hypothesis that approval and confirmation of personal aspects of the self are more important for frequent movers, but approval and confirmation of more collective aspects of the self are more important for nonmovers.

Analogous differences can be found at the level of communities. Oishi and colleagues took advantage of the fact that many U.S. cities have home baseball teams, yet they vary considerably in terms of residential mobility. For example, residents in Tempe, Arizona, are more highly mobile than those in Detroit, Michigan. Residents in mobile cities may support their home baseball team only if the team is doing well and is providing some esteem benefits to residents. But those in relatively stable cities may support their home teams because of their identification with the team. As may be predicted from this reasoning, Oishi, Rothman, and colleagues (2007) found that home game attendance was much more dependent on the team's record in mobile communities than in stable communities.

Voluntary Settlement in the Frontier

Last, but not least, another factor that is related but perhaps partially distinct from all three factors discussed so far is a history of voluntary settlement in the frontier. This factor appears especially relevant in understanding the strong emphasis placed by contemporary American culture on the notion of independence and the social ideology of individualism. Kitayama, Ishii, and colleagues (2006) have argued that when presented with an opportunity to move to a different land, with a hope of economic advancement, people with independent features (e.g., self-initiating, optimistic, and adventurous) are more likely to take part in the opportunity. Moreover, the new land with a frontier ecology may tend to be harsh, with minimal social infrastructures. Under such conditions, the same independent features may help immigrants to survive, flourish, and eventually succeed. For these reasons, voluntary settlement in the frontier may be expected to foster a strongly independent cultural ethos.

This hypothesis applies most obviously to the history of the United States in the past several centuries. Some West Europeans initially settled in the "new continent" during the 15th and 16th centuries. They searched for both religious freedom and economic opportunities. Since then, numerous people have followed suit from all over the world. Furthermore, over the course of the 18th and the 19th centuries, some East Coast residents chose to move westward to open new lands, expelled or even exterminated Native Americans, and along the way created the contemporary United States. This history of voluntary settlement in the frontier is considered to be an important basis of the strongly independent ethos of contemporary U.S. culture.

If this hypothesis is true, North Americans may be expected to be more strongly independent than West Europeans. Moreover, this must be the case, even when one compares Americans with British, who share many factors, including language, religion, and some important aspects of social institutions, with North Americans. In a recent study, Kitayama and colleagues (2009) tested this possibility and found support for it with several implicit measures of independence–interdependence. For example, both North Americans and West Europeans were more likely to experience socially disengaging emotions, such as pride and anger, than socially engaging emotions, such as friendly feelings and guilt, but this tendency was significantly more pronounced among North Americans. Importantly, Kitayama and colleagues tested two distinct groups of West Europeans, namely, Germans and British. As predicted, they found virtually no difference between these two West European groups.

The voluntary settlement hypothesis would also predict that the ethos of independence may be found even in traditionally more interdependent Asian regions that have undergone a similar history of voluntary settlement. With this idea in mind, Kitayama, Ishii, Imada, Takemura, and Ramaswamy (2006) tested residents of a northern island of Japan, called Hokkaido. Hokkaido was a wilderness until approximately 150 years ago. Around that time, the feudal government in mainland Japan collapsed and, at the same time, Russia expanded its territory to the Far East and became a major threat to the new government of Japan. To deal with the situation, the new government sent ex-samurai warriors to Hokkaido to create a small number of settlements, followed by a large number of farmers and peasants. They immigrated in large numbers and by the mid-20th century Hokkaido had become an integral part of Japan.

As may be expected, Kitayama, Ishii, and colleagues (2006) found initial evidence that Hokkaido Japanese are more independent, at least in some respects, compared to their mainland counterparts. For example, the researchers found that Hokkaido Japanese show a dispositional bias in attribution that is as strong as the one typically found in North Americans. As mentioned earlier, mainland Japanese typically show little or no such bias. They also observed that both North Americans and Hokkaido Japanese, but not mainland Japanese, show a strong defense response when their personal, but not social, identity is threatened.

CONCLUSIONS

In this chapter, we have discussed how cultural contexts might influence the human mind. Our analysis is formulated in terms of cultural tasks of independence and interdependence. Different cultures provide an assortment of independent and interdependent tasks. Yet Western cultures tend to provide more and a greater variety of independent tasks. People engaging in these cultures seek to achieve the cultural imperative of independence by selectively adapting and performing some of the tasks. In contrast, Eastern cultures tend to provide more and a greater variety of interdependent tasks. People engaging in these cultures seek to achieve the imperative of interdependence by selectively participating in some of these tasks. Several important implications of the cultural task analysis must be reiterated:

1. People engage in certain tasks of culture repeatedly over time from a very early age, even before they understand cultural ideologies such as independence and interdependence. Psychological influences of culture are therefore likely to be implicit in large part. Here we have provided a brief review of empirical studies illustrating this point by comparing two global cultural regions, the "West" (mostly North America) and the "East" (mostly East Asia).

2. Cultures do vary systematically in terms of their emphasis on independence and interdependence. However, within each culture, people seek to be either independent or interdependent in their own idiosyncratic ways by selectively engaging in some, but not all, tasks provided by their cultures. It follows that there are no systematic individual differences when implicit independence or interdependence is tested within any given cultural group.

3. Enculturation primarily happens at an implicit level; moreover, this can happen very early on. Thus, explicit beliefs may best be seen as an "add-on" to the cultural mode of being that comprises implicit psychological tendencies of independence and interdependence. It follows that cultural differences should be more robust and more systematic at the implicit level than at the explicit level of beliefs.

4. Cultural tasks, and the corresponding imperatives of independence and interdependence, are likely to be formed over generations in the course of the history of any given cultural group as a function of a variety of factors. Here we have reviewed evidence for four of these factors, namely, pathogen prevalence, social mobility, mode of subsistence, and voluntary settlement.

In considering culture's influences on psychological processes, it used to be and to some extent is still quite commonly assumed that individuals become members of a cultural group by acquiring explicit beliefs, values, and ideologies of the culture. Furthermore, once acquired, these beliefs, values, and ideologies are assumed to guide one's behaviors. This model may be called the attitude–behavior model of cultural influence. Much of the contemporary work on priming is also tacitly grounded in this traditional model of cultural influence.

The cultural task analysis is different. This analysis implies that a culture's beliefs, values, and ideologies often are incorporated into the repertoire of cultural tasks. Moreover, these cultural tasks constitute the very environment to which members of any given cultural group must adapt. Culture's influences are therefore unlikely to be mediated by direct learning of the beliefs, values, and ideologies. Instead, they are likely to be achieved through repeated and long-term engagement in the tasks that are available in one's own cultural context. We believe that the notion of cultural context that comprises tasks of culture is novel, with some important implications. As such, we are hopeful that this analysis expands the empirical horizon of the present understanding of the interface between culture and the mind.

REFERENCES

Allen, M. J., & Yen, W. M. (2002). *Introduction to measurement theory*. Long Grove, IL: Waveland Press.

Barry, H., Child, I. L., & Bacon, M. K. (1959). Relation of child training to subsistence economy. *American Anthropologist*, *61*, 51–63.

Berry, J. W. (1967). Independence and conformity in subsistence-level societies. *Journal of Personality and Social Psychology*, *7*, 415–418.

Berry, J. W. (1975). *Cross-cultural research and methodology series: III. Human ecology and cognitive style: Comparative studies in cultural and psychological adaptation.* Oxford, UK: Sage.

Berry, J. W. (1979). A cultural ecology of social behavior. In L. Berkowitz (Ed.), *Advances in experimental social psychology* (Vol. 12, pp. 177–206). New York: Academic Press.

Cantor, N. (1994). Life task problem solving: Situational affordances and personal needs. *Personality and Social Psychology Bulletin, 20,* 235–243.

Chirkov, V. I., Ryan, R. M., Kim, Y., & Kaplan, U. (2003). Differentiating autonomy from individualism and independence: A self-determination theory perspective on internalization of cultural orientations and well-being. *Journal of Personality and Social Psychology, 8*(1), 97–110.

Choi, I., Nisbett, R. E., & Norenzayan, A. (1999). Causal attribution across cultures: Variation and universality. *Psychological Bulletin, 125,* 47–63.

Chua, H. F., Boland, J. E., & Nisbett, R. E. (2005). Cultural variation in eye movements during scene perception. *Proceedings of the National Academy of Sciences USA, 102,* 12629–12633.

Cohen, D., Hoshino-Browne, E., & Leung, A. K.-Y. (2007). Culture and the structure of personal experience. In M. P. Zanna (Ed.), *Advances in experimental social psychology* (pp. 1–67). San Diego, CA: Academic Press.

Cousins, S. D. (1989). Culture and self-perception in Japan and the United States. *Journal of Personality and Social Psychology, 56,* 124–131.

Diamond, J. (1997). *Guns, germs, and steel: The fates of human societies.* New York: Norton.

Edgerton, R. B. (1965). "Cultural" vs. "ecological": Factors in the expression of values, attitudes, and personality characteristics. *American Anthropologist, 67,* 442–447.

Fincher, C. L., Thornhill, R., Murray, D. R., & Schaller, M. (2008). Pathogen prevalence predicts human cross-cultural variability in individualism/collectivism. *Proceedings of the Royal Society B: Biological Sciences, 275,* 1279–1285.

Fiske, A. P., Kitayama, S., Markus, H. R., & Nisbett, R. E. (1998). The cultural matrix of social psychology. In D. T. Gilbert, S. T. Fiske, & G. Lindzey (Eds.), *Handbook of social psychology* (4th ed., pp. 915–981). Boston: McGraw-Hill.

Gray, H. M., Ambady, N., Ishii, K., & Kitayama, S. (2007). *When misery loves company: Effects of sad mood on affiliation goals and attention to relational cues.* Unpublished manuscript, Tufts University.

Greenwald, A. G. (1982). Ego task analysis: A synthesis of research on ego-involvement and self-awareness. In A. H. Hastorf & A. M. Isen (Eds.), *Cognitive social psychology* (pp. 109–147). New York: Elsevier/North Holland.

Hedden, T., Ketay, S., Aron, A., Markus, H. R., & Gabrieli, J. D. E. (2008). Cultural influences on neural substrates of attentional control. *Psychological Science, 19,* 12–17.

Heine, S. J., Kitayama, S., & Hamamura, T. (2007). Different meta-analyses yield different conclusions: A comment on Sedikides, Gaertner, & Vevea. *Asian Journal of Social Psychology, 10*, 49–58.

Heine, S. J., Lehman, D. R., Markus, H. R., & Kitayama, S. (1999). Is there a universal need for positive self-regard? *Psychological Review, 106*, 766–794.

Hoshino-Browne, E., Zanna, A. S., Spencer, S. J., Zanna, M. P., Kitayama, S., & Lackenbauer, S. (2005). On the cultural guises of cognitive dissonance: The case of Easterners and Westerners. *Journal of Personality and Social Psychology, 89*, 294–310.

Imada, T., & Kitayama, S. (2006). *Cultural mode of being: Independence and interdependence in the United States and Japan.* Poster session presented at the annual meeting of the Society for Personality and Social Psychology, Palm Springs, CA.

Imada, T., & Kitayama, S. (2007). *Dissonance and "eyes of others": Unconscious perception of social influence?* Poster session presented at the annual meeting of the Society for Personality and Social Psychology, Memphis, TN.

Inglehart, R., & Baker, W. E. (2001). Modernization, cultural change, and the persistence of traditional values. *American Sociological Review, 65*, 19–51.

Ishii, K., Kobayashi, Y., & Kitayama, S. (in press). Interdependence modulates the brain response to word–voice congruity. *Social, Cognition, and Affective Neuroscience.*

Ishii, K., Reyes, J. A., & Kitayama, S. (2003). Spontaneous attention to word content versus emotional tone: Differences among three cultures. *Psychological Science, 14*, 39–46.

Iyengar, S. S., & Lepper, M. (1999). Rethinking the value of choice: A cultural perspective on intrinsic motivation. *Journal of Personality and Social Psychology, 76*, 349–366.

Keller, H. (2007). *Cultures of infancy.* Mahwah, NJ: Erlbaum.

Kim, H. S., & Sherman, D. K. (2007). Express yourself: Culture and the effect of self-expression on choice. *Journal of Personality and Social Psychology, 92*, 1–11.

Kitayama, S. (2002). Cultural and basic psychological processes—toward a system view of culture: Comment on Oyserman et al. *Psychological Bulletin, 128*, 189–196.

Kitayama, S., Duffy, S., Kawamura, T., & Larsen, J. T. (2003). Perceiving an object and its context in different cultures: A cultural look at New Look. *Psychological Science, 14*, 201–206.

Kitayama, S., Snibbe, A. C., Markus, H. R., & Suzuki, T. (2004). Is there any "free" choice?: Self and dissonance in two cultures. *Psychological Science, 14*, 527–533.

Kitayama, S., Duffy, S., & Uchida, Y. (2007). Self as cultural mode of being. In S. Kitayama & D. Cohen (Eds.), *Handbook of cultural psychology* (pp. 136–174). Guilford Press.

Kitayama, S., & Imada, T. (2008). Defending cultural self: A dual-process model of agency. In T. Urdan & M. Maehr (Eds.), *Advances in motivation and achievement* (Vol. 15). Bingley, UK: Emerald Publishing.

Kitayama, S., & Ishii, K. (2002). Word and voice: Spontaneous attention to emotional utterances in two languages. *Cognition and Emotion, 16*, 29–60.

Kitayama, S., Ishii, K., Imada, T., Takemura, K., & Ramaswamy, J. (2006). Voluntary settlement and the spirit of independence: Evidence from Japan's "Northern frontier." *Journal of Personality and Social Psychology, 91*, 369–384.

Kitayama, S., & Markus, H. R. (1994). Introduction to cultural psychology and emotion research. In *Emotion and culture: Empirical studies of mutual influence* (pp. 1–19). Washington, DC: American Psychological Association.

Kitayama, S., & Markus, H. R. (1999). Yin and yang of the Japanese self: The cultural psychology of personality coherence. In D. Cervone & Y. Shoda (Eds.), *The coherence of personality: Social cognitive bases of personality consistency, variability, and organization* (pp. 242–302). New York: Guilford Press.

Kitayama, S., Markus, H. R., Matsumoto, H., & Norasakkunkit, V. (1997). Individual and collective processes in the construction of the self: Self-enhancement in the United States and self-criticism in Japan. *Journal of Personality and Social Psychology, 72*, 1245–1267.

Kitayama, S., Mesquita, B., & Karasawa, M. (2006). Cultural affordances and emotional experience: Socially engaging and disengaging emotions in Japan and the United States. *Journal of Personality and Social Psychology, 91*, 890–903.

Kitayama, S., & Park, H. (2007). Cultural shaping of self, emotion, and well-being: How does it work? *Social and Personality Psychology Compass, 1*, 202–222.

Kitayama, S., Park, H., Servincer, A. T., Karasawa, M., & Uskul, A. K. (2009). A cultural task analysis of implicit independence: Comparing North America, West Europe, and East Asia. *Journal of Personality and Social Psychology, 97*, 236–255.

Lewis, R. S., Goto, S. G., Kong, L. L., & Lowenberg, K. (2008). Culture and context: East Asian American and European American differences in P3 event-related potentials. *Personality and Social Psychology Bulletin, 34*, 623–634.

Markus, H. R., & Kitayama, S. (1991). Culture and the self: Implications for cognition, emotion, and motivation. *Psychological Review, 98*, 224–253.

Markus, H. R., & Kitayama, S. (2004). Models of agency: Sociocultural diversity in the construction of action. In G. Berman & J. Berman (Eds.), *The 49th Annual Nebraska Symposium on Motivation: Cross-cultural differences in perspectives on self* (pp. 1–57). Lincoln: University of Nebraska Press.

Masuda, T., & Nisbett, R. E. (2001). Attending holistically versus analytically: Comparing the context sensitivity of Japanese and Americans. *Journal of Personality and Social Psychology, 81*, 992–934.

Matsumoto, D. (1999). Culture and self: An empirical assessment of Markus and Kitayama's theory of independent and interdependent self-construal. *Asian Journal of Social Psychology*, 2(3), 289–310.

Miller, D. T., & Ross, M. (1975). Self-serving biases in the attribution of causality: Fact or fiction? *Psychological Bulletin, 82*, 213–225.

Miller, J. G. (1984). Culture and the development of everyday social explanation. *Journal of Personality and Social Psychology, 46*, 961–978.

Miyamoto, Y., & Kitayama, S. (2002). Cultural variation in correspondence bias: The critical role of attitude diagnosticity. *Journal of Personality and Social Psychology, 83*, 1239–1248.

Morris, B. (1991). *Western conceptions of the individual.* Oxford, UK: Berg.

Morris, M. W., & Peng, K. (1994). Culture and cause: American and Chinese attributions for social and physical events. *Journal of Personality and Social Psychology, 67*, 949–971.

Na, J., & Kitayama, S. (2008). *Choice as an antidote for under-performance in ego-involving tasks.* Unpublished manuscript, University of Michigan.

Nisbett, R. E. (2003). *The geography of thought: How Asians and Westerners think differently and why.* New York: Free Press.

Oishi, S., & Diener, E. (2003). Culture and well-being: The cycle of action, evaluation and decision. *Personality and Social Psychology Bulletin, 29*, 939–949.

Oishi, S., Lun, J., & Sherman, G. D. (2007). Residential mobility, self-concept, and positive affect in social interactions. *Journal of Personality and Social Psychology, 93*, 131–141.

Oishi, S., Rothman, A. J., Snyder, M., Su, J., Zehm, K., Hertel, A. W., et al. (2007). The socio-ecological model of pro-community action: The benefits of residential stability. *Journal of Personality and Social Psychology, 93*, 831–844.

Oyserman, D., Coon, H. M., & Kemmelmeier, M. (2002). Rethinking individualism and collectivism: Evaluation of theoretical and assumptions and meta-analyses. *Psychological Bulletin, 128*, 3–72.

Oyserman, D., & Lee, S. W. S. (2007). Priming "culture": Culture as situated cognition. In S. Kitayama & D. Cohen (Eds.), *Handbook of cultural psychology* (pp. 255–280). New York: Guilford Press.

Pickett, C. L., Gardner, W. L., & Knowles, M. (2004). Getting a cue: The need to belong and enhanced sensitivity to social cues. *Personality and Social Psychology Bulletin, 30*, 1095–1107.

Rhee, E., Uleman, J., Lee, H., & Roman, R. (1995). Spontaneous trait-descriptions and ethnic identities in individualistic and collectivistic cultures. *Journal of Personality and Social Psychology, 69*, 142–152.

Rose, J. P., Endo, Y., Windschitl, P. D., & Suls, J. (2008). Cultural differences in unrealistic optimism and pessimism: The role of egocentrism and direct versus indirect comparison measures. *Personality and Social Psychology Bulletin, 34*, 1236–1248.

Sanchez-Burks, J. (2002). Protestant relational ideology and (in)attention to relational cues in work settings. *Journal of Personality and Social Psychology, 83*, 919–929.

Shweder, R. A., & Bourne, E. J. (1982). Does the concept of person vary cross-culturally? In A. J. Marsella & G. M. White (Eds.), *Cultural conceptions of mental health and therapy* (pp. 130–204). London: Reidel.

Singelis, T. M. (1994). The measurement of independent and interdependent self-construals. *Personality and Social Psychology Bulletin, 20*(5), 580–591.

Takano, Y., & Osaka, E. (1999). An unsupported common view: Comparing Japan and the U.S. on individualism/collectivism. *Asian Journal of Social Psychology, 2*, 311–341.

Taylor, C. (1989). *Sources of the self: The making of modern identities.* Cambridge, MA: Harvard University Press.

Taylor, S. E., & Brown, J. D. (1988). Illusion and well-being: A social psychological perspective on mental health. *Psychological Bulletin, 103*, 193–210.

Trafimow, D., Triandis, H. C., & Goto, S. G. (1991). Some tests of the distinction between the private self and the collective self. *Journal of Personality and Social Psychology, 60*, 649–655.

Triandis, H. C. (1989). The self and social behavior in differing cultural contexts. *Psychological Review, 96*, 506–520.

Triandis, H. C. (1995). *Individualism and collectivism.* Boulder, CO: Westview Press.

Uchida, Y., Kitayama, S., Mesquita, B., Reyes, J., & Morling, B. (2008). Is perceived emotional support beneficial?: Well-being and health in independent and interdependent cultures. *Personality and Social Psychology Bulletin, 34*, 741–754.

Uchida, Y., Park, J., & Kitayama, S. (2009). *Implicit independence and interdependence of the self: A cross-cultural study.* Unpublished manuscript, University of Michigan.

Uskul, A. K., Kitayama, S., & Nisbett, R. E. (2008). Eco-cultural basis of cognition: Farmers and fishermen are more holistic than herders. *Proceedings of the National Academy of Sciences USA, 105*, 8552–8556.

Weber, M. (1958). *The Protestant ethic and the spirit of capitalism* (T. Parsons, Trans.). New York: Scribner. (Original work published 1904–1905)

10

Platonic Blindness and the Challenge of Understanding Context

YARROW DUNHAM
MAHZARIN R. BANAJI

In *The Republic*, Plato offers the "Allegory of the Cave," in which he describes humans as generally able to see only the shadows of real things, cast on the cave wall. For Plato, the primary goal of philosophical–scientific advancement is to free us from this limitation, such that we might exit the cave and apprehend the objects of the world in their true form. In his view, veridical perception of external entities is difficult but realizable under conditions of principled inquiry.

To a considerable extent, we all share Plato's intuition that the objects of perception exist independently of our observation of them, and can therefore, at least in principle, be understood in their fundamental nature. But this intuition has fared poorly in the modern epoch, falling out of favor in fields running the gambit from literary theory to particle physics. Across these disparate areas, the notion of an autonomous external reality, definable without reference to the viewer, has crumbled beneath mounting evidence that our descriptions are always inescapably rooted in the specifics of our situation, our context. Thus, old views of a Platonic external reality have given way to a notion of *systems*, in which viewer and viewed are at least in part mutually defined.

This new appreciation of context has played out differently in different fields, and we find it instructive to examine how it has unfolded in sciences that have matured somewhat ahead of our own. Doing so immediately makes clear that when we speak of "contextual influence," we may be speaking of several quite different things. In particular, we see at least two shifts in thinking, both involving a rethinking of the very nature of reality in light of surprising "intrusions" of context.

TWO REVOLUTIONS

A first shift in thinking comes from recognizing the influence of context on the very act of observation. More precisely, it concerns the intrusion of the observer into the system being observed. In the early 1970s, a professor of psychology and seven colleagues gained admission to mental institutions by claiming to hear voices (Rosenhan, 1973). Immediately after admission, these "pseudopatients" reported a cessation of all symptoms, answered all diagnostic efforts with real details from their lives, and behaved normally in all possible respects. Surprisingly, pseudopatients were kept an average of 19 days before being released, in most cases with a diagnosis of "schizophrenia in remission." What explains the inability to "diagnose" sanity, even among expert clinicians at leading institutions? Clearly, part of the answer is that the beliefs of the clinicians colored their perceptions of the patients. Far from an objective state to be observed in a patient, "illness" arose in large part from the process of expectancy-laden observation. Since this seminal demonstration, social psychology has documented dozens more examples, showing in particular that evaluative states, such as attitudes, causally influence external perceptions without in any way disrupting our feeling of confidence that our judgments are "evidence-based"; sure of our own objectivity, we interpret a stigmatized other's behavior as hostile, blind to the fact that our internalized representation of that stigma—in the form of a negative attitude—has railroaded our observations down that very track.

This principle should be familiar from the Heisenbergian revolution in physics, in which the dichotomy between observer and observed collapsed in the face of evidence that *observations* can affect our ability to observe other properties, and may in some cases even change the values of those properties (observing the location of a particle prevents us from observing other aspects of its nature, e.g., its precise momentum or spin). Now, our experiments, indeed our very eyes, are inescapably part of the context within which targets of observation must be understood. Appreciating context in this case involves recognizing that, in these cases, "*observation*" is a verb not a noun, an action with consequences for the observed system.

We can illustrate a second shift in thinking by imagining a fine soufflé. Notice that it in no way resembles its ingredients—the eggs, flour, and sugar that compose its internal structure. What is more, its finished form is not the simple result of combination. Rather, it depends on exposure to a notoriously narrow range of external environments (appropriate mixing, precise time at precise temperature). Each ingredient interacts with the others and with each environmental influence in nonlinear ways, creating a dynamic system complex enough to frustrate mathematical modelers and master chefs alike.

In the psychological context, the traditional Platonic view holds that internal and stable mental states, such as attitudes, interact with external phenomena, such as attitude objects, in an additive fashion that linearly produces behavior. Our liking of chocolate (an attitude) plus our perception of a chocolate bar (an attitude object) leads to consumption of said chocolate (a behavior). However, this sort of model rests on assumptions no more tenable then a culinary model in which all we have to do is sum the reactive properties of eggs, flour, and sugar to produce an optimal soufflé. The shortcomings of this approach are made manifest when we consider the failure of attitudes to predict behavior in anything like the simple way described earlier (e.g., Bohner & Schwarz, 2001).

Speaking of a parallel revolution in genetics, Lewontin (2000) provided the metaphor of the "triple helix," consisting of the two familiar strands of deoxyribonucleic acid interwoven with a third, invisible strand, the environment within which gene expression occurs. Translating this insight to the social-psychological domain requires recognizing that "endogenous" properties, such as attitudes, owe a large part of their causal influence to exogenous factors that interact with them in multifaceted ways. On its own, the endogenous factor is inert until activated by exogenous forces, suggesting not two independent factors but a single interwoven system.

In summary, one shift in thinking about context involves the intrusion of an *observer* into a system previously thought to be definable independently of observation. Back into the cave, where our view will always be situated and therefore in some ways limited. The second revolution is, in a sense, the inverse of the first, involving the intrusion of surrounding *contextual forces* into a system thought to be definable independently of that context. Beyond the properties of our minds and eyes, the shadows on the cave wall can be adequately characterized only with reference to ambient light, surface properties of the wall, and so on. We can change our view but not the fact that we see with particular eyes, from a particular angle.

MIND IN CONTEXT

These transformative ways of thinking in physics and biology have sown fertile seeds in our own discipline; psychology contains many examples of both types of contextual effect. Indeed, social interaction is one of the most striking places to observe the effects of context, as well as our customary blindness to them. This was well appreciated by early founders of social psychology, including Milgram, Asch, Mischel, and others, and context continues to serve as the most intriguing of variables in many influential research programs today. Indeed, this volume is one more testament to the central role of context in the contemporary empirical endeavor.

Yet this volume and others like it (e.g., Shoda, Cervone, & Downey, 2007) also testify to something else: our continued struggle to develop an *intuitive* understanding of context. In other words, why do we—and here we mean to include even those of us who do our work in this area—need constantly to remind ourselves of the central role context plays? In the remainder of this chapter, we provide a range of examples illustrating various forms of contextual influence, drawn primarily from the literature on attitudes. We then take a step back to ask why the lessons suggested by these results are so hard to assimilate into both our everyday and scientific worldviews. Our primary suggestion is that our basic intuitions about the nature of reality lead us to underestimate contextual influence in our explanations. We call this *Platonic blindness*, a blindness created by the ontological assumptions that shape how we habitually see.

THE MIND IS IMPOSED ON THE WORLD

Rosenhan's (1973) experience in psychiatric institutions demonstrated that even expert judgments can be distorted by the assumptions or theories we hold. This principle has now been upheld in dozens of studies showing that evaluative preferences influence subsequent judgments, generally in ways invisible to the actor. In the paradigmatic cases, because we see through a distorting lens, nearly everything we observe fits our preconceptions and so seems to validate the expectations with which we began.

For example, negative attitudes toward black Americans shift interpretations of observed situations in a valence-consistent (i.e., negative) direction. One of the earliest experimental observations of this phenomenon used videos depicting an interaction in which an actor bumped into someone in a manner ambiguous between an aggressive act and an accident; when the actor was a black American, participants were considerably more likely to interpret the act as aggressive and hostile—despite the fact that the videos were identical except for the race of the actor (Duncan, 1976). The implications of this finding are striking: An attitudinal schema inside the head of the observer can make the very same event *look different*. More recently, a field study (Agerström & Rooth, 2009) found that hiring decisions made by real-world human resource managers in Sweden were profoundly influenced by implicit attitudes, such that potential employers higher in implicit bias against Arab Muslims systematically undervalued job applicants from that group. The manager's *subjective* experience is one of merely evaluating the evidence (i.e., the candidate's work experience and other qualifications), but the experimental record reveals that these evaluations are themselves partly the result of attitudinal biases in the head of the evaluator.

This sort of example, in which attitudinal biases affect subsequent processing, is widespread and even penetrates down to basic processes, such as emotion perception. White Americans with negative implicit attitudes toward black Americans, for example, are more prone to see black faces as angry (anger both lingers longer and appears more readily on black than on white faces; Hugenberg & Bodenhausen, 2003). The reverse relationship has also been demonstrated: Emotion influences the perception of racial category membership. For those with negative implicit attitudes toward black Americans, racially ambiguous *angry* faces are more likely to be categorized as black than otherwise identical *happy* faces (Hugenberg & Bodenhausen, 2004). This effect is now known to appear early in development, from the earliest instances of racial categorization (around age 3–4; Dunham & Banaji, 2008). In these cases, a relatively subtle contextual cue (emotional expression) shifts categorical judgments that we might be tempted to think of as based on clear perceptual (i.e., morphological) criteria. Recent meta-analytic evidence allows us to generalize these findings considerably. We now know that subtle implicit attitudes exert a profound and wide-ranging impact on behavior, particularly in the context of discrimination (e.g., Greenwald, Poehlman, Uhlmann, & Banaji, in press).

Other evidence suggests that attitudes are also systematically affected by motivational states. In one striking example of this phenomenon, Ferguson and Bargh (2004) found that objects that can be used to achieve a currently active goal tend to be evaluated more positively ("I like hammers more in the presence of nails I want to drive in"). Similarly, chronic goals to avoid being prejudiced appear to moderate implicit biases against racial outgroups (Barden, Maddux, Petty, & Brewer, 2004; Maddux, Barden, Brewer, & Petty, 2005). In addition, our implicit attitudes toward food stimuli are more positive when we are hungry (Seibt, Hafner, & Deutsch, 2007), highlighting the emergent and goal-directed aspects of evaluation. These findings suggest that internal represented states are themselves a crucial contextual factor, systematically shifting the standard of evaluation in a direction consistent with them.

Across all these examples, objects out in the world are not perceived "as they are," and evaluations of objects are not stable values that can be exactly measured. Rather, perceptions and attitudes are partially constructed and interpreted out of what is already inside our heads. At the broadest level, these cases can be thought of as instances of a confirmation or correspondence bias, in which internal expectancies influence perception, judgment, and action, pulling them in a direction determined by preexisting internally represented attitudinal schemas—the internal context against which social cognition occurs.

ACTION AT A DISTANCE

One of our most cherished notions is that *who we are* is stable, definable by enduring traits and dispositions. For example, one might think of oneself as by nature a messy person, never overly fastidious. How surprising, then, to find out that a lingering scent of citrus (a common element in cleaning products) could lead one to pluck up more diligently the crumbs produced by eating a cookie (Holland, Hendriks, & Aarts, 2005)! This is by no means the only example of a subtle external environmental factor that seems to remake our internal dispositions in surprising ways. Another favorite example of ours is the connection between weather and psychological states. For instance, people express more positive attitudes toward their marriage on sunny days, unless they are asked about the weather prior to the assessment (Schwarz & Clore, 1983).

One difficulty in identifying contextual influences stems from the fact that "context" exists at so many levels at once: The flow of time gives rise to infinite momentary variations, each exerting its own subtle influence, but at the same time we live within more stable "macrocontexts" that constitute our cultural milieu. For example, a tendency to prefer one's ingroup seems to be pervasive in members of the majority. Yet, at least when measured at the implicit level, members of racial and ethnic minorities often do not show ingroup preference (Nosek et al., 2007). Here, the "context" is the broader climate of power relations, a background ecology that reverses the tendency to prefer one's own. These effects emerge early, as early as implicit preferences have been successfully measured (5- to 6-year-old children; Dunham, Baron, & Banaji, 2007). This general backdrop is easily taken for granted, placed under an amorphous rubric of "cultural factors." Yet results like this one suggest that the cultural climate that surrounds us is at least as likely to shape our attitudes as is the literal weather outside.

A step below this macrocontext, the physical environment within which evaluation occurs also exerts an influence on the power and direction of those evaluations. Outgroup targets in a stereotypical context (i.e., black Americans on an inner-city street corner) are judged more negatively than the same targets in a more positive context (i.e., black Americans at a family picnic) (Wittenbrink, Judd, & Park, 2001). And not all such effects are negative; recent work on the malleability of implicit attitudes has also revealed several ways in which contextual influences can make us more positive toward groups we might otherwise be hostile toward. For example, the mere presence of a black American experimenter led white participants to manifest less negative implicit attitudes toward blacks, presumably because the experimenter represented a competent and positive (and therefore counterstereotypical) exemplar who activated more positive aspects of the attitudinal schema (Lowery, Hardin, & Sinclair, 2001). Being cued with positive outgroup exemplars (e.g., Martin Luther King, Jr. and Michael Jordan in the case of black Americans) can similarly decrease the strength of negative implicit evaluations toward those groups (Dasgupta & Greenwald, 2001).

The examples just discussed seem to be primarily unidirectional, in that an environmental factor exerts causal influences on our mental states. However, in most cases, they also rely on internally represented knowledge structures. For example, the effects of exposure to a citrus scent likely depend on a learned association between citrus and cleaning. Closer analysis reveals that, in many cases, external and internal contextual factors reciprocally affect one another. An illustrative example, in the form of a sort of feedback loop, is provided by Chen and Bargh (1997). Activating negative schemas related to black Americans led participants to behave negatively, thereby eliciting negative responses in interaction partners. But because the participants did not recognize their own role in bringing about the negative response, they tended to interpret the other as dispositionally hostile; that is, internal schemas brought about negative behavior, which caused negative responses in others, which were then interpreted as evidence in favor of a negative evaluation of that other. We can easily imagine this phenomenon occurring with respect to other findings we have discussed. For example, the tendency to perceive outgroup faces as angry obviously decreases the quality of intergroup interactions. But systematically "false-alarming" to anger also creates the perception of recurrent evidence in favor of the negative attitude that began the cycle; that is, if one's negative attitude toward black Americans leads one to perceive black Americans as hostile, then this (mis)perception will seem like strong justification for one's negative attitude, creating a self-fulfilling prophecy (e.g., Bargh, Chen, & Burrows, 1996).

Taken together, these examples demand a rejection of the Platonic conception of discrete person and discrete thing. As in other fields, we must move toward ecological thinking, in which the person–environment is conceptualized as a single interdependent system and dispositional states such as attitudes do not have independent reality. Rather, they are the emergent properties of figure–ground interactions between person and context (for elaboration on these themes from a variety of perspectives, see Ferguson & Bargh, 2007; Mischel, 1968; Richardson, Marsh, & Schmidt, Chapter 15, this volume; Schwarz, 2007; Schwarz & Bohner, 2001).

Many of the contextual effects we have discussed operate primarily outside of conscious awareness. Thus, they rarely participate in our own causal explanations of events in the world. This point cannot be overemphasized because it generates a critical gap between our naive psychological explanations and the facts as they are revealed by controlled experiments. Noticing this gap is the first step toward understanding why our intuitive explanations so often underestimate contextual influences, a point to which we now turn.

A CUSTOMARY BLINDNESS

There is an old analogy likening conscious awareness to a flashlight illuminating a slender circle on the wall of a darkened room; wherever we look, there it is. This analogy is helpful in revealing why we tend to overestimate the importance of consciousness, but it does not go far enough. We might add: Yes, and beneath the illuminated surface of wall, extensive wiring and plumbing hum away, causally efficacious but forever outside illumination. We might add: Yes, and the light, limited to certain spectra, fails to reveal many aspects of the target that are no less real than what we see. What we see is surface, one of infinitely many surfaces that could be revealed should different eyes turn toward the same space.

We want to construct accurate theories of behavior, but at least in the context of our everyday lives, we can only incorporate regularities we perceive, regularities constrained by the narrow bandwidth of conscious attention. Thus, our explanations tend to be Platonic in character, based on assumptions of discrete internal and external realities, systematically excluding the sorts of contextual factors now known to influence us. Furthermore, to the extent that our explanations feel successful (an extent that will greatly outstrip their actual efficacy, a point brought home by Nisbett & Wilson as early as 1977), our confidence in them only grows, rendering more contextual explanations less necessary.

Why these limitations? We believe them to be in large part rooted in the shortcuts evolution has provided us to facilitate our understanding of the world. The evolutionary basis of these abilities is clear when we explore the surprising competencies of infants, revealed by revolutionary developmental research undertaken in the last few decades. This shift has centered on a move away from empiricist presuppositions, in which all knowledge is constructed on the basis of direct experience. It is now widely recognized that some initial knowledge, a "preparedness" to learn certain kinds of information given certain kinds of input, is necessary to get knowledge acquisition off the ground (often dubbed *core knowledge*; see Spelke, 2000; Spelke & Kinzler, 2007). For our purposes here, we want to consider how these presuppositions might affect our understanding of objects and events, and how they might relate to our ability or inability to recognize contextual influences.

Both infants and other primates represent core aspects of physical objects, such as their lack of self-generated motion and their solidity. This understanding leads them to be surprised by violations of these expected properties, such as a physical object that moves on its own, or one object passing through another (Aguiar & Baillargeon, 1999; Spelke, 1990). We can conceptualize this knowledge as a causal schema for understanding inanimate physical objects. Of course, some entities in the world routinely violate these guidelines. Take animate entities, such as people and other animals capable of self-generated motion. As it turns out, infants are not surprised when animates behave in this way because they have an independent core knowledge system for reasoning about this class of entities, which we might call core knowledge of *agents*. Interestingly, infants do not think the difference between objects and agents is *merely* the power of self-generated motion. Rather, infants deploy a more complicated schema involving *goals*. For example, upon observing a hand making several reaches for a toy duck instead of a toy truck, infants are surprised if the hand next reaches for the truck, even if the spatial position of the two objects is reversed, such that reaching for the duck now requires a novel path of motion (Woodward, 1998); that is, infants have inferred the presence of a "duck-goal," and so assume that that goal persists even after the duck and truck have switched positions, and this goal violation is more surprising to them than a visually salient change in the path of motion. Thus, infants attribute a stable, internal disposition to the actor, something they will not do in the case of otherwise identically behaving inanimate objects.

Certainly by adulthood we have additional explanatory resources at our command, giving us recourse to theories unavailable to the infant (perhaps the doll that moves on its own is mechanical, perhaps the reach for the duck was based on a false belief), but the mature adult still operates on principles recognizable, in skeletal form, in the first year of life. After all, these are powerful explanatory principles that give us real insight into the workings of the world. That is to say, they largely serve us well. However, to the extent that we rely on their guidance, we are also constrained by them.

The central tenet encoded in core knowledge of objects is *contact causality*, that objects only move or change when contacted by another object. This model is essentially one in which discrete entities are changed only when other discrete entities physically impinge on them. Core knowledge of agents is based around an assumption that goals are stable dispositional states belonging to individuals, by virtue of which we can predict action. As we discussed earlier, however, both of these core principles are routinely violated in psychological life, in which action at a distance and dynamically changing goals, beliefs, and attitudes are rule more than exception. Yet one of our primary means of understanding causality (core knowledge of objects and agents) systematically excludes such influence. The deck is stacked against our perceiving it accurately.

PUTTING THINGS BACK INTO CONTEXT

We have identified two sorts of factors that restrict our ability to grasp contextual influence. First, basic limitations in the scope of conscious attention constrain the causal pathways we can identify and then incorporate into intuitive theory. Second, innate schemas for causal reasoning provide templates that partially structure explanation in ways that restrict or even preclude a sophisticated understanding of subtle contextual influences. Given the central role that contextual factors must play in present and future theory, these considerations raise the possibility that, left to its own course, the gap between lay and scientific theory will only continue to widen.

It may be that nothing will close this gap, that as in a field like physics, the cutting edge of our science will only continue to arc further from our everyday intuitions. But it is equally possible that new revolutions in thinking will enable us to be smarter about context. Paul Churchland (1985) has argued that changes in theory and language can open windows into new perceptual experiences. Focusing on our ability to perceive subtle physiological states, Churchland points out that the global taste of red wine most of us perceive can, on an expert's tongue, be decomposed into more than a dozen distinct elements and their relative concentrations (ethanol, glycol, fructose, acid, tannin, etc.). This ability is greatly aided by, indeed may wholly rely on, the theory and language of wine tasting; that is, distinctions absent in ordinary language (and therefore largely imperceptible), but which in principle are within our discriminatory range, can be made perceptible if the relevant theory and terminology is mastered.

> Suppose we trained our native mechanisms to make a new and more detailed set of discriminations, a set that corresponded not to the primitive psychological taxonomy of ordinary language, but to some more penetrating taxonomy of states drawn from a completed neuroscience. (Churchland, 1985, p. 16)

Substitute an ecological social psychology for a completed neuroscience, and one has a concrete proposal for remaking intuitions in ways more accommodating to context. Our own experience provides some support for this possibility. In particular, we have found the theory of implicit social cognition and, in particular, implicit bias helpful in describing and understanding our own behavior no less than that of our experimental subjects. Alert to the possibility, and armed with the necessary vocabulary, we are considerably more prepared to identify and, if necessary, counteract at least some of the forms of influence we would prefer to do without. The question, then, is whether the theoretical vocabulary of a mature social psychology can stand in for our lay psychological vocabulary, and in so doing call attention to influences previously overlooked.

Testing this possibility requires adopting our theoretical language in our everyday lives, and places the development of a nuanced and precise theoretical vocabulary at center stage. If our considerations are right, if our resistance to contextual explanation is deeply rooted in our natural intuitions, we may need to consider such radical moves. In Wittgenstein's (1922/2006, p. 7) memorable words, "What we cannot speak about we must pass over in silence." All praise, then, for the birth of new words.

REFERENCES

Agerström, J., & Rooth, D. (2009). Implicit prejudice and ethnic minorities: Arab-Muslims in Sweden. *International Journal of Manpower, 30*(1–2), 43–55.

Aguiar, A., & Baillargeon, R. (1999). 2.5-month-old infants' reasoning about when objects should and should not be occluded. *Cognitive Psychology, 39*, 116–157.

Barden, J., Maddux, W. W., Petty, R. E., & Brewer, M. B. (2004). Contextual moderation of racial bias: The impact of social roles on controlled and automatically activated attitudes. *Journal of Personality and Social Psychology, 87*, 5–22.

Bargh, J. A., Chen, M., & Burrows, L. (1996). Automaticity of social behavior: Direct effects of trait construct and stereotype activation on action. *Journal of Personality and Social Psychology, 71*, 230–244.

Bohner, G., & Schwarz, N. (2001). Attitudes, persuasion, and behavior. In A. Tesser & N. Schwarz (Eds.), *Blackwell handbook of social psychology: Intraindividual processes* (pp. 413–435). Oxford, UK: Blackwell.

Chen, M., & Bargh, J. A. (1997). Nonconscious behavioral confirmation processes: The self-fulfilling nature of automatically-activated stereotypes. *Journal of Experimental Social Psychology, 33*, 541–560.

Churchland, P. M. (1985). Reduction, qualia, and the direct introspection of brain states. *Journal of Philosophy, 81*(1), 8–28.

Darley, J. M., & Gross, P. H. (1983). A hypothesis-confirming bias in labeling effects. *Journal of Personality and Social Psychology, 44*, 20–33.

Dasgupta, N., & Greenwald, A. G. (2001). On the malleability of automatic attitudes: Combating automatic prejudice with images of liked and disliked individuals. *Journal of Personality and Social Psychology, 81*, 800–814.

Duncan, B. L. (1976). Differential social perception and attribution of intergroup violence: Testing the lower limits of stereotyping of blacks. *Journal of Personality and Social Psychology, 34*(4), 590–598.

Dunham, Y., & Banaji, M. R. (2008). *The invariance of intergroup bias across the lifespan.* Unpublished manuscript, University of California, Merced.

Dunham, Y., Baron, A. S., & Banaji, M. R. (2007). Children and social groups: A developmental analysis of implicit consistency in Hispanic-Americans. *Self and Identity, 6*, 238–255.

Ferguson, M. J., & Bargh, J. A. (2004). Liking is for doing: Effects of goal pursuit on automatic evaluation. *Journal of Personality and Social Psychology, 88*, 557–572.

Ferguson, M. J., & Bargh, J. A. (2007). Beyond the attitude object: Implicit attitudes spring from object-centered-contexts. In B. Wittenbrink & N. Schwarz (Eds.), *Implicit measures of attitudes* (pp. 216–246). New York: Guilford Press.

Greenwald, A. G., Poehlman, T. A., Uhlmann, E., & Banaji, M. R. (2009). Understanding and using the Implicit Association Test: III. Meta-analysis of predictive validity. *Journal of Personality and Social Psychology, 97*(1), 17–41.

Holland, R. W., Hendriks, M., & Aarts, H. (2005). Smells like clean spirit: Nonconscious effects of scent on cognition and behavior. *Psychological Science, 16*(9), 689–693.

Hugenberg, K., & Bodenhausen, G. V. (2003). Facing prejudice: Implicit prejudice and the perception of facial threat. *Psychological Science, 14*, 640–643.

Hugenberg, K., & Bodenhausen, G. V. (2004). Ambiguity in social categorization: The role of prejudice and facial affect in racial categorization. *Psychological Science, 15*, 342–345.

Lewontin, R. (2000). *The triple helix.* Cambridge, MA: Harvard University Press.

Lowery, B. S., Hardin, C. D., & Sinclair, S. (2001). Social influence on automatic racial prejudice. *Journal of Personality and Social Psychology, 81*, 842–855.

Maddux, W. W., Barden, J., Brewer, M. B., & Petty, R. E. (2005). Saying no to negativity: The effects of context and motivation to control prejudice on automatic evaluative responses. *Journal of Experimental Social Psychology, 41*, 19–35.

Mischel, W. (1968). *Personality and assessment.* New York: Wiley.

Nisbett, R., & Wilson, T. (1977). Telling more than we can know: Verbal reports on mental processes. *Psychological Review, 84*, 231–259.

Nosek, B. A., Smyth, F. L., Hansen, J. J., Devos, T., Lindner, N. M., Ranganath, K. A., et al. (2007). Pervasiveness and correlates of implicit attitudes and stereotypes. *European Review of Social Psychology, 18*, 36–88.

Rosenhan, D. L. (1973). On being sane in insane places. *Science, 179*, 250–258.

Schwarz, N., & Bohner, G. (2001). The construction of attitudes. In A. Tesser & N. Schwarz (Eds.), *Blackwell handbook of social psychology: Intraindividual processes* (pp. 436–457). Oxford, UK: Blackwell.

Schwarz, N., & Clore, G. L. (1983). Mood, misattribution, and judgments of well-being: Informative and directive functions of affective states. *Journal of Personality and Social Psychology, 45*, 513–523.

Schwarz, N. (2007). Attitude construction: Evaluation in context. *Social Cognition, 25*(5), 638–656.

Seibt, B., Hafner, M., & Deutsch, R. (2007). Prepared to eat: How immediate affective and motivational responses to food cues are influenced by food deprivation. *European Journal of Social Psychology, 37*(2), 359–379.

Shoda, Y., Cervone, D., & Downey, G. (Eds.). (2007). *Persons in context: Building a science of the individual.* New York: Guilford Press.

Spelke, E. S. (1990). Principles of object perception. *Cognitive Science, 14*, 29–56.

Spelke, E. S. (2000). Core knowledge. *American Psychologist, 55*, 1233–1243.

Spelke, E. S., & Kinzler, K. D. (2007). Core knowledge. *Developmental Science, 10*(1), 89–96.

Wittenbrink, B., Judd, C. M., & Park, B. (2001). Spontaneous prejudice in context: Variability in automatically activated attitudes. *Journal of Personality and Social Psychology, 81*(5), 815–827.

Wittgenstein, L. (2006). *Tractatus logico-philosophicus.* New York: Hard Press. (Original work published 1922)

Woodward, A. (1998). Infants selectively encode the goal object of an actor's reach. *Cognition, 69*, 1–34.

11

Social Tuning of Ethnic Attitudes

STACEY SINCLAIR
JANETTA LUN

The typical scientific portrait of ethnic prejudice depicts people as striving to control the stereotyping and prejudice they reflexively experience. People are thought to be mired in ethnic biases that are instilled and reinforced by parents, peers, and the media. Though these biases rarely diminish, when circumstances allow, people justify or attempt to control the expression of them. This chapter describes recent research suggesting that ethnic biases are not as rigid as originally construed to be. Rather, they can be quite pliable, fluidly adjusting to the views of others with whom one wants to get along. We begin with a brief history of research on stereotyping and prejudice to support the claim that ethnic prejudice has long been presented as ingrained and resistant to alteration. The second part of the chapter explicates and reviews existing evidence for the view that ethnic prejudice is surprisingly responsive to the interpersonal context.

Since the inception of research on stereotyping and prejudice, social psychologists have documented two seemingly contradictory observations: the pervasiveness of these phenomena and the presence of culturally valued norms that repudiate them. A plethora of research demonstrates that stereotyping and prejudice abound, so much so that they seem to be part of the cultural fabric. Seminal research showed that ethnic stereotypes were widely socially shared and acquired through shared cultural norms rather than idiosyncratic experiences (Katz & Barly, 1933). Despite initial assertions that these stereotypes were becoming less consensual (Gilbert, 1951; Karlins, Coffman, & Walters, 1969), closer examination indicates wide agreement on the content of ethnic stereotypes even now (Devinc & Elliot, 1995; Madon, Guyll, & Aboufadel, 2001). Recent research paints a similar picture, with a Web-based measure that captures individuals' less conscious (i.e., implicit) ethnic attitudes. Data gathered from several thousand people show that 68% of respondents had more generally negative associations toward black than toward white people. Moreover, 72% of respondents were more likely to associate black people rather than white people with weapons, consistent with stereotypes of African American criminality (Nosek et al., 2007).

The pervasiveness of stereotyping and prejudice coexists with cultural norms that object to such bias. The notion that all members of society should be treated equally is thought to be a foundational American ideology (Myrdal, 1944). Moreover, it is one that Americans seem to be increasingly taking to heart. Survey research reveals dramatic increases in white Americans' willingness to endorse principles of integration and job equality over time. For example, in the early 1940s, 68% of white respondents in a national survey indicated that white and black children should attend different schools, compared to 1995, when 96% of whites said such children should attend the same schools. Furthermore, in the early 1940s, 54% of whites surveyed believed whites should be given preference over blacks in hiring. But by the early 1970s, this percentage effectively decreased to zero, causing the elimination of this question from the survey (Bobo, 2001; Schuman, Steeh, Bobo, & Krysan, 1997).

A widely accepted resolution to this apparent contradiction is that individuals are subject to stubborn, ingrained prejudices but attempt to manage these impulses in appropriate contexts (e.g., Crandall & Eshleman, 2003; Dovidio & Gaertner, 1986, 1991). Although theories of this ilk differ in people's presumed awareness of underlying prejudices and proposed strategies for managing them, they share the assumption that most individuals are subject to some amount of stereotyping and/or prejudice that is difficult to reduce in a fundamental way. This resolution can be seen in the early influential work by Gordon Allport (1954), who argued that prejudice and adherence to stereotypes is largely learned during childhood from one's parents. He likened transmission of these biases to a comfortable habit that is passed from generation to generation so subtly and effectively that one could misconstrue the link as hereditary. In adulthood, he further argued, although individuals often behave in accordance with these biases, they learn to engage in "double-talk"; that is, they learn that they must "give lip service to democracy and equality ... and somehow plausibly justify the remaining disapproval that one expresses" (p. 310). In other words, prejudice and stereotyping learned in childhood are undiminished by realization of egalitarian norms in adulthood; rather, individuals learn to manage their expression of stereotypical or prejudiced views appropriately.

"Modern" theories of prejudice retain this basic juxtaposition between ingrained prejudice and efforts to manage it in response to egalitarian norms (e.g., McConahay, 1986). Perhaps the most prominent and clearly articulated of these theories is the *symbolic racism perspective* (Kinder & Sears, 1981; Sears & Henry, 2003, 2005; Sears & Kinder, 1971), which claims that as social norms increasingly condemn the open expression of ethnic prejudice, obvious forms of anti-black prejudice are replaced by a more subtle form, symbolic racism. According to Sears and Kinder (1971), this new form of prejudice is not the abandonment of ingrained negative affect toward African Americans; rather, it is an integration of such affect with ideologies that legitimize it. In describing this notion, for example, they state that negative affective reactions to African Americans are "a longstanding matter within each individual's life, dating from pre-adult acquisition of attitudes and gradually evolving into the 'symbolic racism' currently expressed" (p. 70). Rather than being reduced by adult pressures to appear egalitarian, negative affective reactions toward African Americans are expressed through more palatable ideologies that explain ethnic inequality. Thus, this perspective also contends that early learned prejudice stubbornly withstands consideration of egalitarian norms; in reaction, it simply morphs into a subtle form that *appears* to heed these norms.

Similarly, contemporary social-cognitive research on ethnic stereotyping and prejudice is predicated on the notion that people are subject to inflexible biases that require conscious effort to control. Research on this tradition suggests that people may be unaware of their negative associations toward African Americans after long-term socialization or repeated reinforcement of stereotypes (i.e., implicit ethnic attitudes; Bargh, 1994; Greenwald & Banaji, 1995). Though people are unaware of having these implicit attitudes, such attitudes can influence judgments and behaviors (e.g., Dasgupta, 2004; Dovidio, Kawakami, & Gaertner, 2002; Fazio & Olson, 2003; Olson & Fazio, 2004). This influence is counteracted when individuals are willing and able to reign in their biases via conscious, effortful monitoring of their responses (Devine & Monteith, 1999; Dovidio & Gaertner, 2004). In a prototypical example of this perspective, Devine (1989, p. 15) argued that "nonprejudiced responses are ... a function of intentional, controlled processes and require a conscious decision to behave in a nonprejudiced fashion." Thus, like "modern" theories of prejudice, contemporary social-cognitive perspectives also endow negative associations toward African Americans with inflexibility and inevitability. Although the expressions of these associations can be managed, they are too well-learned to be effectively unlearned (Gregg, Seibt, & Banaji, 2006; Kawakami, Dovidio, Moll, Hermsen, & Russin, 2000).

In summary, a variety of perspectives posit that people are almost ubiquitously subject to ingrained stereotyping and prejudice but manage the expression of these biases in a socially appropriate way. This resolution embraces social psychology's signature emphasis on the power of the social context by suggesting that ingrained biases are often a consequence of long-term exposure to sociocultural influences, and describing the way these biases are situationally managed.

However, recent research indicates that social contexts can play a more direct and immediate role in shaping prejudice and stereotyping than the aforementioned work suggests. In this work, one's level of prejudice and stereotyping is shown to be tied to the apparent beliefs of individuals in the immediate social context, particularly when one wants to get along with the individuals involved. When the beliefs and values apparently held by such people change, individuals' stereotyping and prejudice adjust, or "tune," accordingly. To be clear, this work does not posit that inflexible, ingrained ethnic attitudes are suppressed to adhere to social norms (for such a view, see Crandall & Eshleman, 2003). Prejudice and stereotyping are not squelched or otherwise controlled situationally; rather, they are shown to flexibly adapt to fluctuating social circumstances. In other words, in contrast to the aforementioned work, which suggests that adjustment of prejudice to suit social norms is shallow or effortful, the research we review argues that the social contexts affect "inner representations" of prejudice and stereotyping.

It is interesting to note that results demonstrating individuals' ethnic attitudes toward the apparent beliefs of others are consistent with acknowledgment of the centrality of coordination within dyads and groups for human survival (Caporael, 1997; Dunbar, 1993). Weak, hairless, and characterized by an extended infancy, individual humans could not survive without the protection, resources, and wisdom of their families, work groups, or clan. To the extent that humans are adapted to get along within these relatively small, face-to-face social groupings, it stands to reason that they may have developed the tendency to adapt quickly and efficiently to the prevailing norms within such groupings (see Smith & Collins, Chapter 7, this volume). After all, if their only means of adapting to the views of individuals with whom they want to get along is to manage their attitudes and behaviors effortfully, then group and dyadic coordination would be unduly laborious and taxing.

In the domain of ethnic attitudes, evidence of tuning generally takes one of two forms: tuning toward the consensual views of a group, or tuning toward the views of individuals within dyadic interactions. Though these approaches have different assumptions regarding the type of consensus information to which ethnic attitudes respond (i.e., group or individual), they make parallel points regarding the social basis of ethnic attitudes. In the case of group tuning, ethnic attitudes spontaneously adjust to fit ostensible ingroup norms. Recall that, unlike the aforementioned research, these adjustments are thought to be indicative of inner representations and affective experience rather than outward manifestations of conformity. In the case of dyadic tuning, ethnic attitudes spontaneously adjust to the apparent beliefs of others, particularly those with whom one wants to get along. As such, both lines of research illustrate that ethnic attitudes can easily and fluidly adapt to the apparent views of people in the immediate social context—particularly when one feels a sense of connection to those people.

TUNING TOWARD THE GROUP

The contextualized view of ethnic prejudice has venerable roots in early group norm theory of intergroup attitudes and behavior. The theory suggests that "the individual's directive attitudes, which define and regulate his behavior to other persons, other groups, and to an important extent even to himself, are formed in relation to the values and norms of his reference groups" (Sherif & Sherif, 1953, p. 167). In other words, people construct their attitudes based on the dominant beliefs among members of the group with which they identify (see also Dunham & Banaji, Chapter 10, this volume). This perspective is illustrated by the oft-cited Bennington study on attitude change. Students from highly conservative backgrounds became increasingly liberal after they attended a college that valued liberal norms (Newcomb, 1943). This finding implies that people's ethnic attitudes and behaviors do not have to be the product of a lifetime of socialization but can be the adaptation to ingroup values and norms.

More direct evidence that ethnic prejudice spontaneously tunes toward prevailing group norms is provided by experiments in which people are shown to express different opinions regarding racism depending on the perceived normative context (Blanchard, Crandall, Bringham, & Vaughn, 1994; Crandall, Eshleman, & O'Brien, 2002; Monteith, Deneen, & Tooman, 1996; Stangor, Sechrist, & Jost, 2001). In an early experiment of this nature, students were approached for a brief survey about their race-related opinions, along with a confederate posing as another student participant. The confederate, who always responded first, was instructed to express attitudes that either condoned or condemned racism (e.g., agree that any person who committed a racist act should be expelled). Though there was only a single confederate, the authors expected that the freely disclosed opinion of an ostensible ingroup member would be taken as representative of the local norms. Consistent with the group norm perspective, participants expressed stronger antiracism attitudes when they heard their peer condemn racism than when the peer appeared to condone racism (Blanchard, Lilly, & Vaughn, 1991, Experiment 2). This social norm influence occurred even when participants were asked to privately report their attitudes, suggesting that the effect goes beyond superficial conformity (Blanchard et al., 1994).

Of course, the use of self-report measures or similar techniques makes it difficult for these experiments to overcome the assumption that people are strategically altering their responses to appease norms. However, experiments assessing ethnic attitudes that come to mind automatically, an outcome much less vulnerable to strategic manipulation, yield corresponding findings. In a clever experiment by Sechrist and Stangor (2001), undergraduate participants were led to believe that their stereotypical beliefs about African Americans were shared by a majority (81%) or minority (19%) of students at the same university. Those who thought their beliefs were shared by the majority of students showed greater accessibility of African American stereotypes and sat farther away from an African American confederate (Sechrist & Stangor, 2001). Moreover, even tacit group consensus may shape ethnic attitudes that are automatically available to people. A recent experiment showed that participants had significantly lower implicit prejudice toward blacks when they completed an Implicit Association Test (IAT) with a group of fellow students versus alone (Castelli & Tomelleri, 2008). The authors attributed this difference to the egalitarian norm tacitly elicited by the presence of other students. Supporting this interpretation, the authors found that participants' perception of discrimination as unjust was related to IAT scores for those in the group condition but not in the individual condition. In summary, these research findings provide persuasive evidence that explicit and implicit ethnic attitudes and relevant behavior are constructed based on the dominant beliefs in one's immediate social context.

It is not, however, that people blindly align their beliefs toward the consensus of any group (Kelman, 1961; Sherif & Sherif, 1953). Rather, they align their ethnic attitudes to fit with the consensus among ingroup members, or when they feel a strong connection with a group. The apparent consensus among students at one university influenced college students' prejudice more strongly than the apparent consensus among students at a different university (Stangor et al., 2001). Research guided by self-categorization theory also shows that people who identify with their ingroup are more likely to adapt to prevailing ingroup attitudes and behave in a manner consistent with those attitudes (Terry & Hogg, 1996). These findings demonstrate that ethnic attitudes may be more susceptible to the prevailing beliefs of an ingroup than an outgroup. Furthermore, attitudes may be more influenced when people experience a strong sense of identification with the ingroup.

TUNING WITHIN DYADS

In addition to group consensus, people's ethnic attitudes are also be shaped by consensus developed in dyadic interactions. Much of this work is done within the framework of *shared reality theory* (Hardin & Conley, 2001; Sinclair & Huntsinger, 2005), which postulates that the experience of seeing something the same way another person sees it validates the meaning of that thing. Moreover, being able to achieve such consensus with someone establishes an interpersonal bond with him or her. We have examined the following hypotheses rendered from these assertions: (1) Ethnic attitudes are experienced as a function of the apparent views of an interaction partner; (2) the degree to which a person's ethnic attitudes correspond to the partner's views is moderated by motivation to get along with that person or to acquire knowledge; and (3) social tuning of ethnic attitudes should occur to the extent that it facilitates the achievement of shared understanding within that specific interaction. Though we have found some similar effects using explicit prejudice measures (Huntsinger, 2007), we concentrated on examining fluctuations in implicit ethnic attitudes to avoid the argument that people were merely strategically manipulating their responses.

Are ethnic attitudes experienced as a function of the apparent views of an interaction partner? We began to examine this hypothesis by looking at the effect of an experimenter's ethnicity on people's implicit prejudice. As expected, people experienced less implicit prejudice toward African Americans when the experimenter who administered the task was an African American rather than a European American (Lowery, Hardin, & Sinclair, 2001). We postulated that the reduction reflected presumed greater egalitarianism of the African American versus the European American experimenter. However, one could also argue that the change stemmed from the African American experimenter serving as a counterstereotypical exemplar (Blair, Ma, & Lenton, 2001; Dasgupta & Greenwald, 2001). For this reason, we further clarified our assertion by demonstrating that people also had lower implicit prejudice around a European American experimenter who endorsed egalitarian beliefs than with the same experimenter who did not do so (Sinclair, Lowery, Hardin, & Coangelo, 2005). Thus, people evidently were responding to the apparent beliefs of the other person rather than his or her demographic characteristics.

According to the shared reality perspective, shared reality afforded by tuning social views can bind people together and validate beliefs (Hardin & Conley, 2001). Thus, people are particularly encouraged to tune their beliefs toward those of an interaction partner when they experience the motivation to get along with the partner (*affiliative motivation*) or to acquire knowledge (*epistemic motivation*). To demonstrate the role of affiliative and epistemic motivation in tuning of ethnic attitudes, we typically had participants interact with an experimenter who either appeared to endorse egalitarian beliefs by wearing a T-shirt with the word "Eracism" printed on it or a blank T-shirt. The relevant motivations were measured or manipulated in a variety of ways across experiments. In one instance, for example, affiliative motivation was manipulated by having a European American experimenter behave in a friendly manner to induce a desire to get along (affiliative motivation) or in a rude manner to dispel any chronic presence of such motivation. Then, participants completed a subliminal priming task that measured their implicit prejudice. As expected, participants interacting with the friendly experimenter who ostensibly endorsed egalitarian beliefs experienced lower implicit prejudice toward African Americans than participants who interacted with a friendly experimenter wearing a blank T-shirt. In contrast, the ostensible beliefs of the rude experimenter had no impact on participants' implicit prejudice (Sinclair et al., 2005, Experiment 2). The desire to acquire knowledge (i.e., epistemic motivation) induced similar shifts in implicit prejudice. People who were epistemically motivated because they were chronically uncertain of their ethnic attitudes or primed with uncertainty were also more likely to experience lower implicit prejudice in the presence of the ostensibly egalitarian experimenter (Lun, Sinclair, Whitchurch, & Glenn, 2007).

Recent data also confirm that this dyadic tuning of ethnic attitudes occurs spontaneously, without conscious and effortful manipulation of responses (Sinclair & Huntsinger, 2008). Participants showed no impairment on their performance in a Stroop task after their implicit ethnic attitudes aligned with the views of a likeable experimenter, suggesting that doing so did not consume precious cognitive resources (Baumeister, Muraven, & Tice, 2000; Richeson & Trawalter, 2005). Moreover, using statistical techniques that separate the automatic and control components of responses to implicit attitude measures, Conrey, Sherman, Gawronski, Hugenberg, and Groom (2005) found that perceived views of the interaction partner affected the automatic component but not the controlled component. These findings lend support to the direct role of one's immediate interpersonal context in influencing ethnic prejudice over an argument that the immediate context inspires effortful unlearning or suppression on the part of the individual.

Finally, the assertion that affiliative and epistemic needs are fulfilled through tuning one's beliefs toward those of others in the immediate context leads to the third hypothesis: Social tuning of ethnic attitudes should occur to the extent that it pertains to the interpersonal interaction and facilitates the achievement of shared understanding in that specific interaction. To illustrate this, epistemically motivated participants interacted with an experimenter who appeared to endorse egalitarian beliefs (i.e., wearing a T-shirt that said "Eracism") or with an experimenter who did not indicate her beliefs, or they were asked to read the word "Eracism" on a poster that clearly did not belong to the experimenter. Consistent with the interpersonal nature of social tuning, only those who were epistemically motivated and thought the experimenter endorsed egalitarian beliefs had lower implicit prejudice. No difference in implicit prejudice was observed in the no-belief condition or when the egalitarian belief was merely presented on the poster (Lun et al., 2007, Experiment 3). This finding suggests that ethnic prejudice does not respond to any social cue that happens to be in the environment. Instead, people's views tune specifically toward the perceived beliefs of an interaction partner because only such tuning will facilitate the achievement of interpersonal consensus.

The research summarized here clearly suggests that prejudice and stereotyping fluidly adapt to the apparent views of others in the immediate social context. People's ethnic attitudes become aligned with the prevailing beliefs about racism or ethnic stereotypes within an ingroup (e.g., Blanchard et al., 1994; Sechrist & Stangor, 2001), or the ostensible egalitarian beliefs of an interaction partner with whom one wants to get along (e.g., Sinclair et al., 2005). These findings complement other research suggesting that an individual's other attitudes (see Prislin & Wood, 2005, for a review), behaviors (see Chartrand, Maddux, & Lakin, 2005, for a review), and affective experience (Anderson, Keltner, & John, 2003; Huntsinger, Lun, Sinclair, & Clore, 2009; Oishi & Sullivan, 2006) are profoundly influenced by those of the people with whom they are currently interacting. This collection of research also challenges the common notion that ethnic prejudice is indelibly ingrained in people's minds.

QUESTIONS TO ANSWER

The notion that ethnic attitudes are more pliable than often assumed is tantalizing because it raises new questions about ethnic prejudice. One that immediately comes to mind is how demonstrated pliability coincides with the mass of research suggesting that ethnic attitudes are stubborn, responding to egalitarian social norms with effort, and then only superficially. Perhaps it is the case that people tacitly recognize the disjuncture between egalitarian social norms and widespread stereotyping and prejudice. If so, the apparent stubbornness of prejudice may not stem from ingrained associations but is instead symptomatic of consistent immersion in interpersonal contexts presumed to harbor ethnic bias.

Such speculation is substantiated by the fact that people assume that others, including ingroup members, subscribe to some degree of prejudice and stereotyping of outgroups (Judd, Park, Yzerbyt, Gordijn, & Muller, 2005). This assumption is revealed in the way people communicate about other groups. For example, people are more likely to communicate stereotype-consistent information about a target to an audience because stereotype-consistent information is assumed to promote mutual understanding and help to regulate social relationships with the audience (Clark & Kashima, 2007; Ruscher, 1998; Schaller, Conway, & Tanchuk, 2002). Also, because it is more likely to be communicated, stereotype-consistent information tends to be perceived as socially endorsed (Schaller et al., 2002). If people's day-to-day interactions are with individuals and groups assumed to share social stereotypes, their ethnic attitudes in these interactions should adapt accordingly, thus appearing to be consistently prejudiced. In contrast, the ideal of egalitarianism may not course through the veins of daily social interaction; it is only when individuals are reminded of it that they strive to achieve it. Thus, responses to invoking abstract egalitarian norms are more artificial, controlled, and effortful.

Another question pertains to the relative sway of group versus dyadic consensus in the shaping of ethnic attitudes. In other words, if individuals' ethnic attitudes instinctively harmonize with ingroup members and within dyads characterized by the desire to get along, what happens when apparent views held across these social groupings contrast? On the one hand, consensus with an individual may override group consensus, effectively creating a "you and me against the world" situation (Gerin, Pieper, Levy, & Pickering, 1992). On the other hand, given the evolutionary significance of group memberships (Caporeal, 1997), perhaps consensus with many others trumps consensus with a dissenting individual. Documenting the interplay between group and dyadic tuning of attitudes is integral to designing effective and sustainable environmental interventions aimed at reducing prejudice.

Finally, if ethnic attitudes are situationally constructed within a social context, how does the mind do it? At this point, our answers to this question rely on the theoretical foundations of connectionism or situated cognition and the promise of neuroscience research. The connectionist perspective suggests that attitudes are represented in memory as a pattern of activation in an individual's neural network, which includes activation elicited from relevant contextual cues (situations, goals, mood, etc.; Conrey & Smith, 2007; McClelland & Rumelhart, 1986; Smith, 1996; Smith & DeCoster, 1998; see Smith & Collins, Chapter 7, this volume, for a discussion of situated cognition). Thus, an attitude is not retrieved from memory as a discrete cognitive representation of the attitude object alone; rather, it is an integrative and distributed activation of different representational units reflecting the specific configuration of one's social context. This perspective allows a flexible view of ethnic attitudes that integrates social inputs and individuals' motivation to accommodate the changes brought about when one moves from one social context to another (see Dunham & Banaji, Chapter 10, this volume). Additionally, we are hopeful that the expansion of neuroscience research on stereotyping and prejudice may provide useful inroads to clarify the processes involved. We would be delighted to discover that socially inspired fluctuations in ethnic attitudes are mediated by inferences about others' mental states (e.g., Mitchell, Mason, Macrae, & Banaji, 2006), but it is also conceivable that they are the product of rapid control mechanisms (Correll, Urland, & Ito, 2006).

The understanding that ethnic attitudes are socially pliable commences a new venture in eradicating racism. This perspective redirects people's attention to the importance of understanding ethnic prejudice in the context of social interaction. It also suggests that stereotyping and prejudice can be reduced by exploiting individuals' fundamental desire to get along with others who believe in social equality. Many prescriptions for prejudice can be psychologically demanding for perceivers or burdensome for targets. Individuals afflicted by stereotyping or prejudice must become adept at putting the brakes on their impulses (Devine & Monteith, 1999) or targets should be pleasant and counterstereotypical as they interact with perceivers (Dasgupta & Greenwald, 2001; Sinclair & Kunda, 1999). The emerging work we have discussed suggests that it may also be fruitful to convince people that members of their ingroup, or others with whom they want to get along, genuinely embrace egalitarian beliefs. If this can be done, people will be effortlessly drawn toward embracing such beliefs themselves.

REFERENCES

Allport, G. W. (1954). *The nature of prejudice*. Cambridge, MA: Addison-Wesley.

Anderson, C., Keltner, D., & John, O. P. (2003). Emotional convergence between people over time. *Journal of Personality and Social Psychology*, *84*, 1054–1068.

Bargh, J. A. (1994). The four horsemen of automaticity: Awareness, intention, efficiency, and control in social cognition. In R. S. Wyer, Jr. & T. K. Srull (Eds.), *Handbook of social cognition* (2 vols., 2nd ed., pp. 1–40). Hillsdale, NJ: Erlbaum.

Baumeister, R. F., Muraven, M., & Tice, D. M. (2000). Ego depletion: A resource model of volition, self-regulation, and controlled processing. *Social Cognition, 18*, 130–150.

Blair, I. V., Ma, J. E., & Lenton, A. P. (2001). Imagining stereotypes away: The moderation of implicit stereotypes through mental imagery. *Journal of Personality and Social Psychology, 81, 828–841.*

Blanchard, F. A., Crandall, C. S., Bringham, J. C., & Vaughn, L. A. (1994). Condemning and condoning racism: A social context approach to interracial settings. *Journal of Applied Psychology, 79*, 993–997.

Blanchard, F. A., Lilly, T., & Vaughn, L. A. (1991). Reducing the expression of racial prejudice. *Psychological Science, 2*, 101–105.

Bobo, L. (2001). Racial attitudes and relations at the close of the twentieth century. In N. J. Smelser, W. J. Wilson, & F. M. Mitchell (Eds.), *Racial trends and their consequences* (pp. 264–301). Washington, DC: National Academy Press.

Caporael, L. R. (1997). The evolution of truly social cognition: The core configurations model. *Personality and Social Psychology Review, 1*, 276–298.

Castelli, L., & Tomelleri, S. (2008). Contextual effects on prejudiced attitudes: When the presence of others leads to more egalitarian responses. *Journal of Experimental Social Psychology, 44*(3), 679–686.

Chartrand, T. L., Maddux, W. W., & Lakin, J. L. (2005). Beyond the perception–behavior link: The ubiquitous utility and motivational moderators of nonconscious mimicry. In R. R. Hassin, J. S. Uleman, & J. A. Bargh (Eds.), *The new unconscious* (pp. 334–361). New York: Oxford University Press.

Clark, A. E., & Kashima, Y. (2007). Stereotypes help people connect with others in the community: A situated functional analysis of the stereotype consistency bias in communication. *Journal of Personality and Social Psychology, 93*, 1028–1039.

Conrey, F. R., Sherman, J. W., Gawronski, B., Hugenberg, K., & Groom, C. J. (2005). Separating multiple processes in implicit social cognition: The quad model of implicit task performance. *Journal of Personality and Social Psychology, 89*, 469–487.

Conrey, F. R., & Smith, E. R. (2007). Attitude representation: Attitudes as patterns in a distributed, connectionist representational system. *Social Cognition, 25*, 718–735.

Correll, J., Urland, G. R., & Ito, T. A. (2006). Event-related potentials and the decision to shoot: The role of threat perception and cognitive control. *Journal of Experimental Social Psychology, 42*, 120–128.

Crandall, C. S., & Eshleman, A. (2003). A justification–suppression model of the expression and experience of prejudice. *Psychological Bulletin, 129*, 414–446.

Crandall, C. S., Eshleman, A., & O'Brien, L. T. (2002). Social norms and the expression and suppression of prejudice: The struggle for internationalization. *Journal of Personality and Social Psychology, 82*, 359–378.

Dasgupta, N. (2004). Implicit ingroup favoritism, outgroup favoritism and their behavioral manifestations. *Social Justice Research, 17*, 143–169.

Dasgupta, N., & Greenwald, A. G. (2001). On the malleability of automatic attitudes: Combating automatic prejudice with images of admired and disliked individuals. *Journal of Personality and Social Psychology, 81*, 800–814.

Devine, P. G. (1989). Stereotypes and prejudice: Their automatic and controlled components. *Journal of Personality and Social Psychology, 56*, 5–18.

Devine, P. G., & Elliot, A. J. (1995). Are racial stereotypes really fading?: The Princeton trilogy revisited. *Personality and Social Psychology Bulletin, 21*, 1139–1150.

Devine, P. G., & Monteith, M. J. (1999). Automaticity and control in stereotyping. In S. Chaiken & Y. Trope (Eds.), *Dual-process models and themes in social psychology* (pp. 339–360). New York: Guilford Press.

Dovidio, J. F., & Gaertner, S. L. (1986). Prejudice, discrimination, and racism: Historical trends and contemporary approaches. In J. F. Dovidio & S. L. Gaertner (Eds.), *Prejudice, discrimination, and racism* (pp. 1–34). New York: Academic Press.

Dovidio, J. F., & Gaertner, S. L. (1991). Changes in the expression and assessment of racial prejudice. In H. J. Knopke, R. J. Norrell, & R. W. Rogers (Eds.), *Opening doors: Perspectives on race relations in America* (pp. 119–148). Tuscaloosa: University of Alabama Press.

Dovidio, J. F., & Gaertner, S. L. (2004). Aversive racism. In M. P. Zanna (Ed.), *Advances in experimental social psychology* (Vol. 36, pp. 1–52). San Diego, CA: Academic Press.

Dovidio, J. F., Kawakami, K., & Gaertner, S. L. (2002). Implicit and explicit prejudice and interracial interaction. *Journal of Personality and Social Psychology, 82*, 62–68.

Dunbar, R. I. M. (1993). Coevolution of neocortical size, group size and language in humans. *Behavioral and Brain Sciences, 16*, 682–735.

Fazio, R. H., & Olson, M. A. (2003). Implicit measure in social cognition research: Their meaning and use. *Annual Review of Psychology, 54*, 297–327.

Gerin, W., Pieper, C., Levy, R., & Pickering T. G. (1992). Social support in social interaction: A moderator of cardiovascular reactivity. *Psychosomatic Medicine, 54*, 324–336.

Gilbert, G. M. (1951). Stereotype persistence and change among college students. *Journal of Abnormal and Social Psychology, 46*, 245–254.

Greenwald, A. G., & Banaji, M. R. (1995). Implicit social cognition: Attitudes, self-esteem, and stereotypes. *Psychological Review, 102*, 4–27.

Gregg, A. P., Seibt, B., & Banaji, M. R. (2006). Easier done than undone: Asymmetry in the malleability of implicit preferences. *Journal of Personality and Social Psychology, 90*, 1–20.

Hardin, C. D., & Conley, T. D. (2001). A relational approach to cognition: Shared experience and relationship affirmation in social cognition. In G. B.

Moskowitz (Ed.), *Cognitive social psychology: The Princeton Symposium on the Legacy and Future of Social Cognition* (pp. 3–17). Mahwah, NJ: Erlbaum.

Huntsinger, J. R. (2007). *Mood and automatic processes*. Unpublished doctoral dissertation, University of Virginia, Charlottesville.

Huntsinger, J. R., Lun, J., Sinclair, S. A., & Clore, G. L. (2009). Contagion without contact: Anticipatory mood matching in response to affilitative motivation. *Personality and Social Psychology Bulletin, 35*(7), 909–922.

Judd, C. M., Park, B., Yzerbyt, V., Gordijn, E. H., & Muller, D. (2005). Attributions of intergroup bias and out-group homogeneity to in-group and out-group others. *European Journal of Social Psychology, 35*, 677–704.

Karlins, M., Coffman, T. L., & Walters, G. (1969). On the fading of social stereotypes: Studies in three generations of college students. *Journal of Personality and Social Psychology, 13*, 1–16.

Katz, D., & Barly, K. (1933). Racial stereotypes of one hundred college students. *Journal of Abnormal and Social Psychology, 28*, 280–290.

Kawakami, K., Dovidio, J. F., Moll, J., Hermsen, S., & Russin, A. (2000). Just say no (to stereotyping): Effects of training in the negation of stereotypic association on stereotype activation. *Journal of Personality and Social Psychology, 78*, 871–888.

Kelman, H. C. (1961). Processes of opinion change. *Public Opinion Quarterly, 25*, 57–78.

Kinder, D. R., & Sears, D. O. (1981). Prejudice and politics: Symbolic racism versus racial threats to the good life. *Journal of Personality and Social Psychology, 40*, 414–431.

Lowery, B. S., Hardin, C. D., & Sinclair, S. (2001). Social influence effects on automatic racial prejudice. *Journal of Personality and Social Psychology, 81*, 842–855.

Lun, J., Sinclair, S., Whitchurch, E. R., & Glenn, C. (2007). (Why) do I think what you think?: Epistemic social tuning and implicit prejudice. *Journal of Personality and Social Psychology, 93*, 957–972.

Madon, S., Guyll, M., & Aboufadel, K. (2001). Ethnic and national stereotypes: The Princeton trilogy revisited and revised. *Personality and Social Psychology Bulletin, 27*, 966–1010.

McClelland, J. L., & Rumelhart, D. E. (1986). A distributed model of human learning and memory. In J. L. McClelland & D. E. Rumelhart (Eds.), *Parallel distributed processing: Explorations in the microstructure of cognition* (Vol. 2, pp. 170–215). Cambridge, MA: MIT Press.

McConahay, J. B. (1986). Modern racism, ambivalence, and the Modern Racism Scale. In J. F. Dovidio & S. L. Gaertner (Eds.), *Prejudice, discrimination, and racism* (pp. 91–125). New York: Academic Press.

Mitchell, J. P., Mason, M. F., Macrae, C. N., & Banaji, M. R. (2006). Thinking about others: The neural substrates of social cognition. In J. T. Cacioppo, P. S. Visser, & C. L. Pickett (Eds.), *Social neuroscience: People thinking about thinking people* (pp. 63–82). Cambridge, MA: MIT Press.

Monteith, M. J., Deneen, N. E., & Tooman, G. D. (1996). The effect of social norm activation on the expression of opinions concerning gay men and blacks. *Basic and Applied Social Psychology, 18*, 276–288.

Myrdal, G. (1944). *An American dilemma: The Negro problem and modern democracy*. New York: Harper.

Newcomb, T. M. (1943). *Personality and social change: Attitude formation in a student community*. New York: Dryden.

Nosek, B. A., Smyth, F. L., Hansen, J. J., Devos, T., Lindner, N. M., Ranganath, K. A., et al. (2007). Pervasiveness and correlates of implicit attitudes and stereotypes. *European Review of Social Psychology, 18*, 36–88.

Oishi, S., & Sullivan, H. W. (2006). The predictive value of daily vs. retrospective well-being judgments in relationship stability. *Journal of Experimental Social Psychology, 42*, 460–470.

Olson, M. A., & Fazio, R. H. (2004). Train inferences as a function of automatically activated racial attitudes and motivation to control prejudiced reactions. *Basic and Applied Social Psychology, 26*, 1–11.

Prislin, R., & Wood, W. (2005). Social influence in attitudes and attitude change. In D. Albarracín, B. T. Johnson, & M. P. Zanna, (Eds.), *The handbook of attitudes* (pp. 671–705). Mahwah, NJ: Erlbaum.

Richeson, J. A., & Trawalter, S. (2005). Why do interracial interactions impair executive function?: A resource depletion account. *Journal of Personality and Social Psychology, 88*, 934–947.

Ruscher, J. B.(1998). Prejudice and stereotyping in everyday communication. *Advances in Experimental Social Psychology, 30*, 241–307.

Schaller, M., Conway, L. G., III., & Tanchuk, T. L. (2002). Selective pressures on the once and future contents of ethice stereotypes: Effects of the communicability of traits. *Journal of Personality and Social Psychology, 82*, 861–877.

Schuman, H., Steeh, C., Bobo, L., & Krysan, M. (1997). *Racial attitudes in America: Trends and interpretations*. Cambridge, MA: Harvard University Press.

Sears, D. O., & Henry, P. J. (2003). The origins of symbolic racism. *Journal of Personality and Social Psychology, 85*, 256–275.

Sears, D. O., & Henry, P. J. (2005). Over thirty years later: A contemporary look at symbolic racism. *Advances in Experimental Social Psychology, 37*, 95–105.

Sears, D. O., & Kinder, D. R. (1971). Racial tensions and voting in Los Angeles. In W. Hirsch (Ed.), *Los Angeles: Viability and prospects for metropolitan leadership* (pp. 51–88). New York: Praeger.

Sechrist, G. B., & Stangor, C. (2001). Perceived consensus influences intergroup behavior and stereotype accessibility. *Journal of Personality and Social Psychology, 80*, 645–654.

Sherif, M., & Sherif, C. W. (1953). *Groups in harmony and tension: An integration of studies on intergroup relations*. New York: Octagon.

Sinclair, L., & Kunda, Z. (1999). Reactions to a black professional: Motivated inhibition and activation of conflicting stereotypes. *Journal of Personality and Social Psychology, 77*, 885–904.

Sinclair, S., & Huntsinger, J. (2005). The interpersonal basis of self-stereotyping. In S. Levin & C. van Laar (Eds.), *Claremont Symposium on Applied Social Psychology: Stigma and group inequality: Social psychological approaches*. Mahwah, NJ: Erlbaum.

Sinclair, S., & Huntsinger, J. R. (2008). [The automaticity of social tuning.] Unpublished raw data.

Sinclair, S., Lowery, B. S., Hardin, C. D., & Coangelo, A. (2005). Social tuning of automatic racial attitudes: The role of affiliative motivation. *Journal of Personality and Social Psychology*, *89*, 583–592.

Smith, E. R. (1996). What do connectionism and social psychology offer each other? *Journal of Personality and Social Psychology*, *70*, 893–912.

Smith, E. R., & DeCoster, J. (1998). Person perception and stereotyping: Simulation using distributed representations in a recurrent connectionist network. In S. J. Read & L. C. Miller (Eds.), *Connectionist models of social reasoning and social behavior* (pp. 111–140). Mahwah, NJ: Erlbaum.

Stangor, C., Sechrist, G. B., & Jost, J. T. (2001). Changing racial beliefs by providing consensus information. *Personality and Social Psychology Bulletin*, *27*, 486–496.

Terry, D. J., & Hogg, M. A. (1996). Group norms and the attitude–behavior relationship: A role for group identification. *Personality and Social Psychology Bulletin*, *22*, 776–793.

PART IV

BEHAVIOR

12

The Multiple Forms of "Context" in Associative Learning Theory

MARK E. BOUTON

The concept of context has always been central, at least implicitly, in theories of associative learning. For example, when a learning theorist says that a behavior is controlled by either Pavlovian or operant conditioning, he or she has typically identified a "context" in which the behavior usually occurs (the conditional stimulus, or CS, in the Pavlovian case and a discriminative stimulus, or S^D, in the operant one). Of course, modern learning theory is not merely interested in identifying conditioned and discriminative stimuli in the world. Since at least the 1970s, the broad impact of context on basic learning processes has been widely recognized and has become a major focus of research in the field (e.g., Balsam & Tomie, 1985; Pearce & Bouton, 2001). In this chapter, I review the most important roles that are now attributed to contexts, discuss how they operate, and consider what the "special" characteristics of contexts might be.

In contemporary learning theory, *context* is typically defined as the background stimuli provided by the apparatus (e.g., Skinner box) in which the experiment is conducted. This definition is similar to the one used in the human memory literature, where *context* is often defined as stimuli provided by cues emanating from the room in which the experiment occurs (e.g., Smith, 1988; Smith & Vela, 2001). In either case, the context is a relatively long-duration stimulus that surrounds or embeds the target stimuli that are to be learned about or remembered (whether they are conditioned or discriminative stimuli, or items in a list). In the first part of the chapter, I describe four theoretical roles that have been assigned to this sort of context in the learning theory tradition. For many years, my students and I have been especially interested in one of those roles, namely, the idea that the context determines the current *meaning* of the CS. In the subsequent parts of the chapter I therefore review some of the research that suggests such a role and also identifies other novel context effects. With this as background, I then discuss two theoretical questions that are the focus of much contemporary interest. First, why should the context ever become important in controlling the meaning of a stimulus? (It often has surprisingly little impact.) Second, what stimuli besides apparatus or room cues can play the role of context? The latter question allows me to discuss research on how the passage of *time* might provide contextual change and thus provide a significant part of the context.

THE MULTIPLE ROLES OF CONTEXT IN ASSOCIATIVE LEARNING

It is possible to distinguish several meanings of the term *context* in modern learning theory (Bouton, 2007). In the first and perhaps most straightforward meaning, the term simply denotes a stimulus or setting that elicits behavior directly. Thus, for example, certain settings can trigger emotions in humans (Bouton, 2005; Nelson & Bouton, 2002) or prime "automatic" behaviors or cognitions or habits (e.g., Bargh & Chartrand, 1999). Similarly, in animal learning experiments, rats freeze when they are put in a Skinner box or chamber where they have been shocked before (e.g., Fanselow, 1980). Rats sometimes also exhibit a compensatory conditioned response when they are put in a box that has been associated with a drug (e.g., Siegel, 2005). The compensatory nature of the conditioned response can cancel the effect of the drug when it is delivered and thereby contribute to drug tolerance. In such an instance, drug tolerance is said to be *context-specific*, or mainly evident in the context in which it was learned. In each of these cases, the context is merely a stimulus that elicits behaviors directly, much as the bell elicited salivation in Pavlov's original experiments once it was associated with a food unconditional stimulus (US).

A second role for context builds upon the first. In addition to eliciting behavior on its own, a context that is associated with a US can also *compete* with learning about, and/or judgments about, CSs that occur in them. For example, in a number of influential experiments, Rescorla (e.g., 1968) showed that animals are sensitive to not only the probability of the US in the presence of the CS but also the probability of the US in its *absence*—the overall context in which the CS–US pairings occur. Specifically, rats given an equal number of CS–US pairings showed different levels of conditioned responding to the CS depending on how often the US was also presented when the CS was off. When the two probabilities were equal, there was no conditional responding to the CS at all. Interestingly, human contingency and causal judgments may operate the same way; we judge a CS or an event to be a weak cause of a second event if the probability of the second event in that context is already high (e.g., Baker, Murphy, Mehta, & Baetu, 2005). Theories of conditioning that followed Rescorla's experiments (e.g., Mackintosh, 1975; Pearce & Hall, 1980; Rescorla & Wagner, 1972; Wagner, 1981) have all assumed that when the US occurs in the absence of the CS, it actually occurs in the presence of contextual stimuli. In Rescorla and Wagner's words (1972, p. 88), "To speak of shocks occurring in the absence of the CS is to say they occur in the presence of situational stimuli arising from the experimental environment." Conditioning of these stimuli then allows them to "block" (Kamin, 1969) conditioning of the CS when the CS itself was paired with the US. Modern theories of conditioning now almost universally emphasize context in the sense that the effect of any conditioning trial is assumed to depend on the associative strength of *all* the cues that are present at the same time, including other CSs, as well as the context (see also Denniston, Savastano, & Miller, 2001; Gallistel & Gibbon, 2000). In modern learning theory, learning thus depends fundamentally on the context in which it occurs.

A third role that has often been assigned to the context comes from the memory literature rather than the learning literature: The context is a stimulus that supports memory retrieval. It is widely known that memory in both humans and animals is best when the context that is present during testing matches the context that was present during learning (e.g., Spear, 1978; Tulving & Thomson, 1973). Thus, a change of context leads to retrieval failure, one of the most important causes of forgetting. In principle, this mechanism predicts that changing the room or apparatus context after conditioning will weaken the conditional response to the CS—much as a change in the room context (e.g., Smith, 1979) or a move from land to under water (or vice versa; Godden & Baddeley, 1975) can disrupt memory for words. Interestingly, although a context switch after conditioning can *sometimes* reduce responding to the CS, such a result is actually surprisingly rare (e.g., Bouton, 1993). The same is also true for memory of word lists (e.g., Smith, 1988; Smith & Vela, 2001)—that is, a context switch often has little effect.

A fourth role of context may be related to the retrieval function just described (e.g., Bouton, 1993, 1994). Instead of merely entering into a simple association with the CS or the US, the context may come to signal or "set the occasion" for the relationship between them—the current association between the CS and US. As reviewed in later sections, this role of context becomes important when the CS is associated with different events in different phases of the experiment (e.g., as in extinction, when the CS is paired with the US in one phase, and then with no US in the next). In this sort of situation, the context appears to select between the CS's two available associations (CS–US and CS–no US) and thus disambiguate the current meaning of the CS, much as the verbal context determines the meaning of an ambiguous word (e.g., Bouton, 1991, 1994).

THE SPECIAL INFLUENCE OF CONTEXT IN EXTINCTION

Over the years, my students and I have run many experiments that have identified a central role for the context in extinction (for reviews, see Bouton, 2004; Bouton & Woods, 2008). That role is most easily illustrated by a phenomenon known as the *renewal effect.* In one example of renewal, rats may be given pairings of a tone and mild footshock in one Skinner box, Context A. This, of course, gives the tone the power to elicit fear when it is presented again. If extinction trials (the tone being presented without the shock) are then administered in Context B, the fear behaviors will decline. However, if the tone is then returned to Context A and tested there, fear of the tone returns (it is "renewed"). Similar renewal effects occur when conditioning, extinction, and testing occur in Contexts A, B, and C ("ABC renewal") or Contexts A, A, and B ("AAB renewal"). These and other results suggest that extinction does not destroy the original learning, but instead leaves the CS with two available meanings (e.g., CS–US and CS–no US). As noted earlier, and discussed further below, the context may then work in part by selecting between them (e.g., Bouton, 1994, 2004; Bouton & Bolles, 1985).

Renewal has been demonstrated with a very wide range of methods. It has been demonstrated in many examples of Pavlovian learning in animals, including fear and appetitive conditioning (where the tone is paired with footshock or with food, respectively), taste aversion learning (where the CS is a taste that is paired with illness), and operant learning (where pressing a lever is reinforced by presentation of a positive consequence). As an example of the latter, Crombag and Shaham (2002; see also Crombag, Grimm, & Shaham, 2003) found that rats will learn to press a lever in a Skinner box when the behavior causes intravenous delivery of a mixture of cocaine and heroin. When the response was then extinguished in a different Skinner box, responding was at the same level as it was when extinction was conducted in the same context, but once again, on return to the original context, responding was substantially renewed.

Renewal is also well known in humans. For instance, it is readily observed in laboratory conditioning tasks (e.g., Alvarez, Johnson, & Grillon, 2007; Milad, Orr, Pitman, & Rauch, 2005). Using "virtual reality" technology, Alvarez and colleagues (2007) found that after a tone was paired with shock in one virtual context (e.g., the interior of an airport) and then extinguished in another (e.g., on a city street), electrodermal and fear-potentiated startle responding was renewed when the tone was returned to and tested in the original context. Renewal in humans has practical applications. Since extinction is thought to be involved in many cognitive-behavioral therapies designed to reduce maladaptive thoughts, emotions, and behaviors, the basic interdependence of context and extinction may have implications for clinical lapse and relapse (e.g., Bouton, 2002). Consistent with this possibility, there is evidence that the effects of exposure therapy in one context can be context-dependent; for example, when tested in a second context, anxiety in response to a spider (e.g., Mystkowski, Craske, Echiverri, & Labus, 2006) or cravings and salivation in response to alcohol cues (Collins & Brandon, 2002) can be renewed. Renewal likewise occurs in more explicitly "cognitive" paradigms. For example, Rosas, Vila, Lugo, and Lopez (2001) gave human participants a series of Pavlovian-like trials in which a series of fictitious patients ingested a drug (e.g., "Batim") and then experienced a side effect (e.g., "fever"). The medical cases were said to occur in a particular context—in either the Vanguardia Hospital or the Central Clinic. In a second phase, the same drug was associated with a different side effect in the other context. In a final test, when returned to the original context, the participants expressed the belief that the drug would cause the original side effect. The overall point is that renewal appears to be a fairly general feature of learning that operates over a range of circumstances and species. The context is thus extremely important in determining behavior after extinction.

CONTEXTS AS OCCASION SETTERS

In the Pavlovian renewal experiment, it is possible that the contexts are simple eliciting cues, like Pavlov's bell, just like what I described as the first role of context earlier. For example, in simple ABA renewal, Context A may acquire a direct association with the US during conditioning, and Context B might acquire an inhibitory one (e.g., Rescorla & Wagner, 1972). These associations might then summate with associations to the tone to create the performance we observe. Why is it necessary to explain renewal in some other way? The reason is, although direct associations between a context and a US can certainly be learned under the right conditions, experimenters have failed to detect any evidence that they are necessary to produce the renewal effect; renewal can occur without independent evidence of associations between the US and Context A or inhibitory associations between the US and Context B (e.g., Bouton & King, 1983; Bouton & Swartzentruber, 1986; for a review, see Bouton, 1991). In addition, strong context–US associations do not influence performance to a CS except when responding to the CS has previously been extinguished (e.g., Bouton, 1984; Bouton & King, 1986). Thus, demonstrable associations between the context and the US are neither necessary nor sufficient for a context to influence behavior to a CS. The implication is that contexts do not necessarily control behavior through their direct associations with the US the way that ordinary eliciting CSs do. They are somehow different. We (e.g., Bouton, 1991; Bouton & Swartzentruber, 1986) suggested that in producing the renewal effect, the contexts retrieve or "set the occasion" for the whole CS–US or CS–no US association (see Holland, 1992; Schmajuk & Holland, 1998; Swartzentruber, 1995).

Research on *occasion setting* (e.g., for reviews, see Holland, 1992; Swartzentruber, 1995) is therefore highly relevant. An *occasion setter* is a type of CS that modulates the response elicited by a second CS rather than simply eliciting behavior on its own. Instead of merely being associated with the US, the occasion setter appears to activate the association between the other CS and the US. It is usually studied in procedures in which a "target" CS is paired with the US on some trials but is presented without the US on others. In a "feature-positive discrimination," a second CS (a "feature" CS) occurs on those trials where the target is paired with the US. Thus, there is a mixture of *FT*+ and *T*– trials, where *F* is the feature, *T* is the target, and + and – are trials with the US and without it, respectively. Notice that the presence of the feature allows the subject to discriminate the positive and negative trials, and thus respond appropriately. In a "feature-negative discrimination," the feature CS is added on those trials when the target is *not* paired with the US: *T*+, *FT*–. In this case, the subject learns *not* to respond in the presence of the feature.

As in the basic renewal effect, there is nothing special about feature-positive and feature-negative discriminations in the sense that simple and direct associations to the feature (an excitatory one in the feature-positive case and an inhibitory one in the feature-negative case) can explain them (e.g., Pearce & Hall, 1980; Rescorla & Wagner, 1972; Wagner, 1981). And, in fact, when the feature and target occur simultaneously (coming on and going off at the same times), that is generally how the animal learns them. But Peter Holland discovered (e.g., Ross & Holland, 1981) that if the onset of the feature precedes the onset of target by a mere 10 seconds or so, the feature sets the occasion for responding to the target: It can enable responding to the target CS of the form that only the target–US association can control (e.g., a light feature does not elicit a head-jerking response in rats, but it will cause the rat head jerk to a tone target in a feature-positive [*LT*+, *T*–] discrimination; see also Rescorla, 1985). Holland has suggested that the "serial" presentation of feature-then-target allows occasion setting because the feature is not salient when the target comes on. All that remains of it is a memory trace. Consistent with this idea, Holland (1989) further showed that even simultaneous presentation of feature and target would permit occasion setting if the auditory feature were very weak in volume. Stimuli appear to acquire the occasion setting function rather than the simple eliciting function when they are not salient, or perhaps when they are less salient than the target CS that occurs with them.

This point is relevant to understanding context effects because the typical apparatus context is not especially salient either. For example, in fear conditioning experiments in my own laboratory, the rat is usually put in the experimental chamber for a 90-minute session each day. In those sessions, a 60-second CS might be presented four to eight times, and the animal is usually in the box for at least 20 minutes before the first CS is presented. Thus, as I noted earlier, the context is a long-duration stimulus that embeds or surrounds the CS and the US in time. The long-duration property of the context, and the fact that its onset precedes that of the CS, might serve to reduce its salience by the time the CS itself is presented; the animal might habituate to the context's presence, and pay less attention to it the longer it is present in the background. This fact might make sense of the common finding that, as noted earlier, a context switch after conditioning can have surprisingly little effect on responding to the CS. And other evidence suggests that context-shock and CS-shock associations do not summate when the CS is presented 5 minutes after, as opposed to immediately, when the rat is placed in the chamber (Miller, Grahame, & Hallam, 1990). Indeed, there is evidence that the salience of a long cue is reduced within 2 minutes (Darby & Pearce, 1995). Thus, contextual cues that precede the CS in time might be less salient and likely to control responding to a CS through their direct associations with the US—and more through their occasion-setting capability.

It is worth noting that the distinction between a CS's effectiveness as an eliciting cue on the one hand and as an occasion setter on the other is probably not all-or-none. In many occasion-setting experiments involving the feature-positive (*FT*+, *T*–) discrimination, the occasion-setting feature elicits responses directly despite its additional ability to occasion-set responding to the target. Thus, a feature stimulus can be an eliciting CS and an occasion setter at the same time; the two mechanisms might fade into one another as one changes variables, like the feature salience, that might favor one mechanism or the other. And so it might be with contexts. As mentioned earlier, contexts can in fact elicit direct conditioned responses when they are associated with shock or with drugs (Fanselow, 1980; Siegel, 2005). And there is evidence that contextual cues associated with extinction can also develop direct inhibitory associations with the US under some conditions (e.g., Cunningham, 1979). Woods and Bouton (2006) recently made this point while discussing the effects of D-cycloserine on fear extinction. D-cylcoserine has attracted considerable attention recently as a way to enhance the effects of exposure therapy. The drug is an agonist for a type of brain receptor (the *N*-methyl-D-aspartic acid [NMDA] receptor) that is involved in long-term potentiation, a form of brain plasticity that might underlie many forms of learning. If extinction is new learning, the argument goes, then facilitating the NMDA receptor might also facilitate extinction learning. And it does: D-cycloserine administered during extinction can increase the rate at which extinction is learned (e.g., Walker, Ressler, Lu, & Davis, 2002). However, the drug does not necessarily eliminate the context's fundamental role in extinction: We found that fear extinction was learned quicker with D-cycloserine, but it was still context-specific and vulnerable to relapse in the form of the renewal effect (Bouton, Vurbic, & Woods, 2008; Woods & Bouton, 2006). Based on other known effects of the drug on extinction (Ledgerwood, Richardson, & Cranney, 2003, 2004), we argued that the drug might work by enhancing direct inhibitory conditioning of the context. It is possible that the drug somehow increases the salience of contextual cues, and (consistent with the earlier result) thus favors the learning of direct inhibition, rather than occasion setting, in the extinction context. Either occasion setting or inhibition in the extinction context would reduce responding to the CS, but it would also make extinction performance fundamentally context-specific (see also Morris & Bouton, 2007).

OTHER PROPERTIES OF LONG-DURATION STIMULI

Although the long-duration nature of the context may usually encourage the occasion-setting function, it might also influence the form of the conditioned response that the context elicits when it is directly associated with the US. Learning theorists have long known that the duration of a Pavlovian signal can influence the form of the conditioned response. For example, in rabbit eyeblink conditioning, a mild shock delivered near the rabbit's eye will elicit both an eyeblink response and a fear response (indicated, e.g., by a change in heart rate). With short CSs (typically those that terminate in a US less than 1 second after CS onset), the CS elicits a protective blink of the eye where the US is delivered. With longer CSs (e.g., 6.75 seconds or more), the CS elicits a change of heart rate response suggesting fear instead of the blink (VanDercar & Schneiderman, 1967). Conditioned responses get the organism ready for the upcoming US, and different types of responses are presumably functional at different timescales (e.g., Akins, Domjan, & Gutiérrez, 1994; Timberlake, 2001). Based on this sort of analysis, Bouton, Mineka, and Barlow (2001) proposed that cues signaling a trauma relatively remotely in time might elicit anxiety, a conditioned response designed to cope with trauma on that timescale, whereas CSs that signal the US more closely in time might elicit fear or panic (see also Bouton, 2005). Consistent with this perspective, Waddell, Morris, and Bouton (2006) found that lesions of the bed nucleus of the stria terminalis, a brain area thought to control anxiety rather than fear behaviors (e.g., Walker, Toufexis, & Davis, 2003), abolished conditioning to a CS whose onset occurred 10 minutes before a footshock US was delivered, but had no effect on a CS whose onset occurred 1 minute before the footshock. Thus, long-duration signals may elicit anxiety mediated by the bed nucleus of the stria terminalis, whereas shorter-duration CSs do not.

Waddell and colleagues (2006) further showed that lesions of the bed nucleus of the stria terminalis also abolished conditioning of the context that occurred when the rat received eight footshocks delivered in a 90-minute session. One important effect of such context conditioning is that it can "reinstate" fear to an extinguished CS; if the rat receives several USs after extinction, so that the USs condition the context in which the CS is later tested, the contextual conditioning augments fear of the extinguished CS (e.g., Bouton, 1984; Bouton & King, 1986). Waddell and colleagues also found that the bed nucleus lesion reduced that reinstatement. The implication is that reinstatement occurs because the shocks might cause anxiety to be conditioned to the context, and the presence of anxiety during the test might augment fear of the CS. Interestingly, conditioning of the long-duration context has little effect on fear elicited by CS that has been conditioned (paired with a US) but not extinguished (e.g., Bouton, 1984; Bouton & King, 1986; see also Miller et al., 1990). In contrast, it has a strong effect on a CS that is under the influence of extinction (Bouton, 1984; Bouton & King, 1986). One possibility is that anxiety itself has contextual properties that might retrieve the memory of conditioning (e.g., Bouton, Rosengard, Achenbach, Peck, & Brooks, 1993) or simply change the context from the one that otherwise prevailed during extinction (e.g., García-Gutiérrez & Rosas, 2003).

Either possibility suggests that reinstatement is a special example of the renewal effect.

Some writers have argued that another feature of the apparatus context that makes it different from an ordinary CS is its complexity (e.g., Fanselow, 2007). The typical Skinner box is really composed of a very large assortment of stimuli: It has various tactile features, odors emanating from different locations, and a multitude of visual and auditory cues (e.g., the exhaust fan that typically blows in the background) that all change as the animal moves around in the environment. Fanselow has argued that before the rat can associate such a complex stimulus with footshock, it must first associate these various features and put them together in an integrated representation. Consistent with this possibility, the rat needs a little time in the box before it can learn about it; if the rat is shocked immediately upon placement in a novel apparatus, it will not learn to associate the box with shock (e.g., Fanselow, 1986, 1990). But if the shock is delayed for a minute or two (so the rat has more time to learn about the box), or if the rat is exposed to the box for a minute or two the day before getting placed in the box and immediately shocked, then the rat will readily learn to associate the box with shock (Fanselow, 1990; Kiernan & Westbrook, 1993). Presumably, the extra time in the context allows the animal to interassociate the various cues that compose it (e.g., McLaren, Kaye, & Mackintosh, 1989). Simpler CSs, such as tones and lights, require much less exposure for learning (Fanselow, 2007). Unitizing the different contextual features seems to require the hippocampus; lesions of this part of the brain reduce context conditioning but typically do not influence conditioning of simpler cues, such as tones (e.g., Kim & Fanselow, 1992). Interestingly, a role for hippocampus in the renewal effect, a different example of context learning, is not as clear (e.g., see Corcoran & Maren, 2004; Frohardt, Guarraci, & Bouton, 2000), and there is no evidence that complexity of the context is a factor that favors the occasion-setting function emphasized earlier. But overall, it is worth noting that the contexts used in animal learning experiments are often (1) longer in duration and (2) more complex than typical CSs, such as brief tones and lights, and these two factors do appear to influence how the organism uses them.

WHY AREN'T LEARNING AND MEMORY ALWAYS CONTEXT SPECIFIC?

As noted earlier, one of the most interesting facts about the contextual control of behavior is that the context is not always very important. For example, the contextual conditioning that causes reinstatement of fear to an extinguished CS (as in Waddell et al., 2006) has no impact on CSs that have not been extinguished (Bouton, 1984; Bouton & King, 1986). And we have often seen that a context switch performed after conditioning has surprisingly little effect on behavior elicited by the CS. It is worth noting that the fact that the context switch does not disrupt conditioned responding after conditioning suggests that the renewal effect is more than merely a case of generalization decrement, where (for example) the CS is simply perceived as a different stimulus in the two contexts. (If it were, then the amount of generalization of conditioning and extinction should be equivalent across contexts.) The difference in the importance of the context after conditioning and extinction is also indicated by the ABC and AAB renewal effects, where responding is renewed when the organism is tested in a context that differs from the ones in which both conditioning and extinction occurred. Neither ABC nor AAB renewal would be possible if extinction learning generalized as much to the new context as does conditioning. Extinction is thus clearly more context-specific than simple conditioning. The question to be addressed in this section is why this should be so. Research in animals and humans suggests several tentative answers.

The context-dependence of extinction (but not conditioning) has an interesting parallel in the effects of context in studies of human memory. Although memory for word lists in humans is sometimes weakened when the context is changed (e.g., Godden & Baddeley, 1975; Smith, 1979), such effects are often rather difficult to obtain (see Smith, 1988). In contrast, it is relatively easy to observe a context effect on memory in interference designs in which the participant is given one word list in one context, and another list in a second context (Smith, 1988). Here, memory becomes context-specific, just as it appears to be in animals after an interfering extinction treatment. Smith and Vela (2001) performed a meta-analysis suggesting that the effect of context on remembering a single list is really always there but often diminished by other processes that support memory retrieval at the time of the test. For example, *outshining* refers to the idea that if other cues besides the context can support memory retrieval, and if they are present in both the training and testing context, then they will diminish any context switch effect. Such a process is easy to imagine in an animal experiment, when the animal is tested with a CS in a different context: The animal is responding to a highly salient cue for the US (the CS) that might easily overcome the absence of contextual support in the changed context. According to familiar (competition) principles of conditioning (e.g., Rescorla & Wagner, 1972), the CS is a better predictor of the US than the context, so it is not necessarily surprising for it to control behavior more than the context does.

But something happens in extinction that makes the context relevant. One early idea (Bouton, 1993) was that extinction involves inhibitory learning, and that inhibition conditioned to the CS might be more context-specific than simple excitation. The hypothesis was tested and quickly disconfirmed in several experiments: Conditioned inhibition transfers as readily across contexts as conditioned excitation does (e.g., Bouton & Nelson, 1994; Nelson, 2002; Nelson & Bouton, 1997). Another early idea (Bouton, 1993) was that extinction is context-specific because it is the second thing learned about the CS. Nelson (2002) confirmed the fact that whether the "meaning" of the CS is excitatory or inhibitory is less relevant than whether excitation or inhibition was the first or second thing learned about the CS. In either case, when it was the first the learned, the meaning transferred perfectly across contexts; when it was the second thing learned, it did not. Consistent with this possibility, we know that in counterconditioning designs in which a CS is first paired with shock and then with food pellets (or vice versa), fear conditioning or appetitive conditioning are more context-specific when they are in the second position (Peck & Bouton, 1990). It is as if the learning and memory system encodes the second thing learned about a stimulus as a conditional, context-specific exception to the rule. Bouton (1994) suggested some functional grounds for why the learning and memory system might have evolved this way.

At the present time, it appears that the outcomes of early Phase 2 trials (e.g., the occurrence of no US in extinction when a US is expected) might cause the subject to pay more attention to the context (Bouton, 1993; cf. Pearce & Hall, 1980). We now know, for example, that if a CS has been conditioned and then extinguished in one context, conditioned responding to a second CS that is subsequently conditioned there is now context-specific (Rosas & Callejas-Aguilera, 2007). The extinction treatment seems to encourage the animal to pay attention to the context. We also know that after extinction in one context (e.g., Context B), the context in which the CS was originally conditioned (e.g., Context A) now also controls performance in response to the CS (Harris, Jones, Bailey, & Westbrook, 2000): After extinction, there is more responding to the CS in the original context (A) than in a neutral context (C). Thus, extinction seems to increase attentiveness to other contexts besides the context in which extinction occurs. The possibility has been extended and confirmed in predictive learning experiments with humans (Rosas & Callejas-Aguilera, 2006). In one experiment, each participant was involved in two separate and very different predictive learning tasks that each occurred in different contexts. In one task, fictional foods were paired with gastric distress in one set of contexts (fictitious restaurants), and in the other task, different-colored garden products would make plants flourish and grow in another set of contexts (different farms). Provided that extinction was experienced in the first-learned task, cue–outcome associations in the second task—with completely different cues, outcomes, and contexts—were judged to be weaker when the context was changed. Without extinction in the first task, there was no such context specificity in the second. Thus, extinction or, more generally, a situation where new learning replaces older learning (Nelson & Callejas-Aguilera, 2007), introduces surprise and/or ambiguity, and this causes the organism to pay attention to all contexts.

The major exception to the "second thing learned" rule is a phenomenon known as *latent inhibition* (e.g., Lubow, 1989). In this effect, a CS is first presented a number of times on its own, without being paired with a US. In a second phase, the CS is then paired with a US; the latent inhibition result is slower conditioning with a CS that has been preexposed than with a novel CS. One of the most important things we know about latent inhibition is that it is context-specific; CS preexposure causes less interference when conditioning and preexposure are conducted in different contexts (e.g., Hall & Channell, 1985; Rosas & Bouton, 1997b). Thus, even though preexposure is a first learning experience, its effect is clearly context-specific. Latent inhibition might engage its own idiosyncratic context mechanism, however. When a tone or light CS is presented without a consequence, it is no different from other stimuli that arguably make up the context, such as the intermittent fan noise or odor that the animal occasionally notices in the background. These may ultimately become part of a unitized representation of the context, as discussed earlier. When the CS is subsequently presented and paired with the US, it is difficult to extract the CS from its place in the context. This might make it slow to be effective as a CS; but in a different environment, where the CS has not been absorbed, learning to associate the CS with the US would be easier because the CS has not become integrated with the background. Gluck and Myers (1993) have presented a similar analysis of the consequences of preexposure to a CS.

Hall and Mondragón (1998) have emphasized another possible result of preexposure to the CS in a given context. According to the models of Wagner (1981, 2003; Wagner & Brandon, 1989), an association between the context and the CS would be formed, and such an association would allow the context to retrieve or "prime" the representation of the CS into a secondary state of activation in working memory. Because primed stimuli do not receive a high level of processing in working memory, this would reduce the CS's ability to control responding. Presenting the CS in a different context would eliminate this priming effect, thus making it easier for the organism to learn about the CS, and for the CS to control responding (see Hall & Mondragón, 1998; Honey, Hall, & Bonardi,

1993). If the same mechanism were to develop during CS–US pairings, it would go against any inherent context specificity of responding to the CS; that is, although the context switch might attenuate the conditioned response (because learning is generally context-specific), any tendency for the conditioned response to decrease after a context switch would be offset by the fact that the CS would be liberated from priming and be more ready to control responding. Perhaps consistent with this possibility, we have recently shown that a context switch can actually *increase* fear of a CS after extensive conditioning (Bouton, Frohardt, Sunsay, Waddell, & Morris, 2008; see also Kaye & Mackintosh, 1990). Both attentional and associative processes may come into play and cause some types of learning to be context-specific and other types not.

THE TEMPORAL CONTEXT

As I noted earlier, most studies of context effects in learning and memory laboratories have manipulated the apparatus or room in which learning and remembering occur. There are writers who would prefer to stick with apparatus as the sole definition of *context* (Fanselow, 2007). However, it seems clear that many different kinds of cues—besides the apparatus or room in which the participant in an experiment is asked to learn—can play the same role (e.g., see Bouton, 2002). We just considered context effects evoked by merely cognitive instructions in humans (e.g., Rosas & Callejas-Aguilera, 2006). As another example, drugs can provide internal contexts, and support retrieval and occasion setting through *state-dependent retention* (e.g., Overton, 1985). When rats are given fear extinction while under the influence of alcohol (e.g., Cunningham, 1979; Lattal, 2007) or a benzodiazepine tranquilizer (Bouton, Kenney, & Rosengard, 1990), fear is renewed when the animal is tested outside the drug state. In effect, extinction performance may be as specific to the context provided by the drug as it is to any external apparatus. Other *interoceptive contexts* that may support memory retrieval include hormonal state (e.g., Ahlers & Richardson, 1985); mood state (e.g., Bower, 1981; Eich, 1995, 2007); deprivation state (e.g., Davidson, 1993; see also Balleine, 2001); expectation of events (e.g., Bouton et al., 1993; García-Gutiérrez & Rosas, 2003); recent events, such as recent CS–US or CS–no US trials (e.g., Bouton, Woods, & Pineño, 2004; see also Woods & Bouton, 2007); and perhaps even body temperature (Briggs & Riccio, 2007). In principle, any of these different stimuli may play any of the context roles discussed earlier.

In my own laboratory we have become especially interested in the fact that the passage of time provides an additional source of contextual change (e.g., Bouton, 1993). As time passes, some stimulus correlate (or correlates) of time might change, so that after a retention interval the organism is in a different "temporal context." Thus, as several memory theorists have assumed, the forgetting that occurs over a long retention interval may be due at least in part to a mismatch between the contexts present during learning and testing (e.g., Estes, 1955; McGeoch, 1932; Mensink & Raaijmakers, 1988; Spear, 1978). This perspective provides an explanation of *spontaneous recovery*, the effect (first reported by Pavlov, 1927) in which extinguished responding to the CS recovers if time elapses following extinction: Spontaneous recovery is a renewal effect that occurs when the organism is tested outside the temporal context of extinction (Bouton, 1993). The implication is that both spontaneous recovery and renewal are due to failures to retrieve extinction because of contextual change. Consistent with this possibility, renewal effects resulting from a change of physical context, and spontaneous recovery resulting from a change in temporal context, are both reduced if the organism is given a cue that "reminds" it of extinction at the time of the test (Brooks, 2002; Brooks & Bouton, 1993, 1994). Thus, renewal and spontaneous recovery might result from a common mechanism. Time—or some change in stimulation that correlates with time—is also part of the context that influences memory and learning.

The idea that a retention interval can be treated as a context change is consistent with the broad parallel between retention interval and physical context switch effects that have been noted in the literature (see Bouton, 1993). Learning phenomena that are disrupted by a change of context (e.g., extinction and latent inhibition) are also disrupted by a retention interval, while those that are not affected by a change of physical context (e.g., simple conditioning) are also not as readily affected by retention interval (e.g., Gleitman, 1971; Hendersen, 1985). Bouton (1993) predicted that if the effects of physical context switches and retention intervals are mediated by the same underlying process, then the effect of performing both manipulations simultaneously should be greater than that of manipulating either alone. Put casually, manipulating context and time together should create an even bigger kind of context switch. The biggest retrieval failure should occur when the two manipulations are combined.

This prediction quickly collides with a paradox that David Riccio and his associates have raised for context change accounts of forgetting (e.g., Riccio, Richardson, & Ebner, 1984; Riccio, Rabinowitz, & Alxelrod, 1994). They have noted that generalization between similar stimuli increases as time elapses between training and testing (e.g., Perkins & Weyant, 1958). If humans and other animals thus differentiate less between stimuli over time, how can forgetting be due to subtle context change that occurs over time? My colleagues and I have considered and attempted to resolve the paradox (Bouton, Nelson, & Rosas, 1999; Rosas & Bouton, 1997a, 1998; see also Rosas et al., 2001). We began by noting that the increasing generalization that occurs between stimuli over time itself appears to result from retrieval failure; generalization gradients that have flattened or broadened over time can be resharpened if the subject is given a reminder treatment (e.g., Moye & Thomas, 1982; Zhou & Riccio, 1996). But why? We suggested that physical contexts are always presented within the context of the passage of time; that is, the temporal context is *superordinate* to the physical context. Increased generalization between physical contexts thus occurs because of forgetting due to temporal context change. There is no inherent incompatibility between a context change account of forgetting and increasing generalization over time. There are no theoretical or empirical grounds for supposing that generalization around the temporal context will change over time.

To test the approach, we returned to the "additivity" prediction noted earlier; superordinate or not, manipulating time with physical context should still produce a bigger context change. But we also noted that this hypothesis needs to be tested in a particular way. If generalization between contexts does increase over time (e.g., Rosas & Bouton, 1997a), then the degree to which the perceived physical context changes as a consequence of a context switch after short and long retention intervals is not the same. To make them comparable, we need to remind the animals of the contexts before the test at the long delay. When this is done, the effects of time and physical context change have been shown to be additive in latent inhibition (Rosas & Bouton, 1997a; see also Westbrook, Jones, Bailey, & Harris, 2000) and extinction (Rosas & Bouton, 1998). Rosas and colleagues (2001) also reported completely parallel results in a causal judgment scenario in humans. We interpret these converging results as consistent with the idea that time and context influence memory through a common mechanism: Time and physical context change both cause background (contextual) stimulus change.

We have gone on to study the temporal context in more detail by asking how animals use the passage of time when it is a cue that predicts whether or not the next CS will be paired with the US (Bouton & García-Gutiérrez, 2006; Bouton & Hendrix, 2009). If time plays the role of a contextual stimulus, then animals should readily use it to disambiguate the current meaning of a CS, just as they do with other types of context. Rats were given a series of presentations of a tone CS separated by an intermixed sequence of long and short intertrial intervals (ITIs). For some rats, the tone was paired with a food pellet when it occurred at the end of a long ITI (e.g., 16 minutes), but the tone was presented without food if it occurred after a short ITI (e.g., 4 minutes). In this sort of "long+/short–" discrimination, the rats quickly learn to use time as a context, responding when the tone is presented after a long ITI, but not when it is presented after a short one. Control groups given the same ITIs, but with either ITI ending in tone–pellet and tone–no pellet half the time, respond equivalently after the short and long intervals—so the differential responding in the experimental group clearly indicated contextual control by the ITI. But the interesting new result occurs with the opposite discrimination, in which the *short* ITI signals that the tone will be paired with pellet, but the long ITI signals that it will not (a "short+/long–" discrimination). Here rats learned the discrimination only after extended training; it was far more difficult to learn short+/long– than long+/short–. Thus, there is a marked asymmetry in how animals use time as a context.

To explain the results, we have suggested that the passage of time may generate a series of hypothetical stimuli that occur in a sequence: A, then B, then C, and so forth. In this scheme, during a long ITI, the organism might go through Stimulus A then Stimulus B, and during a shorter interval the animal might only go through Stimulus A, without B. In the temporal element framework, the learnable long+/short– discrimination is one in which the tone CS is paired with the US after AB, but not after A. It is therefore an AB+/A– discrimination, that is, a new type of feature-positive discrimination. In contrast, the difficult short+/long– is a discrimination of the form A+/AB–, a new type of feature-negative discrimination. The crucial insight is that feature-positive discriminations are often learned more rapidly than feature-negative discriminations, a phenomenon known as the *feature-positive effect* (Hearst, 1984; Jenkins & Sainsbury, 1970). At the present time, other ways investigators have modeled the passage of time (e.g., as the number of pulses emanating from a pacemaker accumulated in working memory [Gibbon, Church, & Meck, 1984]; or as a set of oscillators changing between states at different rates [Church & Broadbent, 1990]) do not fare as well in accounting for the characteristics of time when it acts as a contextual stimulus. Thus, studies that investigate the characteristics of time as a context may provide new insights into the psychological processes that underlie timing.

CONCLUSION

To summarize, *context* can take multiple forms in associative learning theory. I started by noting that the term can mean a background stimulus that elicits behavior directly, a stimulus that competes with more obvious CSs for learning and performance, a retrieval cue, or an occasion setter that modulates the strength of the response to CSs that occur in it. The latter function may emerge because long-duration background stimuli are not very salient, and it appears to play an essential role in regulating behavior in extinction. Current research suggests that context becomes important when experience directs the organism's attention to it. And I have also suggested that the *context* can be provided by any of a wide variety of cues, including (for example) interoceptive states and the passage of time—another way in which *context* can take multiple forms. There are, of course, additional roles the context can play in influencing cognition and perception (e.g., Eich, 2007; Smith, 2007). But in associative learning theory alone, *context* can have a number of meanings that have all proven essential in understanding learning and behavior.

ACKNOWLEDGMENTS

This work was supported by Grant No. 2 R01 MH064847 from the National Institutes of Health. I thank Professor Juan M. Rosas for his comments.

REFERENCES

Ahlers, S. T., & Richardson, R. (1985). Administration of dexamethasone prior to training blocks ACTH-induced recovery of an extinguished avoidance response. *Behavioral Neuroscience*, *99*, 760–764.

Akins, C. K., Domjan, M., & Gutiérrez, G. (1994). Topography of sexually conditioned behavior in male Japanese quail (*Coturnix japonica*) depends on the CS–US interval. *Journal of Experimental Psychology: Animal Behavior Processes*, *20*, 199–209.

Alvarez, R. P., Johnson, L., & Grillon, C. (2007). Contextual-specifity of short-delay extinction in humans: Renewal of fear-potentiated startle in a virtual environment. *Learning and Memory*, *14*, 247–253.

Baker, A. G., Murphy, R., Mehta, R., & Baetu, I. (2005). Mental models of causation: A comparative view. In A. J. Wills (Ed.), *New directions in human associative learning* (pp. 11–40). Mahwah, NJ: Erlbaum.

Balleine, B. W. (2001). Incentive processes in instrumental conditioning. In R. R. Mowrer & S. B. Klein (Eds.), *Handbook of contemporary learning theories* (pp. 307–366). Hillsdale, NJ: Erlbaum.

Balsam, P. D., & Tomie, A. (1985). *Context and learning*. Hillsdale, NJ: Erlbaum.

Bargh, J. A., & Chartrand, T. L. (1999). The unbearable automaticity of being. *American Psychologist*, *54*, 462–479.

Bouton, M. E. (1984). Differential control by context in the inflation and reinstatement paradigms. *Journal of Experimental Psychology: Animal Behavior Processes*, *10*, 56–74.

Bouton, M. E. (1991). Context and retrieval in extinction and in other examples of interference in simple associative learning. In L. Dachowski & C. F. Flaherty (Eds.), *Current topics in animal learning: Brain, emotion, and cognition* (pp. 25–53). Hillsdale, NJ: Erlbaum.

Bouton, M. E. (1993). Context, time, and memory retrieval in the interference paradigms of Pavlovian learning. *Psychological Bulletin, 114*, 80–99.

Bouton, M. E. (1994). Conditioning, remembering, and forgetting. *Journal of Experimental Psychology: Animal Behavior Processes, 20*, 219–231.

Bouton, M. E. (2002). Context, ambiguity, and unlearning: Sources of relapse after behavioral extinction. *Biological Psychiatry, 52*, 976–986.

Bouton, M. E. (2004). Context and behavioral processes in extinction. *Learning and Memory, 11*, 485–494.

Bouton, M. E. (2005). Behavior systems and the contextual control of anxiety, fear, and panic. In L. Feldman Barrett, P. M. Niedenthal, & P. Winkielman (Eds.), *Emotion and unconsciousness* (pp. 205–227). New York: Guilford Press.

Bouton, M. E. (2007). Context: The concept in the human and animal memory domains. In H. L. Roediger, Y. Dudai, & S. M. Fitzpatrick (Eds.), *Science of memory: Concepts* (pp. 115–119). Oxford, UK: Oxford University Press.

Bouton, M. E., & Bolles, R. C. (1985). Contexts, event-memories, and extinction. In P. D. Balsam & A. Tomie (Eds.), *Context and learning* (pp. 133–166). Hillsdale, NJ: Erlbaum.

Bouton, M. E., Frohardt, R. J., Sunsay, C., Waddell, J., & Morris, R. W. (2008). Contextual control of inhibition with reinforcement: Adaptation and timing mechanisms. *Journal of Experimental Psychology: Animal Behavior Processes, 34*, 223–236.

Bouton, M. E., & García-Gutiérrez, A. (2006). Intertrial interval as a contextual stimulus. *Behavioural Processes, 71*, 307–317.

Bouton, M. E., & Hendrix, M. (2009). *Intertrial interval as a contextual stimulus: Further analysis of a novel asymmetry in temporal discrimination learning.* Manuscript submitted for publication.

Bouton, M. E., Kenney, F. A., & Rosengard, C. (1990). State-dependent fear extinction with two benzodiazepine tranquilizers. *Behavioral Neuroscience, 104*, 44–55.

Bouton, M. E., & King, D. A. (1983). Contextual control of the extinction of conditioned fear: Tests for the associative value of the context. *Journal of Experimental Psychology: Animal Behavior Processes, 9*, 248–265.

Bouton, M. E., & King, D. A. (1986). Effect of context on performance to conditioned stimuli with mixed histories of reinforcement and nonreinforcement. *Journal of Experimental Psychology: Animal Behavior Processes, 12*, 4–15.

Bouton, M. E., Mineka, S., & Barlow, D. H. (2001). A modern learning theory perspective on the etiology of panic disorder. *Psychological Review, 108*, 4–32.

Bouton, M. E., & Nelson, J. B. (1994). Context-specificity of target versus feature inhibition in a feature-negative discrimination. *Journal of Experimental Psychology: Animal Behavior Processes*, *20*, 51–65.

Bouton, M. E., Nelson, J. B., & Rosas, J. M. (1999). Stimulus generalization, context change, and forgetting. *Psychological Bulletin*, *125*, 171–186.

Bouton, M. E., Rosengard, C., Achenbach, G. G., Peck, C. A., & Brooks, D. C. (1993). Effects of contextual conditioning and unconditional stimulus presentation on performance in appetitive conditioning. *Quarterly Journal of Experimental Psychology*, *46B*, 63–95.

Bouton, M. E., & Swartzentruber, D. (1986). Analysis of the associative and occasion-setting properties of contexts participating in a Pavlovian discrimination. *Journal of Experimental Psychology: Animal Behavior Processes*, *12*, 333–350.

Bouton, M. E., Vurbic, D., & Woods, A. M. (2008). D-cycloserine facilitates context-specific fear extinction learning. *Neurobiology of Learning and Memory*, *90*, 504–510.

Bouton, M. E., & Woods, A. M. (2008). Extinction: Behavioral mechanisms and their implications. In J. H. Byrne (Ed.), *Concise learning and memory: The editor's selection* (pp. 627–648). Oxford, UK: Elsevier.

Bouton, M. E., Woods, A. M., & Pineño, O. (2004). Occasional reinforced trials during extinction can slow the rate of rapid reacquisition. *Learning and Motivation*, *35*, 371–390.

Bower, G. H. (1981). Mood and memory. *American Psychologist*, *36*, 129–148.

Briggs, J. F., & Riccio, D. C. (2007). Retrograde amnesia for extinction: Similarities with amnesia for original acquisition memories. *Learning and Behavior*, *35*, 131–140.

Brooks, D. C. (2000). Recent and remote extinction cues reduce spontaneous recovery. *Quarterly Journal of Experimental Psychology*, *53B*, 25–58.

Brooks, D. C., & Bouton, M. E. (1993). A retrieval cue for extinction attenuates spontaneous recovery. *Journal of Experimental Psychology: Animal Behavior Processes*, *19*, 77–89.

Brooks, D. C., & Bouton, M. E. (1994). A retrieval cue for extinction attenuates response recovery (renewal) caused by a return to the conditioning context. *Journal of Experimental Psychology: Animal Behavior Processes*, *20*, 366–379.

Church, R. M., & Broadbent, H. A. (1990). Alternative representations of time, number, and rate. *Cognition*, *37*, 55–81.

Collins, B. N., & Brandon, T. H. (2002). Effects of extinction context and retrieval cues on alcohol cue reactivity among nonalcoholic drinkers. *Journal of Consulting and Clinical Psychology*, *70*, 390–397.

Corcoran, K. A., & Maren, S. (2004). Factors regulating the effects of hippocampal inactivation on renewal of conditional fear after extinction. *Learning and Memory*, *11*, 598–603.

Crombag, H. S., Grimm, J. W., & Shaham, Y. (2003). Effect of dopamine receptor antagonists on renewal of cocaine seeking by reexposure to drug-associated contextual cues. *Neuropsychopharmacology*, *27*, 1006–1015.

Crombag, H. S., & Shaham, Y. (2002). Renewal of drug seeking by contextual cues after prolonged extinction in rats. *Behavioral Neuroscience, 116*, 169–173.

Cunningham, C. L. (1979). Alcohol as a cue for extinction: State dependency produced by conditioned inhibition. *Animal Learning and Behavior, 7*, 45–52.

Darby, R. J., & Pearce, J. M. (1995). Effects of context on responding during a compound stimulus. *Journal of Experimental Psychology: Animal Behavior Processes, 21*, 143–154.

Davidson, T. L. (1993). The nature and function of interoceptive signals to feed: Toward integration of physiological and learning perspectives. *Psychological Review, 100*, 640–657.

Denniston, J. C., Savastano, H. I., & Miller, R. R. (2001). The extended comparator hypothesis: Learning by contiguity, responding by relative strength. In R. R. Mower & S. B. Klein (Eds.), *Handbook of contemporary learning theories* (pp. 65–118). Mahwah, NJ: Erlbaum.

Eich, E. (1995). Searching for mood dependent memory. *Psychological Science, 6*, 67–75.

Eich, E. (2007). Context: Mood, memory and the concept of context. In H. L. Roediger, Y. Dudai, & S. M. Fitzpatrick (Eds.), *Science of memory: Concepts* (pp. 107–110). Oxford, UK: Oxford University Press.

Estes, W. K. (1955). Statistical theory of spontaneous recovery and regression. *Psychological Review, 62*, 145–154.

Fanselow, M. S. (1980). Conditional and unconditional components of post-shock freezing in rats. *Pavlovian Journal of Biological Sciences, 15*, 177–182.

Fanselow, M. S. (1986). Associative vs. topographical accounts of the immediate shock freezing deficit in rats: Implications for the response selection rules governing species specific defensive reactions. *Learning and Motivation, 17*, 16–39.

Fanselow, M. S. (1990). Factors governing one-trial contextual conditioning. *Animal Learning and Behavior, 18*, 264–270.

Fanselow, M. S. (2007). Context: What's so special about it? In H. L. Roediger, Y. Dudai, & S. M. Fitzpatrick (Eds.), *Science of memory: Concepts* (pp. 101–105). Oxford, UK: Oxford University Press.

Frohardt, R. J., Guarraci, F. A., & Bouton, M. E. (2000). The effects of neurotoxic hippocampal lesions on two effects of context after fear extinction. *Behavioral Neuroscience, 114*, 227–240.

Gallistel, C. R., & Gibbon, J. (2000). Time, rate, and conditioning. *Psychological Review, 107*, 289–344.

García-Gutiérrez, A., & Rosas, J. M. (2003). Context change as the mechanism of reinstatement in causal learning. *Journal of Experimental Psychology: Animal Behavior Processes, 29*, 292–310.

Gibbon, J., Meck, W. H., & Church, R. M. (1984). Scalar timing in memory. In J. Gibbon & L. Allan (Eds.), *Timing and time perception* (pp. 52–77). New York: New York Academy of Sciences.

Gleitman, H. (1971). Forgetting of long-term memories in animals. In W. K.

Honig & P. H. R. James (Eds.), *Animal memory* (pp. 1–44). New York: Academic Press.

Gluck, M., & Myers, C. E. (1993). Hippocampal mediation of stimulus representation: A computational theory. *Hippocampus, 3*, 492–516.

Godden, D. R., & Baddeley, A. D. (1975). Context-dependent memory in two natural environments: On land and underwater. *British Journal of Psychology, 66*, 325–331.

Hall, G., & Channell, S. (1985). Differential effects of contextual change on latent inhibition and on the habituation of an orienting response. *Journal of Experimental Psychology: Animal Behavior Processes, 11*, 470–481.

Hall, G., & Mondragón, E. (1998). Contextual control as occasion setting. In N. Schmajuk & P. C. Holland (Eds.), *Occasion setting: Associative learning and cognition in animals* (pp. 199–222). Washington, DC: American Psychological Association.

Harris, J. A., Jones, M. L., Bailey, G. K., & Westbrook, R.F. (2000). Contextual control over conditioned responding in an extinction paradigm. *Journal of Experimental Psychology: Animal Behavior Processes, 26*, 174–185.

Hearst, E. (1984). Absence of information: Some implications for learning, performance, and representational processes. In H. L. Roitblat, T. G. Bever, & H. S. Terrace (Eds.), *Animal cognition* (pp. 311–332). Hillsdale, NJ: Erlbaum.

Hendersen, R. W. (1985). Fearful memories: The motivational significance of forgetting. In F. R. Brush & J. B. Overmier (Eds.), *Affect, conditioning, and cognition: Essays on the determinants of behavior* (pp. 43–54). Hillsdale, NJ: Erlbaum.

Holland, P. C. (1989). Occasion setting with simultaneous compounds in rats. *Journal of Experimental Psychology: Animal Behavior Processes, 15*, 183–193.

Holland, P. C. (1992). Occasion setting in Pavlovian conditioning. In G. Bower (Ed.), *The psychology of learning and motivation* (Vol. 28, pp. 69–125). Orlando, FL: Academic Press.

Honey, R. C., Hall, G., & Bonardi, C. (1993). Negative priming in associative learning: Evidence from a serial-conditioning procedure. *Journal of Experimental Psychology: Animal Behavior Processes, 19*, 90–97.

Jenkins, H. M., & Sainsbury, R. S. (1970). Discrimination learning with the distinctive feature on positive or negative trials. In D. Mostovsky (Ed.), *Attention: Contemporary theory and analysis* (pp. 239–273). New York: Appleton–Century–Crofts.

Kamin, L. J. (1969). Predictability, surprise, attention, and conditioning. In B. A. Campbell & R. M. Church (Eds.), *Punishment and aversive behavior* (pp. 279–296). New York: Appleton–Century–Crofts.

Kaye, H., & Mackintosh, N. J. (1990). A change of context can enhance performance of an aversive but not of an appetitive conditioned response. *Quarterly Journal of Experimental Psychology, 42B*, 113–134.

Kiernan, M. J., & Westbrook, R. F. (1993). Effects of exposure to a to-be-shocked environment upon the rat's freezing response: Evidence for facilitation, latent inhibition, and perceptual learning. *Quarterly Journal of Experimental Psychology, 46B*, 271–288.

Kim, J. J., & Fanselow, M. S. (1992). Modality-specific retrograde amnesia of fear. *Science, 256*, 675–677.

Lattal, K. M. (2007). Effects of ethanol on the encoding, consolidation, and expression of extinction following contextual fear conditioning. *Behavioral Neuroscience, 121*, 1280–1292.

Ledgerwood, L., Richardson, R., & Cranney, J. (2003). Effects of D-cycloserine on extinction of conditioned freezing. *Behavioral Neuroscience, 117*, 341–349.

Ledgerwood, L., Richardson, R., & Cranney, J. (2004). D-Cycloserine and the facilitation of extinction of conditioned fear: Consequences for reinstatement. *Behavioral Neuroscience, 118*, 505–513.

Lubow, R. E. (1989). *Latent inhibition and conditioned attention theory.* Cambridge, UK: Cambridge University Press.

Mackintosh, N. J. (1975). A theory of attention: Variations in the associability of stimuli with reinforcement. *Psychological Review, 82*, 276–298.

McGeoch, J. A. (1932). Forgetting and the law of disuse. *Psychological Review, 39*, 352–370.

McLaren, I. P. L., Kaye, H., & Mackintosh, N. J. (1989). An associative theory of the representation of stimuli: Applications to perceptual learning and latent inhibition. In R. G. M. Morris (Ed.), *Parallel distributed processing: Implications for psychology and neurobiology* (pp. 102–130). New York: Oxford University Press.

Mensink, G.-J. M., & Raaijmakers, J. G. W. (1988). A model for interference and forgetting. *Psychological Review, 95*, 434–455.

Milad, M. R., Orr, S. P., Pitman, R. K., & Rauch, S. L. (2005). Context modulation of memory for fear extinction in humans. *Psychophysiology, 42*, 456–464.

Miller, R. R., Grahame, N. J., & Hallam, S. C. (1990). Summation of responding to CSs and an excitatory test context. *Animal Learning and Behavior, 18*, 29–34.

Morris, R. W., & Bouton, M. E. (2007). The effect of yohimbine on the extinction of conditioned fear: A role for context. *Behavioral Neuroscience, 121*, 501–514.

Moye, T. B., & Thomas, D. R. (1982). Effects of memory reactivation treatments on postdiscrimination generalization performance in pigeons. *Animal Learning and Behavior, 10*, 159–166.

Mystkowski, J. L., Craske, M. G., Echiverri, A. M., & Labus, J. S. (2006). Mental reinstatement of context and return of fear in spider-fearful participants. *Behavior Therapy, 37*, 49–60.

Nelson, J. B. (2002). Context specificity of excitation and inhibition in ambiguous stimuli. *Learning and Motivation, 33*, 284–310.

Nelson, J. B., & Bouton, M. E. (1997). The effects of a context switch following serial and simultaneous feature-negative discriminations. *Learning and Motivation, 28*, 56–84.

Nelson, J. B., & Bouton, M. E. (2002). Extinction, inhibition, and emotional intelligence. In L. Feldman Barrett & P. Salovey (Eds.), *The wisdom in feeling: Psychological processes in emotional intelligence* (pp. 60–85). New York: Guilford Press.

Nelson, J. B., & Callejas-Aguilera, J. E. (2007). The role of interferente produced by conflicting associations in contextual control. *Journal of Experimental Psychology: Animal Behavior Processes*, *33*, 314–326.

Overton, D. A. (1985). Contextual stimulus effects of drugs and internal states. In P. D. Balsam & A. Tomie (Eds.), *Context and learning* (pp. 357–384). Hillsdale, NJ: Erlbaum.

Pavlov, I. P. (1927). *Conditioned reflexes*. Oxford, UK: Oxford University Press.

Pearce, J. M., & Bouton, M. E. (2001). Theories of associative learning in animals. *Annual Review of Psychology*, *52*, 111–113.

Pearce, J. M., & Hall, G. (1980). A model for Pavlovian conditioning: Variations in the effectiveness of conditioned but not unconditioned stimuli. *Psychological Review*, *87*, 332–352.

Peck, C. A., & Bouton, M. E. (1990). Context and performance in aversive-to-appetitive and appetitive-to-aversive transfer. *Learning and Motivation*, *21*, 1–31.

Perkins, C. C., & Weyant, R. G. (1958). The intertrial interval between training and test trials as determiner of the slope of generalization gradients. *Journal of Comparative and Physiological Psychology*, *51*, 596–600.

Rescorla, R. A. (1968). Probability of shock in the presence and absence of CS in fear conditioning. *Journal of Comparative and Physiological Psychology*, *66*, 1–5.

Rescorla, R. A. (1985). Conditioned inhibition and facilitation. In R. R. Miller & N. E. Spear (Eds.), *Information processing in animals: Conditioned inhibition* (pp. 299–326). Hillsdale, NJ: Erlbaum.

Rescorla, R. A., & Wagner, A. R. (1972). A theory of Pavlovian conditioning: Variations in the effectiveness of reinforcement and nonreinforcement. In A. H. Black & W. K. Prokasy (Eds.), *Classical conditioning II: Current research and theory* (pp. 64–99). New York: Appleton–Century–Crofts.

Riccio, D. C., Rabinowitz, V. C., & Alxelrod, S. (1994). Memory: When less is more. *American Psychologist*, *49*, 917–926.

Riccio, D. C., Richardson, R., & Ebner, D. L. (1984). Memory retrieval deficits based upon altered contextual cues: A paradox. *Psychological Bulletin*, *96*, 152–165.

Rosas, J. M., & Bouton, M. E. (1996). Spontaneous recovery after extinction of a conditioned taste aversion. *Animal Learning and Behavior*, *24*, 341–348.

Rosas, J. M., & Bouton, M. E. (1997a). Additivity of the effects of retention interval and context change on latent inhibition: Toward resolution of the context forgetting paradox. *Journal of Experimental Psychology: Animal Behavior Processes*, *23*, 283–294.

Rosas, J. M., & Bouton, M. E. (1997b). Renewal of a conditioned taste aversion upon return to the conditioning context after extinction in another one. *Learning and Motivation, 28*, 216–229.

Rosas, J. M., & Bouton, M. E. (1998). Context change and retention interval can have additive, rather than interactive, effects after taste aversion extinction. *Psychonomic Bulletin and Review, 5*, 79–83.

Rosas, J. M., & Callejas-Aguilera, J. E. (2006). Context switch effects on acquisition and extinction in human predictive learning. *Journal of Experimental Psychology: Learning, Memory, and Cognition, 32*, 461–474.

Rosas, J. M., & Callejas-Aguilera, J. E. (2007). Acquisition of a conditioned taste aversion becomes context dependent when it is learned after extinction. *Quarterly Journal of Experimental Psychology, 60*, 9–15.

Rosas, J. M., Vila, N. J., Lugo, M., & Lopez, L. (2001). Combined effect of context change and retention interval on interference in causality judgments. *Journal of Experimental Psychology: Animal Behavior Processes, 27*, 153–164.

Ross, R. T., & Holland, P. C. (1981). Conditioning of simultaneous and serial feature-positive discriminations. *Animal Learning and Behavior, 9*, 293–303.

Schmajuk, N. A., & Holland, P. C. (Eds.). (1998). *Occasion-setting: Associative learning and cognition in animals.* Washington, DC: American Psychological Association.

Siegel, S. (2005). Drug tolerance, drug addiction, and drug anticipation. *Current Directions in Psychological Science, 14*, 296–300.

Smith, S. M. (1979). Remembering in and out of context. *Journal of Experimental Psychology: Human Learning and Memory, 5*, 460–471.

Smith, S. M. (1988). Environmental context-dependent memory. In G. M. Davies & D. M. Thomson (Eds.), *Memory in context: Context in memory* (pp. 13–34). New York: Wiley.

Smith, S. M. (2007). Context: A reference for focal experience. In H. L. Roediger, Y. Dudai, & S. M. Fitzpatrick (Eds.), *Science of memory: Concepts* (pp. 111–114). Oxford, UK: Oxford University Press.

Smith, S. M., & Vela, E. (2001). Environmental context-dependent memory: A review and meta-analysis. *Psychonomic Bulletin and Review, 8*, 203–220.

Spear, N. E. (1978). *The processing of memories: Forgetting and retention.* Hillsdale, NJ: Erlbaum.

Swartzentruber, D. (1995). Modulatory mechanisms in Pavlovian conditioning. *Animal Learning and Behavior, 23*, 123–143.

Timberlake, W. (2001). Motivational modes in behavior systems. In R. R. Mowrer & S. B. Klein (Eds.), *Handbook of contemporary learning theories* (pp. 155–209). Hillsdale, NJ: Erlbaum.

Tulving, E., & Thomson, D. M. (1973). Encoding specificity and retrieval processes in episodic memory. *Psychological Review, 80*, 352–373.

VanDercar, D. H., & Schneiderman, N. (1967). Interstimulus interval functions in different response systems during classical discrimination conditioning in rabbits. *Psychonomic Science, 9*, 9–10.

Waddell, J., Morris, R. W., & Bouton, M. E. (2006). Effects of bed nucleus of the stria terminalis lesions on conditioned anxiety: Aversive conditioning with long-duration conditional stimuli and reinstatement of extinguished fear. *Behavioral Neuroscience, 120*, 324–336.

Wagner, A. R. (1981). SOP: A model of automatic memory processing in animal behavior. In N. E. Spear & R. R. Miller (Eds.), *Information processing in animals: Memory mechanisms* (pp. 5–47). Hillsdale, NJ: Erlbaum.

Wagner, A. R. (2003). Context-sensitive elemental theory. *Quarterly Journal of Experimental Psychology, 56B*, 7–29.

Wagner, A. R., & Brandon, S. E. (1989). Evolution of a structured connectionist model of Pavlovian conditioning (AESOP). In S. B. Klein & R. R. Mowrer (Eds.), *Contemporary learning theories: Pavlovian conditioning and the status of traditional learning theory* (pp. 149–189). Hillsdale, NJ: Erlbaum.

Walker, D. L., Ressler, K. J., Lu, K.-T., & Davis, M. (2002). Facilitation of conditioned fear extinction by systemic administration or intra-amygdala infusions of D-cycloserine as assessed with fear-potentiated startle in rats. *Journal of Neuroscience, 15*, 2343–2351.

Walker, D. L., Toufexis, D. J., & Davis, M. (2003). Role of the bed nucleus of the stria terminalis versus the amygdala in fear, stress, and anxiety. *European Journal of Pharmacology, 463*, 199–216.

Westbrook, R. F., Jones, M. L., Bailey, G. K., & Harris, J. A. (2000). Contextual control over conditioned responding in a latent inhibition paradigm. *Journal of Experimental Psychology: Animal Behavior Processes, 26*, 157–173.

Woods, A. M., & Bouton, M. E. (2006). D-cycloserine facilitates extinction but does not eliminate renewal of the conditioned emotional response. *Behavioral Neuroscience, 120*, 1159–1162.

Woods, A. M., & Bouton, M. E. (2007). Occasional reinforced responses during extinction can slow the rate of reacquisition of an operant response. *Learning and Motivation, 38*, 56–74.

Zhou, Y., & Riccio, D. C. (1996). Manipulation of components of context: The context shift effect and forgetting of stimulus attributes. *Learning and Motivation, 27*, 400–407.

13

Threat, Marginality, and Reactions to Norm Violations

DEBORAH A. PRENTICE
THOMAS E. TRAIL

Successful navigation of the social environment requires exquisite sensitivity to the norms that regulate behavior in different contexts. People are supposed to be quiet in libraries and competitive in athletic contests. They are supposed to be extraverted at parties and responsible in the classroom. They are supposed to be self-promoting at work and communal at home. They are supposed to be respectful with their superiors and egalitarian with their friends. In all of these contexts, behavior is governed by social norms that prescribe what is appropriate and describe what is typical. These norms are widely shared and, for the most part, highly functional, in that they enable people to coordinate their activities and meet their goals. Indeed, norms are such a ubiquitous feature of social contexts that people are often unaware of their influence (Cialdini & Trost, 1998).

Social groups also have norms that regulate the behavior of their members; these norms describe and prescribe appropriate behavior for group members (Miller & Prentice, 1996). People are remarkably good at identifying and representing the norms of their social groups accurately, a skill that is all the more impressive given how specific and nuanced these norms can be. Consider, for example, the norms of the Princeton University campus. Here, undergraduate students are supposed to work hard Sunday through Thursday afternoon, play hard beginning Thursday night and continuing on, with some flexibility for academic and athletic obligations, through Saturday night, and then work hard again as soon as they can rouse themselves on Sunday morning. They are supposed to love the university, care about their schoolwork without becoming single-minded, pursue opportunities to travel, and take part in extracurricular and social activities on campus. They are supposed to shine without threatening all of the other students who are trying to shine, and to take themselves seriously, but not too seriously. In short, the campus is governed by a very complex and nuanced set of norms. It is therefore remarkable how quickly students learn the norms, and how closely they observe them in their everyday behavior.

How do people accomplish this feat? How do they learn the norms of their social groups? Observing how other group members behave is certainly one useful source of information. A newcomer to the Princeton campus need only observe the activities of the local inhabitants for a week or two to pick up much of what he or she needs to know. The stated opinions of group members are also very useful, as people are much more likely to give voice to the positions they believe to be normative than to those they believe to be deviant (Berger & Heath, 2005). Taken together, these two sources of information can account for much of the data on the overall accuracy of norm identification, as well as the circumstances under which it goes systematically awry (see Miller & Prentice, 1994, 1996).

The importance of these mechanisms notwithstanding, norm learning does not proceed seamlessly through observation and communication alone. People sometimes misjudge the norms of their groups and violate them unwittingly. They sometimes disregard the norms of their groups and violate them knowingly. They sometimes drift away from group norms as they pursue other ends. Left unchecked, such errant behavior would become acceptable and almost certainly more common, and the resulting heterogeneity within the group would weaken the group's ability to define a collective reality. Thus, social groups must have an effective mechanism for dealing with transgressions of their norms, if they are to retain their power to regulate collective behavior. At least some of these mechanisms operate at the interpersonal level, in interactions between group members.

In this chapter, we investigate the psychological processes that shape these interactions—specifically, the emotional and evaluative reactions people have toward peers who violate group norms. We examine these reactions, drawing primarily on evidence from our own program of research, but also availing ourselves of the insights of others. Taken together, our studies illustrate that reactions to deviates (as well as to conformists) are heavily dependent on the meaning of their behavior in context; that is, they are conditioned on the implications of the behavior for the person enacting it, the person observing it, and the group of which they are both members. Ironically, these reactions are also, in a very important sense, constitutive of the context, in that they help to give the deviant behavior its social meaning. Such is the Janus-like duality of social life that people are simultaneously actors bound by situational constraints and observers whose behavior constrains the actions of others. We begin by outlining social psychology's received wisdom about how people react to deviates, which we call the *group-threat hypothesis*.

THE GROUP-THREAT HYPOTHESIS

The received view of reactions to deviates goes something like this: When people violate the norms of their groups, they receive social punishment from their fellow group members. This punishment might take the form of lower sociometric ratings, negative feedback, assignment to unpleasant tasks, or exclusion from the group (see, e.g., Abrams, Marques, Bown, & Henson, 2000; Eidelman, Silvia, & Biernat, 2006; Iwao, 1963; Schachter, 1951; Smith, Williams, & Willis, 1967). Research on this process has identified two factors that influence the degree of punishment that deviates receive. First, the identity of the observers matters: Punishment is meted out only by members of the group whose norms are violated, not by outgroup members. Indeed, ingroup and outgroup members have much different stakes in the behavior of the deviate: The former see the deviate as a threat to the clarity, functioning, and cohesiveness of their group. They derogate or exclude the deviate in order to dissociate themselves from him or her, to communicate and enforce ingroup norms, and to promote the integrity of the group (e.g., Abrams et al., 2000; Eidelman et al., 2006; Iwao, 1963; Marques, Abrams, Paez, & Martinez-Taboada, 1998; Marques, Abrams, & Serodio, 2001; Smith et al., 1967). Members of outgroups have no investment in another group's norms, and therefore no reason to punish those who violate them.

Second and related, the magnitude of the punishment depends on the severity of the threat deviates pose to the group. When the group is insecure, unstable, or challenged, deviates pose a greater threat and therefore receive stronger derogation (Lauderdale, 1976; Lauderdale, Smith-Cunnien, Parker, & Inverarity, 1984; Marques et al., 2001). When deviates can be excluded from the group, they pose a lesser threat and receive less derogation (Eidelman et al., 2006). Thus, in this formulation, threat to the group is the key variable mediating between violations of group norms and social derogation.

This perspective on reactions to deviates as originating in group threat captures an important, if partial, truth. There is no question that deviates sometimes threaten group norms, and that people will rise up in defense of their group when that group's norms are threatened. Consider, for example, the reactions Democrats are likely to have to a fellow Democrat who supports the War in Iraq. Support for the war does not violate any formal rule of the Democratic Party, but it does run contrary to a very important norm of the Party. Moreover, it aligns with the norms of the outgroup—the Republican Party—and threatens to weaken the Democrats in their ongoing struggle with the Republicans for political supremacy. Thus, we would expect Democrats to react to this war-supporting deviate with derogation, hostility, and rejection. More generally, deviates who violate attitudinal norms, especially those of sociopolitical groups, often receive this kind of treatment, as their deviance challenges a centrally defining norm of the group and often supports the norm of an adversarial outgroup. This is group threat in its purest form. Thus, it is no surprise that much of the empirical support for the group-threat hypothesis comes from studies of reactions to this type of deviate (e.g., Abrams et al., 2000; Marques et al., 2001).

However, many deviates do not fit this template. Consider, for example, the reactions Princeton students are likely to have to a fellow student who does not observe campus norms. This student lives off campus in her own apartment, focuses single-mindedly on her schoolwork, and takes herself extremely seriously. In doing so, she is, by any measure, a deviate; but does she constitute a threat to the group? We would argue no, given her marginal status. This deviate is not a threat to the clarity, functioning, and cohesiveness of the group; she is alone, out of step, and low in status. Her impact on the group is minimal at best. The same is true of many deviates: They are, by definition, alone, out of step, and low in status. Just how much of a threat to the group could they be?

These two examples illustrate a more general point: Deviates come in many different forms. Some of them threaten the group, and others do not. Some of them threaten the individual members of the group, and others do not. Because the field has embraced the group-threat hypothesis, researchers have interpreted all negative reactions to deviates as manifestations of group threat. We believe that this is a serious misreading of the evidence, one that overemphasizes threat and, in particular, threat to the group, as driving all negative reactions to deviates. Moreover, the focus on threat has led researchers to overlook the explanatory potential of what is, in our view, a much more universally significant feature of deviates: their marginality. We propose that the perception of deviates as marginal plays a very important role in the reactions people have to them, including, under some circumstances, hostile and punishing reactions. Threat matters, to be sure, but as a moderator of reactions, not as a mediator. We further propose that the treatment of deviates as marginal has the effect of reinforcing social norms, but at minimal social cost. We now turn to this alternative view, which we term *the marginality hypothesis.*

THE MARGINALITY HYPOTHESIS

The marginality hypothesis is an outgrowth of several years of empirical research on how people feel about and evaluate deviates (see Carranza, Prentice, & Larsen, 2006; Trail & Prentice, 2008; Trail, Prentice, & Carranza, 2008). The goal of this research was to delve into the psychological processes that underlie behavioral responses to deviates; we did not measure behavior itself, but rather the feelings that direct behavior. Our thinking about the marginality hypothesis and the evidence for it have coevolved, as it were, with each additional study leading to elaborations of the theory and reinterpretations of the results of the studies that came before. Thus, we present the theory and the evidence in tandem here.

The evidence comes from a series of experiments that were all variants on a common paradigm. Participants listened to audio recordings of other students making self-referential statements. Each statement was either consistent with prevailing group norms, contrary to prevailing group norms, or irrelevant to group norms. The statements were brief—no more than a sentence or two—but quite evocative, especially in audio form. Participants listened to many of these statements (between 30 and 60 statements, depending on the experiment), and after each one, indicated how the speaker made them feel, their evaluations of the speaker, and their behavioral inclinations toward the speaker. In several of the studies, we also used facial electromyography (facial EMG) to assess participants' spontaneous facial displays while they listened to the statements. Taken together, these measures provide us with a comprehensive view of their reactions to the conforming and deviant targets.

Evaluative and Emotional Reactions to Deviates

How do deviates make people feel? Consider, once again, the reactions Princeton students are likely to have to a fellow student who does not observe campus norms. The group-threat hypothesis suggests that students will see her as a threat to the integrity and functioning of the group, and will react with strong negative affect and evaluations. The marginality hypothesis suggests that they will see her as marginal—a loser—and respond with disdain and derision, but not with strong negative affect. Note that these are both negative reactions, but they are different negative reactions. The first is a response to a strong, negative stimulus, one that has the potential to do considerable harm. The second is a response to a weak, negative stimulus, one that may be irritating or frustrating but not harmful. Which of these predictions better captures reactions to deviant Princeton students?

We addressed this question by presenting Princeton undergraduates with targets who conformed to and deviated from Princeton campus norms. The conformists made statements like the following:

> "I like to go to the 'Street' on Thursday and Saturday nights. Homework is a high priority; I just can't spend all my time on it."
>
> "I had a history class last semester that was so interesting I actually looked forward to doing the readings. Now I think I'm going to be a history major."

The deviates made statements like the following:

> "I wear pretty funky clothes and have a radical hairstyle. Nothing I do follows the current trends, and that's the way I like it."
>
> "I've lived in New Jersey my whole life and have never been further away than St. Louis, Missouri. It's not that I'm against traveling; I've just never had the opportunity."

We collected self-reported evaluations of each target and measures of positive and negative affective responses. We also asked participants how likely they would be to laugh at, tease, and make fun of each target; the composite of these items served as a measure of derision. Finally, we used facial EMG to measure activity over the *frontalis medialis*, *corrugator supercilii*, *orbicularis oculi*, and *zygomaticus major*, while participants listened to the statements (see Trail et al., 2008, Study 1, for more details).

The results of this study provided support for the marginality hypothesis. Participants evaluated deviates more negatively than they evaluated conformists, and showed much more derision toward them. However, they did not show any differences in self-reported positive or negative affect toward the two types of targets, nor any target differences in activity over the *corrugator supercilii*, the "frown muscle," which has been shown to be responsive to negative affect (see, e.g., Cacioppo, Petty, Losch, & Kim, 1986). This pattern of results is much more consistent with a view of deviates as marginal than with a view of them as threatening. Moreover, participants showed greater activity over the *zygomaticus major*, the "smile muscle," in response to deviates as compared with conformists, and these smiles were genuine, Duchenne smiles, indicative of positive affect (see Cacioppo et al., 1986). This difference in smiling was fully mediated by derision (but not by self-reported positive affect toward the targets), suggesting that these were not warm, friendly smiles but rather mocking, derisive smiles. This result, too, is what we would expect if participants viewed deviates as marginal.

Threatening versus Nonthreatening Deviates (and Conformists)

Having established that deviates do not necessarily threaten the group, we hasten to add that they certainly can threaten the group. The existing literature on reactions to deviates provides many examples in which they do. Members of decision-making groups who refuse to modify their position to reach a group consensus threaten the group (e.g., Schachter, 1951). Members of social groups who adopt the attitudinal positions of opposing groups threaten the group (e.g., Marques et al., 2001). For example, African Americans who do not support Affirmative Action policies threaten the group (e.g., Ibekwe, 2004). We would expect these threatening deviates to elicit a uniformly negative affective reaction in observers, in line with the group-threat hypothesis. Specifically, we would expect to see higher negative affect, lower positive affect, higher activity over the *corrugator supercilii*, and lower activity over the *zygomaticus major* in response to threatening compared to nonthreatening deviates. Still, we would expect observers to be sensitive also to the marginality of threatening deviates—that is, to see them as threatening losers, not as threatening winners. This perception of marginality should manifest itself in a tendency to deride these deviates as well.

We tested these predictions by presenting Princeton undergraduates with two types of deviant targets, one of which derogated the group, and the other of which did not. The two types of targets were designed to be equivalent in how much they departed from group norms, and indeed, participants rated themselves as equally (dis)similar to both. The difference was in their stated attitude toward the group . The nonthreatening deviates did not reference the group or its norms explicitly; they used the same statements that deviates used in the study we just described. The threatening deviates made statements that explicitly derogated the group and its norms. The following are examples of statements made by threatening deviates:

"Even though I'm at Princeton, I still have a thing for Harvard. I'm making sure to get good grades so that I can go to Harvard Law School after I'm done here."

"I drank a lot when I first got here, but then I realized it was a waste of time. My grades and my social life have both improved a lot since I stopped spending so much time at the 'Street.'"

We again collected self-reported evaluations and affect ratings, and measured facial EMG activity (see Trail et al., 2008, Study 2, for more details).

The results of this study showed the expected differences in reactions to the two types of deviates. Participants reacted to threatening deviates with more negative affect and less positive affect than they showed in response to nonthreatening deviates. They also showed more activity over the *corrugator supercilii* and less activity over the *zygomaticus major* in response to threatening than to nonthreatening deviates, although neither of these effects was reliable. They evaluated threatening deviates somewhat more negatively than nonthreatening deviates, but showed equivalent (and high) levels of derision toward both types of targets. Thus, participants appear to have seen both threatening and nonthreatening deviates as marginal, though their affective reactions registered the difference in the harm these two types of deviates could do to the group.

Of course, deviates are not the only sources of potential threat in the ingroup; conformists can also be quite threatening, though more to their fellow group members than to the group itself. Consider a Princeton undergraduate who perfectly embodies the campus norms: He is a stellar student and a varsity athlete, too; an officer in his eating club, who also volunteers at the local soup kitchen; a world traveler, who speaks six different languages and has a great sense of style. He is a "tall poppy" (Feather, 1994), a "rate-buster" (Levine, 1992), a "pronorm deviate" (Abrams et al., 2000; Abrams, Marques, Bown, & Dougill, 2002). How will other students react to him? We would expect them to feel threatened, not because he challenges the group norms, but because he challenges their standing within the group. Thus, they should react to him with negative affect. But will they view him as marginal, too? On the one hand, as a hyperconformist, he should be the most central and least marginal member of the group. Yet he would certainly be atypical, and that might be enough to give him marginal status.

We examined reactions to extreme conformists by presenting Princeton undergraduates with two types of conforming targets, one of which exceeded ordinary expectations and the other of which did not. The ordinary conformists used the same statements conformists used in the first study we presented; the extreme conformists made statements like the following:

> "I start each day by reading a couple of newspapers online and then going to the gym to work out. It's worth getting up early to start the day out right."
>
> "People warned me that it would be hard to be a student-athlete, but so far, I have a 3.9 GPA and I haven't had to miss a single practice. In fact, I've never played better."

We again collected self-reported evaluations and affect ratings, and measured facial EMG activity (see Trail et al., 2008, Study 2, for more details).

The results of this study indicated that participants perceived extreme conformists as both threatening and marginal. They rated themselves as much less similar to these targets than to the ordinary conformists and reacted with more negative affect, less positive affect, more negative evaluations, and more derision. Indeed, their reactions looked very much like their reactions to the threatening deviates, with one important exception: Participants did not register any negative affect on their faces. They did not register any positive affect, either: Activity over the *corrugator supercilii* and the *zygomaticus major* in response to these targets was no different than the activity shown in response to neutral targets. The only facial reaction they showed in response to extreme conformists was a narrowing of the eyes (i.e., increased activity over the *orbicularis oculi*), which is typically interpreted as a sign of arousal or interest (Witvliet & Vrana, 1995). The disjunction between their strongly negative self-reported reactions and their poker faces is interesting; we would venture to suggest that it may have something to do with the fact that extreme conformists are not just threatening and marginal, but also high in status. We are planning additional studies to investigate this possibility.

Further Efforts to Disentangle Threat from Marginality

Thus far, we have critiqued the group-threat hypothesis primarily by interrogating the link between deviance and group threat; that is, we have argued that the marginality hypothesis is more generally useful for understanding reactions to deviates because marginality is more of a constant across deviates than is group threat. Now we seek to interrogate the necessity and sufficiency of group threat as an explanation for why deviates receive more social punishment than do conformists. Our argument, in a nutshell, is that although social punishment is indeed a response to threat, that threat need not target the group; people will punish anyone who threatens them, provided that they think they can get away with it. And here is where the marginality hypothesis comes in: It suggests that deviates are punished more often than conformists not because they are necessarily more threatening (though sometimes they are more threatening), but because their marginality makes them more vulnerable targets.

Women who violate gender norms provide an excellent vehicle with which to develop this argument. Numerous studies have found that women who demonstrate stereotypically masculine attributes are evaluated more negatively than are equally masculine men (e.g., Crawford, 1988; Heilman, Wallen, Fuchs, & Tamkins, 2004; Rudman, 1998). Moreover, women who inhabit stereotypically masculine roles elicit lower evaluations of satisfaction, effectiveness, and deservedness of promotion relative to their male counterparts (e.g., Butler & Geis, 1990; Eagly, Makhijani, & Klonsky, 1992). These findings, and many others like them, suggest that masculine women receive more social punishment than do equally masculine men. The question is, why? Theoretical accounts have stressed masculine women's status as deviates and argue that because they violate gender norms, people see and respond to them as a threat (e.g., Burgess & Borgida, 1999; Glick & Fiske, 1999; Heilman, 2001; Janoff-Bulman & Wade, 1996).

Consider an alternative view. Studies of reactions to masculine women have typically focused on masculine qualities such as dominance, agency, competitiveness, and self-promotion. These qualities are quite threatening interpersonally, regardless of the gender of the person who manifests them. Thus, people almost certainly register both men and women who possess these qualities as threatening targets. Why, then, would they treat the women more harshly than they treat the men? The marginality hypothesis has a straightforward answer to this question: Masculine women, because of their deviant and therefore marginal status, are more vulnerable targets for negative treatment. If this hypothesis is correct, then we should expect to find no differences in emotional and evaluative reactions to masculine men and women—no differences in the threat they evoke—despite the well-documented differences in the treatment they receive.

We examined how threatening people find masculine men and women to be in a series of studies of reactions to gender-norm deviates. These studies included six types of targets, created by crossing three types of characteristics—dominant (masculine), communal (feminine), and neutral (norm-irrelevant)—with two genders. The following are statements made by dominant targets (with the male version spoken by a man and the female version spoken by a woman):

"I've always been a gifted natural athlete. My coach warns me to be careful about my ego, but I think my ego works in my favor—especially when I'm on the field."

"I don't mind stepping on a few toes in order to get things done. If someone doesn't like my ideas, I have no problem doing whatever I can to get that person out of the picture."

The following are statements made by communal targets:

"I'm a total romantic. My favorite daydream is one where I meet my perfect match while I'm on my junior year abroad—while strolling on the Champs Élysées, or sunbathing on a Greek island."

"I have the ability to sacrifice my own wants for the sake of others; I can sometimes go overboard in this direction, which isn't good, I know. But that doesn't happen too often."

Each participant listened to targets of all six types and rated each target, across two studies, on a wide range of affective and evaluative dimensions. In one of the studies, we also collected measures of facial EMG activity (see Carranza et al., 2006, for more details).

The results confirmed our expectation that dominant men and women would threaten and threaten equally. Both of these targets elicited strong negative evaluations, negative affect, avoidance tendencies, derision, and activity over the *corrugator supercilii.* Men tended to rate dominant men less negatively than women did, which we take as evidence that men were more tolerant of dominance in men than were women. In fact, women expressed more negative affect, stronger avoidance tendencies, and more derision toward dominant men than toward dominant women. Thus, if anything, women found the dominant men more threatening than the dominant women. There was no evidence in the reactions of male or female participants to support the claim that dominant women were especially threatening.

What of the communal male targets? The literature did not provide us with a clear set of expectations regarding the threat potential of these targets. Indeed, previous studies of reactions to feminine men are few and far between, and those that have been published have yielded inconsistent findings. Studies of men with feminine qualities in masculine roles have shown no evidence that these targets are devalued (e.g., Eagly et al., 1992; Rudman & Glick, 2001). Yet, the developmental literature suggests that feminine boys receive strong social sanctions from both their peers and their fathers (see Carranza et al., 2006, for a review). Thus, we anticipated that communal men would be seen as marginal, at least by other men, and would be evaluated negatively and derided as a result. Whether they would also elicit the negative affect and avoidance tendencies associated with threat was an open question.

The answer to that question turned out to be "yes." Men were clearly threatened by the communal male targets: They showed more negative affect and more derision, weaker approach tendencies and stronger avoidance tendencies, and more negative evaluations of these targets compared to both their own reactions to communal female targets and to women's reactions to communal male targets. However, men's reactions to these deviates were not strongly negative in an absolute sense; they evaluated communal men only slightly (though reliably) more negatively than neutral targets. Men showed increased activity over both the *corrugator supercilii* and the *zygomaticus major* in response to communal male compared to communal female targets, with the former difference mediated by negative affect and the latter difference mediated by derision. Women reacted very positively to communal men, just as positively as they reacted to communal women. They, too, showed increased activity over the *zygomaticus major* in response to communal men, though their smiles were more amused than derisive.

Taken together, these results suggest that both men and women who violate gender norms are threatening, but for different reasons. Communal men are threatening because they are deviant, whereas dominant women are threatening because they are dominant. Indeed, the group-threat hypothesis provides a very good explanation for the data on communal men: These deviates receive more negative reactions from ingroup than from outgroup members, implicating the group, and those negative reactions include negative affect and avoidance, implicating threat. The male group identity—manhood, if you will—appears to be threatened by communal sentiments and behaviors. Womanhood, on the other hand, does not appear to be threatened by dominant sentiments and behaviors. There is no evidence to support the group-threat hypothesis in the data on reactions to dominant women. There is, however, evidence that dominant women, like their male counterparts, are threatening to women and men alike. This threat, combined with the marginality that deviance confers, may explain the strong social sanctions these women typically receive (see Rudman & Fairchild, 2004, for experimental evidence consistent with this view). Indeed, according to the marginality hypothesis, threatening deviates will always receive stronger social sanctions than threatening conformists, regardless of whether the threat stems from their deviance, their personal qualities, their behavior, or outcomes in which they are implicated, and regardless of whether they threaten the group or individuals.

Does Deriding Deviates Feel Good?

When we first began studying reactions to deviates, we were surprised to see participants smiling in response to deviant targets. Our surprise waned when, study after study, we continued to see them smiling, especially in response to deviant targets who were not highly threatening. The fact that this smiling involves activity over the *orbicularis oculi* suggests that these are genuine Duchenne smiles, signaling true positive affect (Cacioppo et al., 1986). What causes our participants to smile pleasurably when they evaluate deviates? We have three candidate answers:

1. Their smiling reflects a positive response to the target. This is the most straightforward explanation and the one that maps most closely onto how facial EMG data in interpersonal perception studies are typically interpreted (see, e.g., Vanman, Paul, Ito, & Miller, 1997). However, it seems unlikely given the plethora of empirical evidence we have accumulated showing negative evaluations of and derisive inclinations toward even nonthreatening deviant targets. Still, it is possible that participants feel positively toward these targets even while they evaluate them negatively, and that our self-report measures are simply too insensitive to pick up this positive feeling.

2. Their smiling reflects a positive response to an errant group member whom they want to bring back into the fold. Interpersonally, this smiling may function to offset the negative response that deviant behavior elicits, and to repair and reestablish a positive relationship between group members. This explanation seems quite plausible in theory, and is broadly consistent with the marginality hypothesis. However, it seems less likely as an account for smiling in our experimental paradigm, where there was no relationship between deviate and observer.

3. Their smiling reflects a positive response to deriding deviates. This possibility, too, is consistent with the marginality hypothesis, consistent with the finding that undermining deviates boosts implicit self-esteem (Rudman & Fairchild, 2004), and consistent with the vast literature on the pleasures of downward social comparison (Wood, 1989). Indeed, deviates would seem a particularly valuable source of downward social comparison, in that they enable one to demonstrate one's knowledge of group norms, one's commitment to the group, and one's superior standing in the group, all at the same time. Thus, we conducted two studies designed specifically to examine how deriding deviates makes people feel.

In these studies, we again gave Princeton undergraduates the task of evaluating their peers by listening to self-referential statements. This time, some of our participants evaluated students who made statements that conformed to campus norms (intermingled with an equal number of students who made neutral statements) and other participants evaluated students who made statements that deviated from campus norms (again, intermingled with an equal number of students who made neutral statements). Thus, in these studies, the status of the targets as conformist or deviant was manipulated between participants. The conforming and deviant targets used the same statements that conforming and deviant targets used in our initial study. We again collected self-reported evaluations and affect ratings after each target, and then, at the end of the session, asked participants to complete measures of their identification with Princeton, their state self-esteem, and their mood (see Trail & Prentice, 2008, for more details).

The results suggested that deriding deviates has positive psychological consequences, especially for men. Across both studies, participants showed reliably stronger identification with Princeton after evaluating deviates than after evaluating conformists. This effect was fully mediated by the extent to which they derided the targets. Men also showed higher social self-esteem and appearance self-esteem after evaluating deviates than after evaluating conformists. Derisive responses to the targets correlated with positive mood across conditions and genders. Taken together, these results indicate that derision feels good, and that deriding deviates strengthens connections to the group and, for men, feelings about the self.

These findings have important implications for understanding the general attitude that people take toward the deviant members of their groups. Previous research has emphasized the inclination to avoid, reject, and exclude deviates, to redraw group boundaries to push deviates out. This attitude may well characterize people's stance toward threatening deviates. But nonthreatening deviates may engender an entirely different attitude. Indeed, to the extent that deriding these targets makes people feel good, they may want to have deviates around. They may even seek out opportunities to evaluate deviant group members and may prefer this task to the task of evaluating conformists. We are currently planning additional studies to investigate this possibility.

CONCLUDING REMARKS

People who violate group norms elicit negative evaluative and behavioral responses from their peers, and those negative responses have the effect of strengthening group norms. These two empirical facts have led social psychologists to embrace the group-threat hypothesis as a general model of the psychological processes that underlie these outcomes. The group-threat hypothesis has a number of intuitively appealing qualities: It is parsimonious, attributing a commonly observed effect (negative evaluative and behavioral responses) to a single causal mechanism (contending with group threat). It is simple, positing that behavior that is motivated by a desire to protect the group has the consequence of protecting the group. Best of all, it is true—deviates do threaten the group and receive social sanctions as a result—but only some of the time.

In this chapter, we have proposed the marginality hypothesis as a general account for reactions to deviates. This hypothesis posits that marginality (and not group threat) is a common feature of all deviates that shapes the emotional and evaluative reactions people have to them. Our empirical studies of this hypothesis have yielded three major insights. First, not all deviates are threatening; some are simply marginal. The former receive strongly negative, avoidant responses; the latter receive mixed valence, derisive responses. Second, within the category of threatening deviates, not all of them threaten the group; some of them threaten individuals (through their personal qualities, the outcomes they produce, etc.). Those that threaten the group elicit negative affect and avoidance only from fellow group members; those that threaten individuals elicit these reactions from everyone. Third, deriding deviates has psychological benefits, including stronger connections to the group and, for men, more positive feelings about the self. These findings reveal reactions to deviates to be much more complex, group-specific, and context-dependent than previous research has suggested.

How do we reconcile this view of reactions to deviates as variable and contingent with the wealth of evidence that deviates are systematically devalued and derogated? We attribute the apparent inconsistency to two sources. First, previous research has assessed reactions to deviates using a narrow range of measures, most of them self-reported evaluations. On these measures, we, too, find lower ratings of deviates than conformists across the board. The variability we find occurs on other measures—primarily affective measures, both implicit and explicit. Second, even though the nature and magnitude of the threat deviates pose is contingent on a host of factors, the consistency of their marginality means that they virtually always elicit more negative reactions than do their conforming counterparts; that is, even when a deviate and a conformist are equally threatening, the deviate, because of his or her social vulnerability, will be treated more harshly.

In closing, we return to the issue with which we began this chapter: the role that sanctioning deviates plays in the maintenance of social norms. In line with the group-threat hypothesis, the accepted view of this process has emphasized the importance of strong social sanctions for bringing deviates into line. The problem with this view is that strong social sanctions are quite costly—to the recipient always, to the sanctioner often, and to the social fabric of the group. We believe that the more modulated negative reactions that we find, reactions in which only highly threatening deviates receive harsh treatment, and negative evaluations are often mixed with signs of positive affect, are actually better calibrated to reinforce group norms while minimizing social cost. Note that this does not mean that the functionality of these reactions explains their existence—indeed, we believe that the reinforcement of group norms is often an unintended consequence of scapegoating a deviate in response to some unrelated threat. Still, the marginal status of deviates is sufficient to ensure that they will receive negative social feedback, and that the norms of the group will be in safe hands.

REFERENCES

Abrams, D., Marques, J. M., Bown, N., & Dougill, M. (2002). Anti-norm and pro-norm deviance in the bank and on the campus: Two experiments on subjective group dynamics. *Group Processes and Intergroup Relations*, *5*(2), 163–182.

Abrams, D., Marques, J. M., Bown, N., & Henson, M. (2000). Pro-norm and anti-norm deviance within and between groups. *Journal of Personality and Social Psychology*, *78*(5), 906–912.

Berger, J. A., & Heath, C. (2005). Idea habitats: How the prevalence of environmental cues influences the success of ideas. *Cognitive Science*, *29*(2), 195–221.

Burgess, D., & Borgida, E. (1999). Who women are, who women should be: Descriptive and prescriptive gender stereotyping in sex discrimination. *Psychology, Public Policy, and Law*, *5*(3), 665–692.

Butler, D., & Geis, F. L. (1990). Nonverbal affect responses to male and female leaders: Implications for leadership evaluations. *Journal of Personality and Social Psychology*, *58*(1), 48–59.

Cacioppo, J. T., Petty, R. E., Losch, M. E., & Kim, H. S. (1986). Electromyographic activity over facial muscle regions can differentiate the valence and intensity of affective reactions. *Journal of Personality and Social Psychology*, *50*(2), 260–268.

Carranza, E., Prentice, D. A., & Larsen, J. T. (2006). *Who threatens and why?: Interpersonal reactions to dominant and communal women and men*. Unpublished manuscript, Princeton University.

Cialdini, R. B., & Trost, M. R. (1998). Social influence: Social norms, conformity, and compliance. In D. T. Gilbert, S. T. Fiske, & G. Lindzey (Eds.),

The handbook of social psychology (4th ed., Vol. 2, pp. 151–192). New York: McGraw-Hill.

Crawford, M. (1988). Gender, age, and the social evaluation of assertion. *Behavior Modification, 12*(4), 549–564.

Eagly, A. H., Makhijani, M. G., & Klonsky, B. G. (1992). Gender and the evaluation of leaders: A meta-analysis. *Psychological Bulletin, 111*(1), 3–22.

Eidelman, S., Silvia, P. J., & Biernat, M. (2006). Responding to deviance: Target exclusion and differential devaluation. *Personality and Social Psychology Bulletin, 32*(9), 1153–1164.

Feather, N. T. (1994). Attitudes toward high achievers and reactions to their fall: Theory and research concerning tall poppies. In M. P. Zanna (Ed.), *Advances in experimental social psychology* (Vol. 26, pp. 1–73). San Diego, CA: Academic Press.

Glick, P., & Fiske, S. T. (1999). Sexism and other "isms": Independence, status, and the ambivalent content of stereotypes. In W. B. Swann, Jr. & J. H. Langlois (Eds.), *Sexism and stereotypes in modern society: The gender science of Janet Taylor Spence* (pp. 193–221). Washington, DC: American Psychological Association.

Heilman, M. E. (2001). Description and prescription: How gender stereotypes prevent women's ascent up the organizational ladder. *Journal of Social Issues, 57*(4), 657–674.

Heilman, M. E., Wallen, A., Fuchs, D., & Tamkins, M. (2004). Penalties for success: Reactions to women who succeed at male gender-typed tasks. *Journal of Applied Psychology, 89*(3), 416–427.

Ibekwe, A. I. (2004). *Affirmative action and anti-normative attitudes: The effects on perceived evaluations from in-group and out-group members.* Unpublished manuscript, Princeton University.

Iwao, S. (1963). Internal versus external criticism of group standards. *Sociometry, 26*(4), 410–421.

Janoff-Bulman, R., & Wade, M. B. (1996). The dilemma of self-advocacy for women: Another case of blaming the victim? *Journal of Social and Clinical Psychology, 15*(2), 143–152.

Lauderdale, P. (1976). Deviance and moral boundaries. *American Sociological Review, 41*(4), 660–676.

Lauderdale, P., Smith-Cunnien, P., Parker, J., & Inverarity, J. (1984). External threat and the definition of deviance. *Journal of Personality and Social Psychology, 46*(5), 1058–1068.

Levine, D. I. (1992). Piece rates, output restriction, and conformism. *Journal of Economic Psychology, 13*(3), 473–489.

Marques, J., Abrams, D., Paez, D., & Martinez-Taboada, C. (1998). The role of categorization and in-group norms in judgments of groups and their members. *Journal of Personality and Social Psychology, 75*(4), 976–988.

Marques, J., Abrams, D., & Serodio, R. G. (2001). Being better by being right: Subjective group dynamics and derogation of in-group deviants when generic norms are undermined. *Journal of Personality and Social Psychology, 81*(3), 436–447.

Miller, D. T., & Prentice, D. A. (1994). Collective errors and errors about the collective. *Personality and Social Psychology Bulletin, 20*(5), 541–550.

Miller, D. T., & Prentice, D. A. (1996). The construction of social norms and standards. In E. T. Higgins & A. W. Kruglanski (Eds.), *Social psychology: Handbook of basic principles.* New York: Guilford Press.

Rudman, L. A. (1998). Self-promotion as a risk factor for women: The costs and benefits of counterstereotypical impression management. *Journal of Personality and Social Psychology, 74*(3), 629–645.

Rudman, L. A., & Fairchild, K. (2004). Reactions to counterstereotypic behavior: The role of backlash in cultural stereotype maintenance. *Journal of Personality and Social Psychology, 87*(2), 157–176.

Rudman, L. A., & Glick, P. (2001). Prescriptive gender stereotypes and backlash toward agentic women. *Journal of Social Issues, 57*(4), 743–762.

Schachter, S. (1951). Deviation, rejection, and communication. *Journal of Abnormal and Social Psychology, 46*(2), 190–207.

Smith, C. R., Williams, L., & Willis, R. H. (1967). Race, sex, and belief as determinants of friendship acceptance. *Journal of Personality and Social Psychology, 5*(2), 127–137.

Trail, T. E., & Prentice, D. A. (2008). *The psychological benefits of deriding deviates.* Unpublished manuscript, Princeton University.

Trail, T. E., Prentice, D. A., & Carranza, E. (2008). *The derisive smile.* Unpublished manuscript, Princeton University.

Vanman, E. J., Paul, B. Y., Ito, T. A., & Miller, N. (1997). The modern face of prejudice and structural features that moderate the effect of cooperation on affect. *Journal of Personality and Social Psychology, 73*(5), 941–959.

Witvliet, C. V., & Vrana, S. R. (1995). Psychophysiological responses as indices of affective dimensions. *Psychophysiology, 32*(5), 436–443.

Wood, J. V. (1989). Theory and research concerning social comparisons of personal attributes. *Psychological Bulletin, 106*(2), 231–248.

14

Behavior as Mind in Context

A Cultural Psychology Analysis of "Paranoid" Suspicion in West African Worlds

GLENN ADAMS
PHIA S. SALTER
KATE M. PICKETT
TUĞÇE KURTIŞ
NIA L. PHILLIPS

> Just because you're paranoid doesn't mean they aren't after you.
>
> — ATTRIBUTED TO KURT COBAIN (among others)

Like some other contributors to this book (Kitayama & Imada, Chapter 9), we approach the theme of "mind in context" from the perspective of cultural psychology (CP). This theme is central to the concept of *culture*, which we define as *explicit and implicit patterns of historically derived and selected ideas and their material manifestations in institutions, practices, and artifacts* (Adams & Markus, 2004, based on Kroeber & Kluckhohn, 1952, p. 357). In contrast to popular associations of culture with group, this statement explicitly defines culture as structures of mind in context: "patterns of ideas ... and their material manifestations" in everyday worlds. Associated with this definition is a conception of culture not as membership in rigidly bounded groups, but rather as engagement with flexible structures of mind in context distributed across unbounded worlds.

The key to our discussion of *behavior* as mind in context comes from the second half of this definition: *Cultural patterns may be considered both products of action and as conditioning elements of further action* (also based on Kroeber and Kluckhohn, 1952, p. 357; see Adams & Markus, 2004). Although theory and research in psychology typically portray behavior as the end product of experience, a CP analysis implies a more dynamic conception in which behavior—and its intentional counterpart, action (Bruner, 1990)—is also a "conditioning element" of further experience. As such, behavior and its observable sediment constitute *intentional worlds*: structures of mind in context that not only bear psychological traces of previous behavior and action, but also direct subsequent behavior and action toward particular ends.

"Mind in Context" as Cultural Psychology

A CP analysis illuminates the theme of "mind in context" in two important senses that we have represented in Figure 14.1. The top arrow of Figure 14.1 refers to the *cultural constitution of psychological experience*: the idea that human experience is not the simple expression of inborn genetic programming, but instead requires *incorporation* or *embodiment* (literally, taking into the body) of structures of mind in context. These structures are not merely interpretative frames applied after the fact to make sense of experience, but instead are *constitutive* of behavior and experience; that is, behavior and experience would not emerge as they do without the ecological scaffolding that structures of mind in context provide. The implication is that to understand observed regularities of psychological functioning one must understand the often ignored structures of mind in context—including cultural models (Holland & Quinn, 1987), social representations (Moscovici, 1984), and discursive repertoires (Potter & Wetherell, 1987)—that provide the ecological scaffolding for these regularities.

The bottom arrow of Figure 14.1 refers to the *psychological constitution of cultural worlds*: the idea that the world is not a natural object separate from human action, but instead is a psychological product. In the course of everyday experience, people continually reproduce structures of mind in context, into which they *inscribe* and *objectify* their beliefs and desires (Berger & Luckmann, 1966; Moscovici, 1984). Rather than an inert mass, the observable sediment of people's behavior carries a psychological charge that exerts independent influence on subsequent action. The implication is something like *mind in society* (Vygotsky, 1978): the idea that the structure of mind is not limited to brain architecture but also extends to psychological traces of behavioral

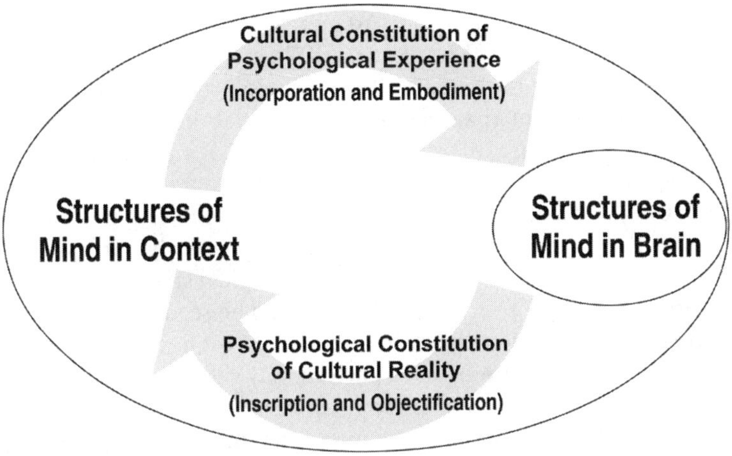

FIGURE 14.1. Mutual constitution of mind and context. The structures of mind in brain that are the typical focus of psychological research exist in a dynamic relationship of mutual constitution with structures of mind in context. These ecological structures of mind in context function as intentional worlds (Shweder, 1990): deposits of behavioral sediment that not only reflect beliefs and desires implicit in previous action (bottom arrow) but also direct subsequent behavior and action toward particular ends (top arrow).

sediment deposited in everyday worlds (see Gosling, Ko, Mannarelli, & Morris, 2002; Morling & Lamoreaux, 2008)

To summarize, the structures of mind in brain that are the typical focus of psychological research exist in a dynamic relationship of mutual constitution—the idea that "psyche and culture … make each other up" (Shweder, 1990, p. 1)—with structures of mind in context. Looking backward, these structures of mind in context represent the psychological sediment of previous behavior and experience. Looking forward, these structures of mind in context provide the ecological scaffolding for subsequent behavior and experience. Underlying structures of mind in context typically remain invisible or unrecognized in mainstream psychological research. The task of a CP analysis is to illuminate them.

OVERVIEW OF EMPIRICAL EXAMPLES

To illustrate this approach to "mind in context" we consider three cases of apparently "paranoid" suspicion in West African worlds: caution about intimate relationship (Adams, 2005), an outbreak of penis-shrinking panic (Adams & Dzokoto, 2007), and suspicion of racism in a vaccination campaign (Obadare, 2005). These cases resemble paranoid behavior to the extent that they involve people's unwarranted concern that they are the target of malice; however, a CP analysis involves two steps that suggest reconsideration of the "paranoid" label (Adams & Salter, 2007). The first step is to *normalize* apparently paranoid behavior; rather than lack of contact with reality, apparently paranoid behavior may reflect normal engagement with ecological structures of mind in context that promote concern about malice. The second step is to *denature* the sense of freedom from malice; rather than the natural expression of inborn programming, this pattern may reflect structures of mind in context that insulate people from concern about malice. Table 14.1 provides an overview of the structures of mind in context associated with both naturalizing (left column) and denaturing (right column) steps for each of the three empirical cases.

BEWARE OF FRIENDS: *CAUTIOUS APPROACHES TO RELATIONSHIP*

If one walks through a taxi stand in various West African worlds, one is likely to find cars with stickers or painted slogans (e.g., "Beware of friends" or "I am afraid of my friends, even you") that advise caution about personal relationship. Resonating with these bits of mind in context, research consistently reveals that people across a variety of West African worlds report a smaller network of friends, express doubts about intimate disclosure, and express greater concern about enemies in intimate spaces than do people across diverse American worlds (Adams, 2005; Adams & Plaut, 2003). How is one to understand these differences?

The tendency in psychological science is to view caution about relationship, to the degree observed in West African settings, as an abnormal deviation from natural reality. Indeed, within mainstream psychology and the worlds that it reflects, the claim to be the target of hidden enemies is a sign of paranoia (with connotations of delusion). Similarly, research in mainstream psychology has emphasized the importance of emotional intimacy and self-disclosure for relationship well-being and production of closeness (Altman & Taylor, 1973; Laurenceau, Barrett, & Pietromonaco, 1998). From this perspective, one might regard the reluctance to share intimate information observed in many West African worlds as a suboptimal form of relationship (e.g., avoidant attachment)

TABLE 14.1. Structures of Mind in Context That Underlie (Responses to) Apparently "Paranoid" Suspicion

Normalizing "paranoid" suspicion in West African worlds	Denaturing lack of suspicion in North American worlds
Example 1: Cautious approaches to relationship	Turning the lens: Open approaches to relationship
• Embedded-interdependent selfways (Adams & Dzokoto, 2003; Carrier, 1999; Markus et al., 1997) • Relational models: authority ranking and communal sharing (Fiske, 1991) • Practices of secrecy associated with concerns about exposure (Shaw, 2000) • Arranged marriage focused on complementary roles; lifelong residence with extended kin (Adams et al., 2004)	• Voluntaristic-independent selfways (Adams & Dzokoto, 2003; Carrier, 1999; Markus et al., 1997) • Relational models: market pricing and equality matching (Fiske, 1991) • Practices of self-expression and affective individualism (Bellah et al., 1985; O'Conner, 1998; Oliker, 1998) • Companionate marriage based on romantic love; neolocal residence with nuclear family (Adams et al., 2004)
Example 2: Mass episodes of genital-shrinking panic	Turning the lens: Biomedical model of illness
• Habits associated with embedded-interdependent selfways: holistic perception (Nisbett et al., 2001); somatization of affect (Dzokoto & Okazaki, 2006); and sense of openness to interpersonal influence (Reisman, 1986). • Practices and artifacts that "objectify" or "make real" sorcery and witchcraft (Geschiere, 1997; Kirby, 1993; Meyer, 2003)	• Habits associated with voluntaristic-independent selfways: analytic perception (Nisbett et al., 2001); dualistic separation of mind and body; and sense of imperviousness to interpersonal influence (Adams, 2005). • Tools for diagnosis and treatment of distress (e.g., DSM-IV; see Adams & Salter, 2007)
Example 3: Perception of racism in health care systems	Turning the lens: Denial of racism in U.S. society
• Collective memory of colonialism and awareness about past incidents of racism (Adams et al., 2006; Eiser & Ellis, 2007) • Community discourse and social representations about present incidents of racism (Turner, 1994) • Official apology of the U.S. government for Tuskegee Syphilis Experiment (White House Office of the Press Secretary, 1997)	• Atomistic pedagogies of racism as individual bias or prejudice (Adams et al., 2008) • Sanitized representations of history that "white out" unflattering acts of past racism (Salter & Adams, 2009) • Color-blind or glorifying constructions of U.S. identity (Phillips & Adams, 2009)

(Collins & Read, 1990; Dion & Dion, 1985; Mikulincer & Nachshon, 1991). Alternatively, one might interpret practices of caution as a form of *self-silencing* (Jack, 1991): inhibition and suppression (rather than indulgence and expression) of personal thoughts and feelings. Research has associated self-silencing with decreased relationship satisfaction, especially among women in heterosexual relationships (see Harper & Welsh, 2007; Jack, 1991).

Normalizing Caution

Rather than consider it a manifestation of abnormality, a CP approach explains caution about relationship in West African settings as a sign of normal sensitivity to structures of mind in context: *embedded-interdependent* selfways that promote both a sense of rootedness in context and an experience of relationship as an ecological affordance (i.e., inherent in the structure of everyday life; see Adams, Anderson, & Adonu, 2004; Markus, Mullally, & Kitayama, 1997). Embedded-interdependent selfways are not just a set of ideas about connection, but also include the "material manifestation" of ideas in concrete realities such as limited social and spatial mobility; the daily practice of eating together from communal bowls; institutions associated with arranged, often polygamous marriage (see Dodoo, 1998); and lifelong communal coresidence in extended-family compounds. These structures of mind in context promote "thick" or "sticky" forms of relationship characterized by dense, overlapping networks and mutual obligations of material support. These structures promote caution about relationship because they imply limitations on people's capacity to choose connections or to insulate themselves from the potential friction that accompanies embeddedness.

In worlds where embedded interdependent selfways provide the ecological scaffolding for experience, the construction of emotional intimacy through self-disclosure may be less imperative for well-being than mainstream research suggests (Chen, 1995). One reason has to do with lack of motivation. The dense networks of connection associated with worlds of embedded interdependence render practices of mutual disclosure unnecessary for the production of common ground. Instead, common ground may arise as a by-product of interaction with a relatively constant, interrelated set of people (Holtgraves, 1997). Another reason has to do with concerns about privacy and self-protection. The overlapping nature of relationship networks in worlds of embedded interdependence affords the possibility that violations of privacy due to revelation of secrets will cause more harm than would occur if one's relationships were compartmentalized and distributed across widely dispersed networks. In these settings, psychological well-being may be associated with structures of mind in context that promote guarded management of information rather than open disclosure (Shaw, 2000).

Likewise, the implications of silence for relationship satisfaction may be less damaging in worlds where embedded-interdependent selfways provide the ecological scaffolding for experience. For example, research among women in a Turkish setting indicates a positive correlation between apparent "self-silencing" and satisfaction in romantic relationships (Kurtiş, 2009). A likely source of this correlation lies in the structures of mind in context—including a strong emphasis on relationship, family integrity, loyalty, and conflict avoidance (Imamoğlu, 1987; Kağitçibaşi, 1973, 1984)—associated with embedded-interdependent selfways that inform traditional Turkish worlds. Self-silencing may be valuable to the extent that inhibition of personal needs and opinions reduces the potential for interpersonal friction that can have particularly disastrous consequences in worlds of embedded interdependence. Traditional gender roles further legitimize the status of silence among Turkish women, making self-silencing a normative practice and therefore less hazardous for personal and relationship well-being.

In short, a CP analysis suggests that relationship tendencies of caution and guarded silence observed in West African settings are not manifestations of pathology. Instead these tendencies reflect particular structures of mind in context: the ecological scaffolding for relationship associated with embedded-interdependent selfways.

Turning the Analytic Lens: Denaturing Openness

Besides providing a "normalizing" account of caution about relationship in West African worlds, an equally important contribution of a CP analysis is to denature the open approach to relationship (and associated sense of freedom from enemies) that masquerades as "natural" in mainstream psychology. Contrary to the portrayal as simple human nature, a CP analysis links this way of being to structures of mind-in-context: *voluntaristic-independent* selfways that promote both a sense of insulation from context and an experience of relationship as the tenuous creation of inherently separate selves (Adams et al., 2004). Again, voluntaristic-independent selfways are not just a set of ideas about separation, but also include the "material manifestation" of ideas in such concrete realities as mobility-affording transportation and communication infrastructure, the practice of "leaving home" in young adulthood, the daily practice of eating from individual place settings, and residence in self-contained apartment units. Resonating with what Fiske (1991) called a *market-pricing* (MP) *model* of relationship, these structures of mind in context promote an experience of the social world as a relatively frictionless "free market" populated by unfettered "free agents" who are both enabled and compelled to arrange their own connections. People feel free not only to construct a broad network of friends but also to avoid negative consequences of connection (including personal enemies).

From this perspective, apparently standard patterns of relationship observed in mainstream psychology—including the prominence of emotional intimacy, self-disclosure, and their implications for well-being and closeness—are not a simple expression of their natural importance. Instead these patterns reflect structures of mind in context associated with voluntaristic-independent selfways. One set of structures concern practices of self-expression associated with *affective individualism*: a value emphasis on exploration, expression, and indulgence of unique, individual feelings (Baumeister, 1987; Bellah, Madsen, Sullivan, Swindler, & Tipton, 1985; Kim, 2002; Kim & Sherman, 2007). Another set of structures concerns relatively direct communication styles. The relatively thin forms of relationship that prevail in settings of voluntaristic independence do not afford a deep sense of "common ground" that permits people to leave much unsaid (Holtgraves, 1997). As a result, people must create common ground through processes of mutual disclosure (O'Conner, 1998; Oliker, 1998). Similarly, because local worlds do not afford a sense of inherent commonality and interdependence, people attempt to create commonality through joint purchases, jointly designed living space, or other practices of place making that produce material interdependence (Lohmann, Arriaga, & Goodfriend, 2003). Rather than consider these practices as inherent motivations for self-expression wired into brain architecture, one can interpret such practices of self-disclosure and domestic place making as cultural innovations for the production of emotional intimacy. As such, these practices provide important means to ensure connection and satisfaction in worlds where voluntaristic-independent selfways provide the ecological scaffolding for experience.

Extension: The Importance of Attractiveness in Everyday Life

As the preceding section illustrates, a CP analysis applies the theme of mind in context to explain not only to explain apparently abnormal phenomena observed in exotic, "other" cultures, but also apparently "natural" phenomena observed in the familiar settings that dominate mainstream research. From this perspective, many relationship phenomena reported in the typical psychology study are not, as mainstream scientific accounts are inclined to portray them, natural expressions of inborn tendencies encoded in brain architecture. Instead, they are ecologically grounded habits of relationship that are continually reconstituted as people necessarily tune themselves to structures of mind in context. Having illuminated these structures of mind in context, it becomes easier to see them at work in other relationship phenomena.

For example, consider one of the best-known relationship phenomena in social psychology: the importance of attractiveness in everyday life. Decades of research have documented that attractive people experience better outcomes than do unattractive people (see Langlois et al., 2000). Standard accounts typically locate these effects in evolved brain structures (e.g., Buss, 1989; Thornhill & Gangestad, 1999). In contrast, a CP perspective suggests that attractiveness effects also reflect local selfways and other structures of mind in context. The relationship between attraction and life outcomes may be greatest in worlds where voluntaristic-independent selfways provide the ecological scaffolding for experience. In worlds that afford people freedom (and compel them) to choose their own relationships, preference (as a determinant of choice) and attraction (as a determinant of preference) gain importance in relationship life. Attraction may be less important in worlds of embedded interdependence, where the thicker or stickier nature of relationship means that personal choice and preference have less impact on life outcomes.

In support of these ideas, research suggests that the relationship between attractiveness and self-reported life outcomes is greater not only (1) in North American settings than in West African settings but also (2) in friend than in family relationships, and (3) in urban than in rural spaces (see Anderson, Adams, & Plaut, 2008, Study 1; Plaut, Adams, & Anderson, in press). Likewise, research suggests that *physical attractiveness stereotyping*—the tendency to rate anticipated outcomes of attractive people more positively than those of unattractive people—is not only greater in the United States than in Ghanaian settings and in urban rather than rural spaces but also (within Ghanaian settings) is greater among people "primed" to think about personal characteristics than personal connections (Anderson et al., 2008, Study 2). Rather than a natural property of mind in brain, this research suggests that the importance of attractiveness for life outcomes reflects structures of mind in context associated with voluntaristic-independent selfways.

DISAPPEARING PENISES: GENITAL-SHRINKING PANIC

If one stays in West African settings for an extended period, one is likely to encounter something like the episode of *genital-shrinking panic* (GSP) that occurred at several sites in Ghana during January 1997 (Dzokoto & Adams, 2005).[1] In its typical presentations, GSP refers to the mass occurrence of distress in which men fear that their penises are shrinking due to magical theft. People in the 1997 episode typically attributed the motivation for such theft to the desire for money, either by holding stolen genitalia for ransom or by using them as ingredients for the production of "money medicine." In any case, the accusation of penis theft placed the accused thief in mortal danger from beatings that bystanders often administered as "instant justice" (see Adams & Dzokoto, 2007; Dzokoto & Adams, 2005; Mather, 2005).

Normalizing Genital Shrinking Panic

As with cautious approaches to relationship, outsider accounts are likely to frame GSP incidents as cases of paranoid behavior to the extent that they involve irrational fear of harm. Indeed, for people in highly educated worlds, the belief that people could steal penises through sorcery or witchcraft seems like exactly the sort of "superstitious nonsense"—reflecting delusion or lack of contact with reality—that science combats (Jackson, 1998). In contrast, a CP perspective suggests that what predisposes people to GSP is not paranoid delusion, superstitious ignorance, or lack of contact with reality, but normal sensitivity to structures of mind in context.

Cultural Grounding of Genital-Shrinking Panic

These structures of mind in context include specific concepts or institutions. As hinted in the previous paragraph, a prevailing construction of reality that underlies concerns about both penis theft and malicious false accusation is the set of concepts referred to in English as *witchcraft*, *sorcery*, or *juju* (see de-Graft Aikins, 2004; Geschiere, 1997; Meyer, 2003). These concepts propose not only magical means through which penis theft might occur but also the existence of malicious enemies who seek to do harm (whether through magical or nonmagical means). Regardless of whether people typically "believe in" them, witchcraft and sorcery are prominent local concepts that are readily available for people to appropriate when—as in the case of GSP—doing so helps them make sense of everyday events.

In addition, the reference to mind in context includes more general cultural models. For example, research associates the embedded-interdependent selfways to which we referred in the previous section with several habits of being that may actively foster penis-shrinking experience (Dzokoto & Adams, 2005). These habits include a sense of openness to interpersonal influence and automatic tuning to social context (Riesman, 1986); "holistic" perceptual habits that direct attention to contextual sources of experience (see Nisbett, Peng, Choi, & Norenzayan, 2001); and *somatization*: the tendency to experience negative affect in bodily rather than psychological forms (e.g., Ryder et al., 2008). These habits of mind are not superficial interpretations applied to more basic experience; instead they play a *constitutive* role in GSP, such that mass episodes would not occur without the scaffolding that these models and representations provide (Good, 1994). To the extent that people inhabit spaces where these habits of mind are (or become) prominent, they are (or become) more likely to experience GSP.

Dynamic Reproduction of Genital-Shrinking Panic Reality

So far, this discussion of GSP has emphasized processes of incorporation or embodiment, represented by the top arrow in Figure 14.1, by which patterns of mind inscribed in local worlds come to shape psychological experience. However, an adequate account of GSP and its relationship to structures of mind in context must also direct attention to the processes of inscription or objectification, represented by the bottom arrow in Figure 14.1, by which everyday belief and behavior reproduce cultural reality.

One way in which beliefs about GSP create their own reality is an intrapersonal version of self-fulfilling prophecy.[2] In this version, episodes of GSP activate ecological structures of mind in context that promote a charged atmosphere of heightened sensitivity to potential malice. In this charged atmosphere, an otherwise innocuous event can trigger a man's concern that he is the target of penis tampering. This concern can arouse intense anxiety and somatic reactions, especially in relatively plastic organs like genitalia, which the man is likely to interpret as confirmation rather than a consequence of his anxious beliefs. This interpretation is likely to create more anxiety, which increases the physiological response of shrinking, which creates more anxiety, and so on, in a self-fulfilling spiral (see Oyebode, Jamieson, Mullaney, & Davison, 1986).

Another way in which beliefs about GSP create their own reality is an interpersonal version of self-fulfilling prophecy akin to behavioral confirmation of stereotypes and other interpersonal expectations (Snyder, 1984). In this version, ecological structures of mind in context associated with GSP include an atmosphere of interpersonal suspicion that has self-fulfilling consequences. If a man meets a woman in town and appears reluctant to return her greeting, this behavioral performance constitutes an instance of mind in context associated with distrust. Based on her observation of the man's behavioral performance, the woman may infer that he dislikes her, and she may respond with suspicion-laden behavior of her own. Her behavioral performance further reproduces ecological structures of mind in context associated with distrust, which the man may interpret as confirmation of his initial suspicions, without recognizing his role in eliciting her response. The man's interpretation may lead to further performances of suspicion, triggering more suspicion-laden responses, and so on, in a self-fulfilling spiral.

Resonating with most work, our example has portrayed behavioral confirmation as a dyadic process. To appreciate implications for the theme of mind in context, one must extend the analysis beyond the level of dyadic interaction (Claire & Fiske, 1998). Behavioral performances of suspicion do more than produce isolated dyads of dislike; in addition, they reproduce ecological structures of mind in context that promote suspicion and GSP among extradyadic observers.

Likewise, one must extend the analysis of behavioral confirmation beyond confirmation of stereotypes or other expectations to consider implications for the reproduction of reality in general. Each time people invoke concepts such as *sorcery*, they not only reproduce those concepts in their original domains of relevance (e.g., erectile dysfunction), but also often extend them to new domains (e.g., school examinations and international soccer matches; Geschiere, 1997, p. 4). Likewise, whether people believe claims of penis theft (and participate in administration of instant justice) or construe claims as false accusation (and intervene heroically to rescue the accused person), their actions constitute behavioral artifacts that serve as informational social influence or emergent norms to guide others' subsequent responses (Deutsch & Gerard, 1955; Stahl, 1982). In general, people's behavioral responses to individual cases of GSP often reinscribe and reconstitute the structures of mind in context that are constitutive of GSP experience in the first place. This idea has three important implications.

First, processes of inscription and objectification represented by the bottom arrow of Figure 14.1 are essential to the "epidemic" character of GSP episodes. In the initial stages of an episode, the structures of mind in context that promote GSP may be relatively inactive, such that only people who are especially situated to experience GSP do so. However, the subsequent behavior of these "early adopters" strengthens or activates the facilitating structures of mind in context that underlie GSP, such that they eventually promote GSP experience among people who were originally less situated to experience it. Without this active reconstitution of the structures of mind in context that are constitutive of GSP, it is unlikely that GSP would impact so many people.

Second, processes of inscription and objectification help to illuminate the collective nature of GSP. What makes GSP *collective* is not its "group" character (i.e., that it occurred in mass episodes rather than isolated cases) but instead the extent to which each person's distress is afforded by the fertile common ground that the behavioral sediment of other people's experience provides. Rather than the aggregate of multiple, isolated individuals constructing similar experience from the same raw materials, mass episodes occur because each person constructs an experience by using the scaffolding provided by the accumulated, material sediment of others' behavior.

Third, this reference to behavioral sediment helps to illuminate the idea of "mind in society." The structures of mind in context that provide fertile common ground for GSP are not only embodied in individual subjectivity but also are objectified in everyday worlds (Berger & Luckmann, 1966; Moscovici, 1984). Rather than transmission from one individual to another across a psychological vacuum, the process of social influence associated with GSP flows through ecologically inscribed structures of mind in context.

Turning the Analytic Lens: Denaturing the Biomedical Model

Besides providing a normalizing account of GSP in West African settings, the second task of a CP analysis is to provide a denaturing account that illuminates the typically invisible structures of mind in context that inform responses to GSP in mainstream health science. Perhaps the most important of these structures is the prevailing *biomedical* model of health and illness. The key points associated with this model include a construction of health as freedom from suffering; an emphasis on biochemical and physiological processes; and a corresponding inattention to social-psychological determinants of well-being, illness, diagnosis, and healing.

Rather than a culture-neutral reflection of natural reality, the biomedical model resonates with the atomistic or independent selfways characteristic of "modern" societies: structures of mind in context that propose abstraction of person from social context and locate the roots of experience in the internal properties of existentially separate individuals. Although this particular cultural foundation provides conceptual advantages for understanding biochemical and physiological manifestations of health and illness, it creates problems for understanding other manifestations. Resonating with the topic of this section, one problem with the biomedical model is that it tends to obscure the extent to which embodied beliefs—and the ecological structures of mind in context to which embodied beliefs are continuously tuned—are constitutive of bodily experience. As a result, mainstream health science has difficulty accommodating phenomena such as placebo effects (Harrington, 1999) or mass psychogenic illness (Colligan, Pennebaker, & Murphy, 1982), in which belief plays a central role.

Resonating with the topic of the next section, another problem with the biomedical model is that its internal gaze and atomistic focus obscure structural, socioeconomic, and geopolitical forces associated with socio-ecological variation in health and disease (see Mirowsky & Ross, 2003; Williams & Collins, 1995). Regardless of individual scientists' intentions, an atomistic focus on physiological processes constitutes a politically consequential "intentional world" that, by ignoring structural determinants of ill health (e.g., malnutrition and poverty), contributes to the reproduction of disease and discomfort in marginalized spaces (see Hepworth, 2006). From this perspective, an adequate health science requires greater attention to the structures of mind in context that influence not only the experience but also the study of health and illness (see Adams & Salter, 2007).

SUSPICION OF VACCINE TAMPERING: FAILURE OF THE GLOBAL POLIO ERADICATION INITIATIVE

In 1988, worldwide health organizations launched a global initiative to eradicate poliomyelitis virus (Global Polio Eradication Initiative, *www.polioeradication.org*). Although the campaign came close to its goal, it stalled (and eventually reversed) in the face of popular resistance to vaccination drives in northern Nigeria. At issue were concerns that doses of oral polio vaccine (OPV) were contaminated with HIV or were designed to render female children infertile as means of population control (Ajiya, 2003). As with suspicion of enemies and incidents of GSP, acts of OPV refusal constitute paranoid behavior to the extent that they appear to involve irrational fear of harm. Indeed, international health organizations generally framed people's suspicions as "unfounded concerns," which they hoped that health workers could alleviate by exposing people to "correct" knowledge (WHO News, 2004). In contrast to such relatively pathologizing characterizations of OPV refusal, a CP analysis emphasizes two points (Adams & Salter, 2007).

Normalizing Suspicion of Vaccine Tampering

First, without endorsing claims of vaccine tampering or advocating vaccine refusal, a CP approach normalizes suspicion of vaccine tampering. Rather as "unfounded concern," these suspicions have a reasonable foundation in structures of mind in context associated with collective memory of racism (Adams & Salter, 2007; see Whaley, 2001). People who refuse OPV may do so not because of ignorance or delusion, but because they are more educated about past incidents of racism than are people who accept OPV. These incidents include documented cases of medical racism, such as the Tuskegee Syphilis Study (Freimuth et al., 2001), sterilization practices designed to control population growth among people of African descent (Mass, 1977), or practices for research in African settings that the same researchers would find unacceptable in European or U.S. settings (Lurie & Wolfe, 1997).

Turning the Analytic Lens: Denaturing Denial of Racism

Second, a CP analysis denatures scientific common sense. Rather than unbiased reflection of truth, trust in the nonracist character of medical science or other mainstream institutions may reflect faith, denial, or outright ignorance. From this perspective, mainstream reactions to OPV refusal are not based on neutral reading of events but instead reflect an "unfounded" inclination by the medical and scientific establishment to deny pervasive racism and remnants of colonialism.

Empirical evidence relevant to this point comes from our research on group differences in perception of racism in U.S. society. Relative to people from a variety of historically oppressed groups, white Americans tend to deny the extent to which racism is responsible for events in U.S. society. In part, this group difference in perception of racism reflects divergent motivational pressures. White Americans are motivated to deny the ongoing significance of racism to preserve a sense of collective self-worth and to defend the legitimacy of a status quo from which they derive benefits (Adams, Tormala, & O'Brien, 2006; Branscombe, Schmitt, & Harvey, 1999). However, even when people genuinely strive for an honest assessment, group differences can also result because different communities inhabit and reproduce different ecologies of mind in context that promote divergent judgments about the ongoing significance of racism. We have investigated this idea with respect to three different manifestations of mind in context.

Representations of Racism

One manifestation concerns representations of racism itself. Relative to people from various oppressed groups, white Americans are motivated to endorse an *atomistic* conception of racism as a problem of individual bias but are less likely to endorse a *sociocultural* conception of racism as a problem inherent in the very fabric of American society (Adams, O'Brien, & Nelson, 2006; Bobo, 2001). To investigate the consequences of these different conceptions, we constructed tutorials that took raw material from mainstream research—for example, discussions of stereotype threat (Steele, 1997) and automatic racism (Devine, 1989)—and presented it in one of two ways (Adams, Edkins, Lacka, Pickett, & Cheryan, 2008). Drawing heavily upon existing pedagogy, the *standard* tutorial presented the topic of racism in a relatively atomistic fashion as the product of biased individuals.[3] In contrast, the *sociocultural* tutorial presented the topic of racism as something embedded in the fabric of U.S. society. Rather than portray racism as widespread individual bias, it portrayed the pervasive nature of automatic racism as the tuning of the individual mind to ecologically inscribed associations and shared realities of racism (see Sinclair & Lun, Chapter 11, this volume). Rather than consider racism as an afterthought to a discussion of stereotyping and prejudice, it emphasized the key insight of stereotype threat research: how the oppressive impact of racism is not limited to cases of individual bias but also includes a "threat in the air" that harms motivation and performance even in the absence of biased treatment (Steele, 1997).

We then conducted two experiments—one online (Study 1) and the other in a classroom lecture setting (Study 2)—in which we randomly assigned white American participants to standard tutorial, sociocultural tutorial, or no-tutorial control conditions (Adams et al., 2008). After a few days, participants completed dependent measures. Results confirmed that participants in the sociocultural tutorial condition perceived greater racism in ambiguous events (e.g., the use of indigenous people as mascots by sports teams) and showed greater support for antiracist policies (e.g., reparations for slavery) than did participants in the other two conditions.

Representations of History

Another manifestation of mind in context concerns the forms of historical knowledge that inform judgments about racism. In one paradigm, we have used a signal detection procedure to assess the relationship between knowledge of historically documented racist incidents (e.g., the Tuskegee Syphilis Study) (Freimuth et al., 2001) and perception of racism in ambiguous current events (e.g., high rates of poverty in African American communities) (Nelson, Adams, Branscombe, & Schmitt, 2008; Salter, 2008). Results generally reveal that, regardless of race, perception of racism is positively related to accurate historical knowledge. However, white Americans score lower on the measure of historical accuracy than do black Americans, and this difference in knowledge of past racism partially accounts for group differences in perception of present racism in U.S. society.

In other research, we consider the consequences of engagement with different representations of the historical past. In one study, white American participants rated their familiarity with historical facts in one of three conditions: celebratory representations of black history that emphasize past achievements of black Americans, critical representations that emphasize past instances of racism, and mainstream representations of U.S. history that render people of African descent invisible. Participants exposed to critical representations not only perceived greater racism in U.S. society but also indicated greater support for policies designed to ameliorate racial inequality than did participants in the other two conditions (Salter & Adams, 2009).

Representations of American Identity

Yet another instance of mind in context that underlies variability in perception of racism concerns different representations of American identity. In one project, we investigated representations of American identity that differ in ideology regarding the multiethnic nature of U.S. society (see Wolsko, Park, Judd, & Wittenbrink, 2000). *Color-blind* representations of American identity deny racial and ethnic difference, and downplay the significance of ethnic and racial identity in U.S. society. In contrast, *multicultural* representations of American identity celebrate cultural differences and acknowledge the ongoing significance of ethnic and racial identity in U.S. society. We conducted both a correlational study, in which we measured endorsement of these representations (Phillips & Adams, 2009; Study 1), and an experiment in which we manipulated exposure to these representations (Phillips & Adams, 2009; Study 2). Across both studies, results indicated that color-blind representations of American identity were associated with greater strength of American identification and stronger denial of racism than were multicultural representations.

Implications for the Theme of "Mind in Context"

The preceding discussion of research on racism denial illuminates the theme of "mind in context" in the sense of the top arrow of Figure 14.1: the cultural constitution of psychological experience. Rather than reflecting a coolly rational perception of objective reality, this research suggests that white American tendencies to perceive little racism in ambiguous events reflect structures of mind in context—including representations of racism, history, and American identity—that promote a tendency to understate the impact of racism in U.S. society.

However, this discussion also hints at a more provocative sense of "mind in context" related to the idea of "mind in society." Mainstream psychology takes it almost as given that whether the natural expression of genetically encoded instructions or the incorporation of ecologically represented structures, psychological processes happen inside individuals. In contrast, research on racism denial suggests the extent to which psychological processes also extend into the structure of everyday worlds. We consider this idea in relation to four psychological processes.

Memory

Psychologists have typically studied memory as individual representation. Although some have investigated sociocultural influences on memory (see Bartlett, 1932; Wang & Ross, 2007), no less authoritative a source than the *Handbook of Social Psychology* locates its chapter on memory in a section titled "Intrapersonal Phenomena" (Smith, 1998). In contrast, a CP analysis suggests that one consider how memory also exists as ecological structures of mind in context (see Smith & Collins, Chapter 7, this volume). The ecological location of memory is particularly clear with respect to representations of history and collective memory (Wertsch, 2002). People do not have firsthand knowledge of past events; instead, their knowledge of the past comes from representations of history inscribed in cultural products (e.g., commemorative holidays, museums, official monuments, and textbooks) (Kurtiş, Adams, & Yellow Bird, in press; Loewen, 1999; Rowe, Wertsch, & Kosyaeva, 2002; Wertsch, 2002). However, the ecological location of memory is also evident in the apparently intrapersonal phenomenon of autobiographical memory. Rather than individual reconstruction, *autobiographical memory* is a joint product that people actively construct in collaboration with listeners through culturally embedded conversational practices and other structures of mind in context (e.g., Wang & Brockmeier, 2002).

Identity

Given its link to memory, one can consider the extent to which identity is not merely limited to intrapersonal representations but also exists as ecological structures of mind in context inscribed in everyday cultural worlds. At the level of individual self, Pasupathi (2001) details how culturally saturated conversational practices influence the stories people tell about experiences, which in turn influence what they remember about those experiences and how they reconstruct personal identity. More generally, McAdams (2001) proposes a conception of personal identity as a *life story*: a psychosocial construction, "coauthored by the person ... and the cultural context within which that person's life is embedded and given meaning" (p. 101). Life stories are loosely based on biographical facts but go far beyond such facts as people integrate across diverse experiences to construct stories that make sense—both to themselves and to their audiences—according to culturally embedded narrative practices, understandings of the life course, and other ecological structures of mind in context (McAdams, 2001). These perspectives emphasize that personal identity is not simply a personal project but also rests on sociocultural structures of mind in context that provide ecological scaffolding for personal identity.

At the level of collective self, ecological structures of social identity include not only social representations of history (i.e., collective memory; Liu & Hilton, 2005), but also practices ("official" languages), artifacts (national flags), institutions (print media), and other structures of mind in context through which people imagine community with distant others (Anderson, 1983; Billig, 1995). These structures of mind in context are perhaps clearest in the case of national identity (Reicher & Hopkins, 2001). Despite similar etymological roots, *national* identities are not *natural*; rather, they are continually reconstructed in innumerable acts of banal nationalism (e.g., reproducing national boundaries by imposing them on satellite maps of weather patterns; Billig, 1995). More generally, people actively coauthor a sense of racial/ethnic, gender, and other social identities based partly on not only biographical "facts" (e.g., skin color or particular genitalia), but also social representations of identity and other structures of mind in context (Duveen, 2001; Philogene, 2001). Different representations of identity—icons like *Chief Wahoo* or Disney's *Pocahontas*, labels like *First Nations* or *Indian*—are not superficially different versions of the same thing; instead, they constitute somewhat different realties that have divergent implications for everyday experience (Adams, Fryberg, Garcia, & Delgado-Torres, 2006; Fryberg, Markus, Oyserman, & Stone, 2005). Research comparing effects of color-blind versus multicultural representations of American identity on racism perception is an example of this idea (Phillips & Adams, 2009; see preceding section).

Motivation

As the link between memory and identity suggests, memory processes are subject to ego-defensive motivational pressures. At the level of individual self, people remember their life story in ways that reflect and promote positive personal identity (e.g., Wilson & Ross, 2003). At the level of collective self, people remember historical events in ways that reflect and promote positive social identities (Sahdra & Ross, 2007; Wohl, Branscombe, & Klar, 2006). A CP analysis adds to these observations by illuminating implications for the idea of mind in context. When people act based on preferences for identity-enhancing versions of the past, they reinscribe identity-enhancing representations of history in everyday worlds (i.e., the process represented by the bottom arrow of Figure 14.1). In other words, they produce ecological structures of motivation in context that bear traces of their understandings and desires.

This idea is evident in an investigation of displays for Black History Month (BHM) in Kansas City area schools (Salter & Adams, 2009). In one study, we observed that schools with majority white populations were more likely than schools with majority black populations (1) to use commercially available, "prepackaged" BHM displays; (2) to link BHM to larger issues of cultural diversity rather than civil rights; and (3) to deemphasize struggles against racism. Evidence from a second study suggests that these differences were not coincidental. When we exposed white American undergraduates to photographs of these BHM displays, they rated displays from majority-white schools to be more attractive and more familiar than the displays from majority-black schools. Briefly stated, these results suggest that the ecologies of memory and identity characteristic of the majority-white schools were not accidental, but instead resonated with white American preferences and motivations.

There is a small but potentially powerful way in which a discussion of motivation as mind in context differs from the preceding discussion of memory and identity. In the case of memory and identity, one might argue—consistent with the reductionist and individualist roots of social psychology (see Farr, 1996)—that associated structures of mind in context are, at most, external storage of psychological content. People may draw upon these external stores in the process of remembering and constructing identity, but (the argument goes) the processes of memory and identity per se occur within individual minds.

Although one can dispute this reductionist interpretation even in the case of memory and identity (see Wertsch, 2002), its inadequacy is especially clear in the case of motivation. To illustrate, consider a person confronted with judgments about possible racism in U.S. society. Even if she manages to approach the judgments in a nondefensive fashion, she must nevertheless draw upon mainstream representations of history and other ecologically inscribed structures of collective memory. Informed by these ecological structures of memory, she is likely to conclude that racism plays little role. Yet the question remains: To what extent was her judgment the product of defensive motivations? In contrast to the standard analysis of motivation as an individual process, a CP analysis suggests that even if the woman managed to set aside ego-defensive motivations and evaluated evidence in an evenhanded fashion, her judgment is nevertheless motivated to the extent that the ecological structures of collective memory (also known as representations of history) that inform her judgment bear the identity-enhancing desires of the people who reproduced them (and silence other, more damning representations; Cohen, 2001). In other words, the motivational forces that inform her judgment are not reducible to an individual motivation to deny racism. Instead, these motivational forces reside outside her individual subjectivity, inscribed and objectified in everyday worlds as ecological structures of memory and identity that promote collectively "desired" action.

Intention

When we design courses that portray racism as individual bias (Adams et al., 2008; Pickett, 2007) or recount celebratory versions of history (Salter & Adams, 2009; see Loewen, 1995), we may not intend to promote denial of racism or opposition to corrective policy. Even so, our behavior reinscribes structures of mind in context that—regardless of our individual intentions—promote these outcomes. Reflecting the bottom arrow of Figure 14.1, people reproduce cultural worlds (e.g., psychology lectures about prejudice or BHM bulletin boards) that infuse their particular understandings and desires into everyday reality. Reflecting the top arrow of Figure 14.1, these ecological structures of mind in context subsequently afford denial of racism and opposition to corrective policy, even among people who might self-consciously intend otherwise.

In CP terms, one can say that atomistic constructions of racism or celebratory constructions of history constitute *intentional worlds* (Shweder, 1990): ecological structures of mind in context that systematically direct experience toward particular ends. As in the discussion of motivation, the *intention* in "intentional worlds" need not reside in the individual subjectivity of the person reciting atomistic definitions of racism or reproducing celebratory constructions of history (as in the case of kids playing with plastic "cowboys and Indians"; see Yellow Bird, 2004). Instead, the intention exists as a psychological trace, implicit in the behavioral sediment that previous waves of actors have deposited into everyday cultural worlds.

CONCLUSION: MIND IN CONTEXT AS INTENTIONAL WORLDS

The concept of intentional worlds provides a powerful way to think about the theme of mind in context. Ecological perspectives and discussions of automaticity have highlighted the extent to which features of everyday worlds structure experience, typically outside of individual awareness (Bargh & Chartrand, 1999; McArthur & Baron, 1983). However, these perspectives have tended to talk about everyday worlds as natural facts that are more or less independent of human agency. In other words, these perspectives have emphasized one sense of "mind in context": the extent to which the structures of mind in brain come to *reflect* the structure of everyday worlds. However, they typically have not emphasized the idea of "mind in society": how mind not only reflects but also *resides in* the structure of everyday worlds (Heft, 2007; Hodges & Baron, 2007).

In contrast, a CP perspective highlights the *intentional* character of everyday worlds: not necessarily in the sense of "consciously or purposefully designed" (although, as with formal education systems, this is often so; see Cheney, 1987), but instead in the sense of "directive." Reflecting the bottom arrow of Figure 14.1, this intentional character means that everyday worlds are not just natural. Instead, they are human products, constituted by layers of behavioral sediment that bear the understandings, desires, and other psychological traces of their (re)producers. Reflecting the top arrow of Figure 14.1, this intentional character means that everyday worlds are not neutral. Instead, they carry a psychological charge that influences experience toward particular ends, regardless of whether their producers intend to imbue them with any charge.

In keeping with the individualist and reductionist roots of the science, we social psychologists have tended to be wary of talk about collective manifestations of mind. Instead, we have typically retreated to atomistic philosophical positions that portray social-psychological phenomena as the aggregate of separate individual experience.[4] Although this portrayal distorts understanding of psychological functioning in general, it is clearly inadequate for understanding phenomena such as GSP episodes, the motivated nature of racism denial, and the racism inherent in mainstream representations of American history. These phenomena require the more collective notion of mind associated with the concept of intentional worlds—not as a metaphysically dubious, superordinate entity with its own subjectivity and consciousness but instead as psychological traces of behavior deposited in everyday worlds as ecological structures of mind in context. Conceived in this way, the notion of mind in context promises a truly social psychology that escapes the constraints of ontological and epistemological individualism.

NOTES

1. The most recent case to receive attention in Western media was an outbreak of GSP in the Democratic Republic of the Congo in April 2008 (Bavier, 2008). Besides the similarity of reported cases to those that we describe in this chap-

ter, a remarkable feature of these reports—for example, the fact that they appeared in forums, such as the section of the Reuters website named "Oddly Enough"—is the extent to which they reproduced stereotypes of primitive superstition and otherness. The incidents even figured prominently on the Comedy Central television network news production, *The Daily Show with Jon Stewart* (April 28, 2008), where an attitude of ridicule coexisted with (self-) censure for the attitude of ridicule: "We mentioned a big story coming out of the Congo—no, not the ongoing, Civil War–based, horrific violence—I am talking about something causing a much bigger international uproar. . . . There is a penis theft panic in the Congo!"

2. Although apparently an intrapersonal process, it is important to emphasize its collective nature. The self-fulfilling power of penis-shrinking belief to create its own behavioral reality is greatest in settings in which the structures of mind in context associated with the belief are or have become strong.
3. This atomistic conception is evident in the titles of textbook chapters and psychology courses that deal with racism and oppression. For example, an online survey of instructors for undergraduate social psychology courses (Pickett, 2007) revealed that the titles of units relevant to racism and oppression overwhelmingly referred to prejudice (95%), stereotypes or stereotyping (46%), and discrimination (33%). No titles included the terms *race* or *racism*. Likewise, the same survey revealed that instructors' definitions of racism most commonly referred to discrimination (53%), prejudice (34%), attitudes (32%), and stereotyping (32%). Only a few respondents (11%) referred to collective or institutional forms of racism.
4. For extended discussions of ideas in this paragraph, see Farr (1996) and Stryker (1997).

REFERENCES

Adams, G. (2005). The cultural grounding of personal relationship: Enemyship in North American and West African worlds. *Journal of Personality and Social Psychology, 88*, 948–968.

Adams, G., Anderson, S. L., & Adonu, J. K. (2004). The cultural grounding of closeness and intimacy. In D. Mashek & A. Aron (Eds.), *The handbook of closeness and intimacy* (pp. 321–339). Mahwah, NJ: Erlbaum.

Adams, G., & Dzokoto, V. A. (2007). Genital-shrinking panic in Ghana: A cultural-psychological analysis. *Culture and Psychology, 13*, 83–104

Adams, G., Edkins, V., Lacka, D., Pickett, K. M., & Cheryan, S. (2008). Teaching about *racism*: Pernicious implications of the standard portrayal. *Basic and Applied Social Psychology, 30*, 349–361.

Adams, G., Fryberg, S., Garcia, D. M., & Delgado-Torres, E. U. (2006). The psychology of engagement with Indigenous identities: A cultural perspective. *Cultural Diversity and Ethnic Minority Psychology, 12*, 493–508.

Adams, G., & Markus, H. R. (2004). Toward a conception of culture suitable for a social psychology of culture. In M. Schaller & C. S. Crandall (Eds.), *The psychological foundations of culture* (pp. 335–360). Mahwah, NJ: Erlbaum.

Adams, G., O'Brien, L. T., & Nelson, J. C. (2006). Perceptions of racism in Hurricane Katrina: A liberation psychology analysis. *Analyses of Social Issues and Public Policy, 6*, 215–235.

Adams, G., & Plaut, V. C. (2003). The cultural grounding of personal relationship: Friendship in North American and West African worlds. *Personal Relationships, 10*, 333–348.

Adams, G., & Salter, P. S. (2007). Health psychology in African settings: A cultural psychological analysis. *Journal of Health Psychology, 12*, 539–551.

Adams, G., Tormala, T. T., & O'Brien, L. T. (2006). The effect of self-affirmation on perceptions of racism. *Journal of Experimental Social Psychology, 42*, 616–626.

Ajiya, B. (2003, November 11). Yobe governor educates royal fathers on polio vaccines HIV/AIDS [Electronic version]. *Vanguard*. Retrieved May 2006 from *news.biafranigeriaworld.com/archive/2003/nov/11/238.html*

Altman, I., & Taylor, D. A. (1973). *Social penetration: The development of interpersonal relationships*. New York: Holt, Rinehart & Winston.

Anderson, B. (1983). *Imagined communities: Reflections on the origin and spread of nationalism*. London: Verso.

Anderson, S. L., Adams, G., & Plaut, V. C. (2008). The cultural grounding of personal relationship: The importance of attractiveness in everyday life. *Journal of Personality and Social Psychology, 95*, 352–368.

Bargh, J. A., & Chartrand, T. L. (1999). The unbearable automaticity of being. *American Psychologist, 54*, 462–479.

Bartlett, F. C. (1932). *Remembering: A study in experimental and social psychology*. Cambridge, UK: Cambridge University Press.

Baumeister, R. F. (1987). How the self became a problem: A psychological review of historical research. *Journal of Personality and Social Psychology, 52*, 163–176.

Bavier, J. (2008, April 23). Lynchings in Congo as penis theft panic hits capital. [Electronic version]. *Reuters*. Retrieved April 28, 2008, from *africa.reuters.com/odd/news/usnl22903232.html.*

Bellah, R., Madsen, R., Sullivan, W., Swindler, A., & Tipton, S. (1985). *Habits of the heart: Individualism and commitment in American life*. New York: Harper & Row.

Berger, P. L., & Luckmann, T. (1966). *The social construction of reality: A treatise in the sociology of knowledge*. New York: Anchor Books.

Billig, M. (1995). *Banal nationalism*. London: Sage.

Bobo, L. D. (2001). Racial attitudes and relations at the close of the twentieth century. In N. J. Smelser, W. J. Wilson, & F. Mitchell (Eds.), *America becoming: Racial trends and their consequences* (pp. 264–301). Washington, DC: National Academy Press.

Branscombe, N. R., Schmitt, M. T., & Harvey, R. D. (1999). Perceiving pervasive discrimination among African Americans: Implications for group identification and well-being. *Journal of Personality and Social Psychology, 77*, 135–149.

Bruner, J. (1990). *Acts of meaning*. Cambridge, MA: Harvard University Press.

Buss, D. M. (1999). Sex differences in human mate preferences: Evolutionary hypotheses tested in 37 cultures. *Behavioral and Brian Sciences*, *12*, 1–49.

Carrier, J. G. (1999). People who can be friends: Selves and social relationships. In S. Bell & S. Coleman (Eds.), *The anthropology of friendship* (pp. 1–38). Oxford, UK: Berg.

Chen, G. (1995). Differences in self-disclosure patterns among Americans versus Chinese. *Journal of Cross-Cultural Psychology*, *26*, 84–91.

Cheney, L.V. (1987). *American memory: A report on the humanities in the nation's public schools*. Washington, DC: National Endowment for the Humanities.

Claire, T., & Fiske, S. T. (1998). A systemic view of behavioral confirmation: Counterpoint to the individualist view. In C. Sedikides, J. Schopler, & C. Insko (Eds.), *Intergroup cognition and intergroup behavior* (pp. 205–231). Mahwah, NJ: Erlbaum.

Cohen, S. (2001). *States of denial: Knowing about atrocities and suffering*. London: Polity Press.

Colligan, M. J., Pennebaker, J. W., & Murphy, L. R. (Eds.). (1982). *Mass psychogenic illness: A social psychological analysis*. Hillsdale, NJ: Erlbaum.

Collins, N. L., & Read, S. J. (1990). Adult attachment, working models, and relationship quality in dating couples. *Journal of Personality and Social Psychology*, *58*, 644–663.

de-Graft Aikins, A. (2004). Strengthening quality and continuity of diabetes care in rural Ghana: A critical social psychological approach. *Journal of Health Psychology*, *9*, 295–309.

Deutsch, M., & Gerard, H. (1955). A study of normative and informational influence upon individual judgment. *Journal of Abnormal and Social Psychology*, *51*, 629–636.

Devine, P. G. (1989). Stereotypes and prejudice: Their automatic and controlled components. *Journal of Personality and Social Psychology*, *56*, 5–18.

Dion, K. K., & Dion, K. L. (1985). Defensiveness, intimacy, and heterosexual attraction. *Journal of Research in Personality*, *12*, 479–487.

Dodoo, F. N. A. (1998). Marriage type and reproduction decisions: A comparative study in sub-Saharan Africa. *Journal of Marriage and the Family*, *60*, 232–242.

Duveen, G. (2001). Representations, identities, resistance. In K. Deaux & G. Philogène (Eds.), *Representations of the social* (pp. 257–271). Oxford, UK: Blackwell.

Dzokoto, V. A., & Adams, G. (2005). Understanding genital-shrinking epidemics in West Africa: *Juju*, *Koro*, or mass psychogenic illness? *Culture, Medicine, and Psychiatry*, *29*, 53–78.

Dzokoto, V. A., & Okazaki, S. (2006). Happiness in the eye and in the heart: Somatic referencing in West African emotion lexica. *Journal of Black Psychology*, *32*, 117–140.

Eiser, E. R., & Ellis, G. (2007). Cultural competence and the African American experience with health care: The case for specific content in cross-cultural education. *Academic Medicine*, *82*, 176–183.

Farr, R. M. (1996). *The roots of modern social psychology, 1872–1954*. Cambridge, UK: Blackwell.

Fiske, A. P. (1991). *Structures of social life: The four elementary forms of human relations: Communal sharing, authority ranking, equality matching, market pricing*. New York: Free Press.

Freimuth, V. S., Quinn, S. C., Thomas, S. B., Cole, G., Zook, E., & Duncan, T. (2001). African Americans' views on research and the Tuskegee Syphilis Study. *Social Science and Medicine*, *52*, 797–808.

Fryberg, S. A., Markus, H. R., Oyserman, D., & Stone, J. M. (2008). Of warrior chiefs and Indian princesses: The psychological consequences of American Indian mascots. *Basic and Applied Psychology*, *30*, 208–218.

Geschiere, P. (1997). *The modernity of witchcraft: Politics and the occult in postcolonial Africa*. Charlottesville: University of Virginia Press.

Good, B. J. (1994). *Medicine rationality and experience: An anthropsological perspective*. Cambridge, UK: Cambridge University Press.

Gosling, S. D., Ko, S. J., Mannarelli, T., & Morris, M. E. (2002). A room with a cue: Personality judgments based on offices and bedrooms. *Journal of Personality and Social Psychology*, *82*, 379–398.

Harper, M. S., & Welsh, D. P. (2007). Keeping quiet: Self-silencing and its association with relational and individual functioning among adolescent romantic couples. *Journal of Social and Personal Relationships*, *24*, 99–116.

Harrington, A. (Ed.). (1999). *The placebo effect: An interdisciplinary exploration*. Cambridge, MA: Harvard University Press.

Heft, H. (2007). The social constitution of perceiver-environment reciprocity. *Ecological Psychology*, *19*, 85–105.

Hepworth, J. (2006). The emergence of critical health psychology: Can it contribute to promoting public health? *Journal of Health Psychology*, *11*, 331—341.

Hodges, B. H., & Baron, R. M. (2007). On making social psychology more ecological and ecological psychology more social. *Ecological Psychology*, *19*, 79–84.

Holland, D., & Quinn, N. (1987). *Cultural models of language and thought*. New York: Cambridge University Press.

Holtgraves, T. (1997). Styles of language use: Individual and cultural variability in conversational indirectness. *Journal of Personality and Social Psychology*, *73*, 624–637.

Imamoğlu, E. O. (1987). An interdependence model of human development. In Ç. Kağitçibaşi (Ed.), *Growth and progress in cross-cultural psychology*. Lisse: Swets & Zeitlinger.

Jack, D. C. (1991). *Silencing the self: Women and depression*. Cambridge, MA: Harvard University Press.

Jackson, M. (1998). *Minima ethnographica: Intersubjectivity and the anthropological project*. Chicago: University of Chicago Press.

Kağitçibaşi, Ç. (1973). Psychological aspects of modernization in Turkey. *Journal of Cross-Cultural Psychology*, *4*, 157–174.

Kağitçibaşi, Ç. (1984). Socialization in traditional society: A challenge to psychology. *International Journal of Psychology, 19*, 145–157.

Kim, H. S. (2002). We talk, therefore we think?: A cultural analysis of the effect of talking on thinking. *Journal of Personality and Social Psychology, 83*, 828–842.

Kim, H. S., & Sherman, D. K. (2007). "Express yourself": Culture and the effect of self-expression on choice. *Journal of Personality and Social Psychology, 92*, 1–11.

Kirby, J. P. (1993). The Islamic dialogue with African traditional religion: Divination and health care. *Social Science and Medicine, 36*, 237–247.

Kroeber, A. L., & Kluckhohn, C. K. (1952). *Culture: A critical review of concepts and definitions.* New York: Random House.

Kurtiş, T. (2009). *Self-silencing and well-being among Turkish women.* Unpublished master's thesis, University of Kansas, Lawrence.

Kurtiş, T., Adams, G., & Yellow Bird, M. (in press). Generosity or genocide?: Identity implications of silence in American Thanksgiving commemorations. *Memory.*

Langlois, J. H., Kalakanis, L., Rubenstein, A. J., Larson, A., Hallam, M., & Smoot, M. (2000). Maxims or myths of beauty?: A meta-analytic and theoretical review. *Psychological Bulletin, 126*, 390–423.

Laurenceau, J-P., Barrett, L. F., & Pietromonaco, P. R. (1998). Intimacy as an interpersonal process: The importance of self-disclosure, and perceived partner responsiveness in interpersonal exchanges. *Journal of Personality and Social Psychology, 74*, 1238–1251.

Liu, J. H., & Hilton, D. J. (2005). How the past weighs on the present: Social representations of history and their role in identity politics. *British Journal of Social Psychology, 44*, 537–556.

Loewen, J. W. (1995). *Lies my teacher told me: Everything your American history textbook got wrong.* New York: Touchstone.

Loewen, J. W. (1999). *Lies across America: What our historic sites get wrong.* New York: Simon & Schuster.

Lohmann, A., Arriaga, X. B., & Goodfriend, W. (2003). Close relationships and placemaking: Do objects in a couple's home reflect couplehood? *Personal Relationships, 10*, 437–449.

Lurie, P., & Wolfe, S. M. (1997). Unethical trials of interventions to reduce perinatal transmission of the human immunodeficiency virus in developing countries. *New England Journal of Medicine, 337*, 853–856.

Markus, H. R., Mullally, P., & Kitayama, S. (1997). Selfways: Diversity in modes of cultural participation. In U. Neisser & D. A. Jopling (Eds.), *The conceptual self in context: Culture, experience, self-understanding* (pp. 13–61). Cambridge, UK: Cambridge University Press.

Mass, B. (1977). Puerto Rico: A case study of population control. *Latin American Perspectives, 4*, 66–81.

Mather, C. (2005). Accusations of genital theft: A case from Northern Ghana. *Culture, Medicine, and Psychiatry, 29*, 33–52.

McAdams, D. P. (2001). The psychology of life stories. *Review of General Psychology, 5*, 100–122.

McArthur, L. Z., & Baron, R. M. (1983). Toward an ecological theory of social perception. *Psychological Review, 90*, 215–238.

Meyer, B. (2003). Ghanaian popular cinema and the magic in and of film. In B. Meyer & P. Pels (Eds.), *Magic and modernity: Interfaces of revelation and concealment* (pp. 200—222). Stanford, CA: Stanford University Press.

Mikulincer, M., & Nachshon, O. (1991). Attachment styles and patterns of self-disclosure. *Journal of Personality and Social Psychology, 61*, 321–331.

Mirowsky, J., & Ross, C. E. (2003). *Education, social status, and health.* New Brunswick, NJ: Aldine.

Morling, B., & Lamoreaux, M. (2008). Measuring culture outside the head: A meta-analysis of individualism–collectivism in cultural products. *Personality and Social Psychology Bulletin, 12*, 199–221.

Moscovici, S. (1984). The phenomena of social representations. In R. M. Farr & S. Moscovici (Eds.), *Social representations* (pp. 3–69). Cambridge, UK: Cambridge University Press.

Nelson, J. C., Adams, G., Branscombe, N. R., & Schmitt, M. T. (2008). *The role of historical knowledge in endorsement of race-based conspiracy beliefs.* Unpublished manuscript, University of Kansas, Lawrence.

Nisbett, R. E., Peng, K. P., Choi, I., & Norenzayan, A. (2001). Culture and systems of thought: Holistic versus analytic cognition. *Psychological Review, 108*, 291–310.

Obadare, E. (2005). A crisis of trust: History, politics, religion, and the polio controversy in Northern Nigeria. *Patterns of Prejudice, 39*, 265–284.

O'Conner, P. (1998). Women's friendships in a post-modern world. In R. G. Adams & G. Allan (Eds.), *Placing friendship in context* (pp. 117–135). Cambridge, UK: Cambridge University Press.

Oliker, S. J. (1998). The modernization of friendship: Individualism, intimacy, and gender in the nineteenth century. In R. G. Adams & G. Allan (Eds.), *Placing friendship in context* (pp. 18–42). Cambridge, UK: Cambridge University Press.

Oyebode, F., Jamieson, R., Mullaney, J., & Davison, K. (1986). Koro—a psychophysiological dysfunction? *British Journal of Psychiatry, 148*, 212–214.

Pasupathi, M. (2001). The social construction of the personal past and its implications for adult development. *Psychological Bulletin, 127*, 651–672.

Phillips, N. L., & Adams, G. (2009, May). *The racism of identity: Implications of different constructions of "American."* Paper presented at the annual meeting of the Association for Psychological Science, San Francisco.

Philogene, G. (2001). From race to culture: The emergence of the African American. In K. Deaux & G. Philogene (Eds.), *Representations of the social* (pp. 113–128). Oxford, UK: Blackwell.

Pickett, K. M. (2007). [Content of racism and oppression lessons in social psychology courses]. Unpublished raw data.

Plaut, V. C., Adams, G., & Anderson, S. L. (in press). Does beauty buy well-being?: It depends on where you're from. *Personal Relationships.*

Potter, J., & Wetherell, M. (1987). *Discourse and social psychology: Beyond attitudes and behaviour.* London: Sage.

Reicher, S., & Hopkins, N. (2001). *Self and nation.* London: Sage.
Riesman, P. (1986). The person and the life cycle in African social life and thought. *African Studies Review, 29,* 71–138.
Rowe, S. M., Wertsch, J. V., & Kosyaeva, T. Y. (2002). Linking little narratives to big ones: Narrative and public memory in history museums. *Culture and Psychology, 8,* 96–112.
Ryder, A. G., Yang, J., Zhu, X., Yao, S., Yi, J., Heine, S. J., et al. (2008). The cultural shaping of depression: Somatic symptoms in China, psychological symptoms in North America? *Journal of Abnormal Psychology, 117,* 300–313.
Sahdra, B., & Ross, M. (2007). Group identification and historical memory. *Personality and Social Psychology Bulletin, 33,* 384–395.
Salter, P. S. (2008). *Perception of racism in ambiguous events: A cultural psychology analysis.* Unpublished master's thesis, University of Kansas, Lawrence.
Salter, P. S., & Adams, G. (2009, February) *Representations of black history as instruments of liberation and oppression.* Paper presented at the annual meeting of the Society for Personality and Social Psychology, Tampa, FL.
Shaw, R. (2000). "Tok af, lef af": A political economy of Temne techniques of secrecy and self. In I. Karp & D. A. Masolo (Eds.), *African philosophy as cultural inquiry* (pp. 25–49). Bloomington: Indiana University Press.
Shweder, R. A. (1990). Cultural psychology: What is it? In J. Stigler, R. Shweder, & G. Herdt (Eds.), *Cultural psychology: Essays on comparative human development* (pp. 1–46). Cambridge, UK: Cambridge University Press.
Smith, E. R. (1998). Mental representation and memory. In D. Gilbert, S. Fiske, & G. Lindzey (Eds.), *Handbook of social psychology* (4th ed., Vol. 1, pp. 391–445). New York: McGraw-Hill.
Snyder, M. (1984). When belief creates reality. *Advances in Experimental Social Psychology, 18,* 62–113.
Stahl, S. M. (1982). Illness as an emergent norm or doing what comes naturally. In M. J. Colligan, J. W. Pennebaker, & L. R. Murphy (Eds.), *Mass psychogenic illness: A social psychological analysis* (pp. 183–198). Hillsdale, NJ: Erlbaum.
Steele, C. M. (1997). A threat in the air: How stereotypes shape intellectual identity and performance. *American Psychologist, 52,* 613–629.
Stryker, S. (1997). In the beginning there is society: Lessons from a sociological social psychology. In C. McGarty & S. A. Haslam (Eds.), *The message of social psychology: Perspectives on mind in society* (pp. 315–327). Cambridge, MA: Blackwell.
The Daily Show with Jon Stewart. (2008, April 28). Penis theft panic update. Video clip retrieved September 1, 2008, from *www.thedailyshow.com/video/index.jhtml?videoId=167140&title=penis-theft-panic-update.*
Thornhill, R., & Gangestad, S. W. (1999). Facial attractiveness. *Trends in Cognitive Science, 3,* 452–460.
Turner, P. A. (1994). *I heard it through the grapevine: Rumor in African-American culture.* Berkeley: University of California Press.

Vygotsky, L. S. (1978). *Mind in society: The development of higher psychological processes*. Cambridge, MA: Harvard University Press.

Wang, Q., & Brockmeier, J. (2002). Autobiographical remembering as cultural practice: Understanding the interplay between memory, self, and culture. *Culture and Psychology, 8*, 45–64.

Wang, Q., & Ross, M. (2007). Culture and memory. In H. Kitayama & D. Cohen (Eds.), *Handbook of cultural psychology* (pp. 645–667). New York: Guilford Press.

Wertsch, J. V. (2002). *Voices of collective remembering*. New York: Cambridge University Press.

Whaley, A. L. (2001). Cultural mistrust and mental health services for African Americans: A review and meta-analysis. *Counseling Psychologist, 29*, 513–531.

White House Office of the Press Secretary. (1997, May 16). *Remarks by the President in apology for study done in Tuskegee*. Retrieved November 1, 2008, from *clinton4.nara.gov/textonly/new/remarks/fri/19970516-898.html*.

WHO News. (2004). Two countries re-infected with polio as Nigeria state resumes vaccinations. *Bulletin of the World Health Organization, 82*(9), 717.

Williams, D. R., & Collins, C. (1995). U.S. socioeconomic and racial differences in health: Patterns and explanations. *Annual Review of Sociology, 21*, 349–386.

Wilson, A. E., & Ross, M. (2003). The identity function of autobiographical memory: Time is on our side. *Memory, 11*, 137–149.

Wohl, M. J. A., Branscombe, N. R., & Klar, Y. (2006). Collective guilt: Justice-based emotional reactions when one's group has done wrong or been wronged. *European Review of Social Psychology, 17*, 1–37.

Wolsko, C., Park, B., Judd, C. M., & Wittenbrink, B. (2000). Framing interethnic ideology: Effects of multicultural and color-blind perspectives on judgments of groups and individuals. *Journal of Personality and Social Psychology, 78*, 635–654.

Yellow Bird, M. (2004). Cowboys and Indians: Toys of genocide, icons of colonialism. *Wicazo Sa Review, 18*, 33–48.

15

Challenging the Egocentric View of Coordinated Perceiving, Acting, and Knowing

MICHAEL J. RICHARDSON
KERRY L. MARSH
R. C. SCHMIDT

A major goal of cognitive and psychological science is to understand the systematic and coordinated patterns of everyday behavior. Whether we are trying to understand the coordinated actions that characterize behaviors such as locomotion, reaching or grasping, or the perceptions of environmental objects, surfaces, or events, understanding the regularity of behavior, its flexibility and stability, the conditions under which it does or does not occur, and the processes or mechanisms by which it comes to be, calls for explanation—to determine causality. Traditionally, cognitive and psychological scientists have sought to confine the causality of all behavior by looking inward, thus reducing the system of interest to "entities" or modules in the mind or brain. In doing so, much of cognitive and psychological science has become exceedingly *egocentric* in focus, attempting to understand human perceiving and acting by isolating the centralized mental, computational, or representational processes that might account for it. Thus, the *context* of agency, of mind, and that which surrounds it and gives it *material* being, has been largely ignored. This is true not only for the activity of individuals but also the many joint or social actions in which individuals engage each day, such as when two or more people are moving furniture together, rowing a canoe, or simply walking and talking. Indeed, traditional explanations of interpersonal and social action are centered on not only the mental processes of mind and brain but also the distinct processes of solitary minds and solitary brains.

Over the past few decades, however, a growing number of psychologists and cognitive scientists have started to question this traditional approach, acknowledging that a purely egocentric perspective of behavioral order is untenable, and that perceiving, acting, and even knowing are embodied and embedded, context-dependent processes (e.g., Beer, 1995; Brooks, 1995; Clark, 1997; Gibbs, 2006; Gibson, 1979; Hutchins, 1995; Thelen & Smith, 1994; Turvey & Shaw, 1979, 1999; Turvey, Shaw, Reed, & Mace, 1981; Varela, Thompson, & Rosch, 1991; Warren, 2006; Wilson, 2002). The term *embodied* is used to convey how the tangible physical reality of an agent's existence, more specifically, its body and action system, matters—and not just in a superficial way, by serving as inferential input to centralized cognitive processes, but rather in fundamentally defining the constituents of mind, as well as the meaning that motivates and constrains an agent's perceptions and actions. Similarly, the term *embedded* is used to convey how an agent's mind, its perceptions of the world, and its actions in that world, are intimately bound to and dependent on environmental context. The environment is not merely viewed as "conditional input," which can color mental inferences made about the world, but is understood to play a mutual role in the causal organization of behavior. Accordingly, the embodied–embedded approach seeks to challenge the classically defined separations between mind and body, between perception and action, and between animal and environment, arguing that such separations are, at best, scientifically nonobvious, arbitrary, and ill-defined. In other words, the organizational processes that underlie behavioral order are not locally or centrally defined within the mind or brain but are distributed across mind, body, and environment—across an animal–environment system. Consistent with this embodied-embedded approach is the belief that human and animal behavior is dynamically *self-organized*, resulting from the multitude of physical and informational "couplings" that exist between animal and environment. At odds with the linear, bottom up, mechanistic notion of causality, this self-organized dynamical systems approach rejects the idea of there being "root causes" of phenomena (that ordered behavior is managed or controlled by an isolated entity or inner source), proposing instead that the coordinated structures, patterns, and properties of behavior are an emergent consequence of the reciprocal relations that exist between an animal and its environment.

Here, we make the claim that studying the mind, body, and environment as a unitary whole, as an animal–environment system, is not only important for understanding the systematic and coordinated patterns of behavior but also is in some instances necessary. We do so by describing recent research on environmental and interpersonal coordination, and the perception of both solo and social affordances. It is our proposal that such research provides support for this claim by demonstrating how the patterning of certain perceptual–motor behaviors results from causal processes that extend beyond the mind or brain and involve the physical and lawful properties of both body and world. In order to provide a more tangible framework for why this research is viewed as challenging the traditional, egocentric approach to behavioral order, we first describe what we mean by *egocentric*, drawing parallels between the geocentric notions of the physical world order that confined the scientific understanding of the universe prior to Galileo. Furthermore, we briefly highlight how such egocentrism is so pervasive in cognitive and psychological science that it continues to underlie many contemporary approaches to perceiving, acting, and knowing.

THE EGOCENTRIC VIEW OF HUMAN BEHAVIOR

The notion that the organization of behavior results from internal, isolated, and locally defined cerebral processes is deeply rooted in traditional approaches to cognitive science. The pervasive spirit of this centralist perspective, namely, that the causal nexus of human behavior is mental cognition, and the brain, however, does not stem from the theorizing of psychologists and cognitive scientists alone but also reflects the implicit certainty of almost all mainstream scientists, including those not directly concerned with psychological phenomena (e.g., physicists, chemists, and biologists). Until recently, even implied challenges to this apparent certainty would have been met with puzzled bemusement. However, resistance to views that challenge standard scientific thinking, regardless of their accuracy, is not a new phenomenon, and there are many examples of such resistance occurring throughout the history of science. Perhaps the most well-known instance of this concerns how, with one simple observation in the early 17th century—that Jupiter had moons, and that these moons did not revolve around the Earth but around Jupiter itself—Galileo was forced to challenge the geocentric view of the universe[1] and, in doing so, was condemned not only by religious leaders (leading to his conviction of heresy and being placed under house arrest), but also by much of the scientific community.

Although Galileo's rejection of the geocentric view of the universe seemed ridiculous at the time, we now know that he (like Copernicus and Kepler before him) was largely correct, and that the Earth, like the other planets in the solar system, can be understood as revolving around the sun.[2] In addition to the religious context that dominated the scientific community during Galileo's time, it is not difficult to understand why, scientifically, a heliocentric view of the universe was also so controversial, as it rejected the unquestioned belief that the Earth or more importantly, man was of central significance. Indeed, renouncing the geocentric view of the universe seemed to run counter to the egocentric perspective that a typical observer is confronted with each and every day—for instance, the observed rising and falling of the sun and moon (Langford, 1998). Yet many of the earthly behaviors that appear mysterious from an egocentric perspective (and apparently the work of some force beyond the purview of scientific reasoning), such as the changing seasons, tides, and weather, suddenly appear lawful, mandatory, and coherent once an egocentric view is rejected. Indeed, attempting to understand such earthly phenomena without acknowledging the Earth's noncentrality is what requires recourse to other, nonobservable, causes—an internal or external controller that dictates how such things occur (Humphrey, 1933; see Turvey & Shaw, 1979).

Interestingly, it is this same egocentric perspective that often makes it difficult to conceive that understanding human behavior might also require a nonegocentric approach. The vista that results from the positioning of the eyes, the resonating tones and muscle activation that spoken language creates in the head, the physical distance between the "me" and the "you," all seem to proclaim the localized centrality of the mind and brain (for other examples, see also Chapter 10 by Dunham and Banaji in this volume). In this respect, the traditional egocentric view of human behavior is analogous to the geocentric view of the universe. This analogy is illustrated in Figure 15.1. Note the passive centrality of both Earth and brain (mind), whereby the essential importance of man and the mental, respectively, are endorsed by separating each from the context of its material surroundings. Moreover, the environment and environmental objects, including other conspecifics (i.e., other planets or animals, respectively), are viewed as peripheral to behavior and meaning. The Cartesian separation between mind and body, between perception and action, and between animal and environment that took hold in 18th, 19th, and 20th centuries is both a consequence and a champion of such egocentrism.

THE MODERN PERSISTENCE OF EGOCENTRISM

The modern endeavor to comprehend the organization of behavior as the result of a purely symbolic, representation based, information-

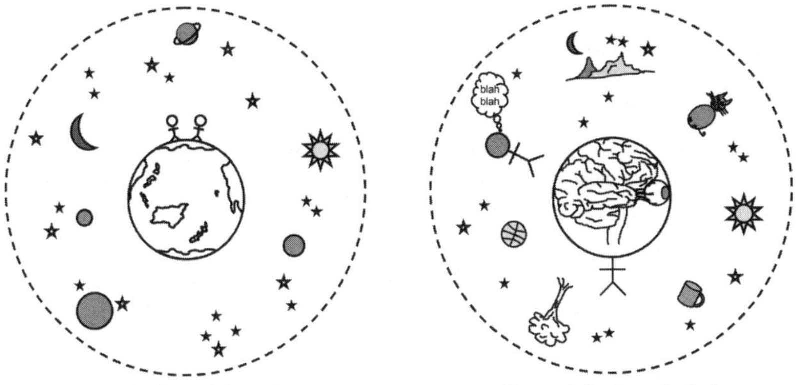

FIGURE 15.1. The geocentric view of the universe and the analogous egocentric view of the human mind.

processing system is the best example of how Cartesian egocentrism underlies contemporary theories of behavioral order. The appeal of approaching the organization of behavior in this way is that the cause of behavior, of perceiving and acting, can be attributed to a centralized computational process whereby a system inputs, stores, manipulates, computes, and outputs information by means of symbolic or representational structures (von Eckardt, 1993). Additional motivation for the centralized information-processing approach is that it implicates "mindful" *disembodied* entities or phenomena as the cause of behavior, such that any material substrate that allows for the computation of symbolic or representational structures can provide an effective framework for studying and understanding behavioral order.[3] Moreover, it allows scientists virtually to ignore the physical body or environmental context. As a result, perception, although important, is viewed as subservient to centralized cognitive–computational processing, with the environment (its objects, events, and surfaces) being reduced to system inputs or stimuli. Similarly, observable actions and movements are viewed as a subservient or secondary consequence of centralized cognitive–computational processing and are simply reduced to system outputs or responses (Gibson, 1966, 1979; Hurley, 1998; Turvey & Shaw, 1979).

The growing appreciation that human and animal behavior is embodied and embedded, and that cognition is situated (see Chapter 7 by Smith and Collins in this volume), is in part a reaction to the philosophical problems that a disembodied computational–representational approach entails, such as the origin and grounding of representational structures, as well as the problem of an internal "knower" or homunculus (e.g., Fodor, 2000; Haugeland, 1998; Searle, 1980; Shaw, 2003; Turvey & Shaw, 1979). The pragmatic frustration of many scientists who have been unable to develop artificially intelligent, robust, or adaptive robotic agents using a purely disembodied computational–representational approach has also played a significant role in motivating the embodied–embedded perspective (e.g., Beer, 1997; Brooks, 1986, 1991; Clark, 1997; Pfeifer & Lida, 2005). The embodied–embedded approach has also gained considerable momentum due to the growing body of empirical research that demonstrates the influence of action and sensorimotor processes on many cognitive activities (e.g., memory, language comprehension) that were previously viewed as being internal activities of mind (e.g., Barsalou, 1999; Dijkstra, Kaschak, & Zwaan, 2007; Wilson, 2001). Perhaps most noteworthy is the abundance of recent work directly aimed at challenging the traditional perception–action dualism, illustrating instead how perception and action are tightly coupled and cannot be understood as completely modular processes (e.g., Knoblich & Flach, 2003; Prinz, 1997; Proffitt, 2006). However, despite many contemporary researchers rejecting the traditional notions that perception and action are causally subservient to centralized mental or neural processes, and the idea that the physical body and environment are of little consequence for understanding the systematic and coordinated patterns of behavior, the underlying thread of egocentrism often remains.

Evidence of this implicit egocentrism can be found in the recent arguments that perception and action are inherently linked because they share the same internal representational domain. Drawing ground from motor theories of movement (e.g., James, 1892; Viviani & Stucchi, 1992) and speech perception (e.g., Liberman, Cooper, Shankweiler, & Studdert-Kennedy, 1967), this kind of "common-coding" hypothesis holds that the representational codes of perceived events are written in the same representational language as to-be-produced events (Hommel, Müsseler, Aschersleben, & Prinz, 2001; see also Bargh & Chartrand, 1999, and Chartrand & Bargh, 1999, for examples of how this kind of "common-coding" approach has been used in social psychological research). Although adopting this kind of approach has advanced our theoretical understanding of perception and action considerably (as well as mind and cognition in general), like traditional approaches to perceiving and acting, this approach still places the causal explanation of behavioral order firmly inside the head and mind (and, ultimately, the brain). Moreover, despite arguing against the classic perception–action dualism, knowing and acting remain largely separate, only indirectly linked via representational processes. Thus, not only does such an approach remain egocentric in focus but it also continues to reinforce the very thing that it strives to undermine—the irrelevance of body and environment in cognition. Related research aimed at demonstrating the *interaction* of sensorimotor states on traditionally defined cognitive process (i.e., memory, social knowing, affective evaluations, and emotions) reflects the same implicit egocentrism, reinforcing the classic dualisms by theoretically presupposing that such cognitive phenomena exist as centrally defined, trait- or state-like corporeal processes.

Consistent with these kinds of common-coding or interactionist[4] accounts of behavioral order are some of the recent conclusions drawn by researchers investigating *mirror neurons*, the cells that were discovered in area F5 of the premotor cortex of macaque monkeys, and that fire when a monkey both executes and observes a particular action (Di Pellegrino, Fadiga, Fogassi, Gallese, & Rizzolatti, 1992; Gallese, Fadiga, Fogassi, & Rizzolatti, 1996). Following the discovery of mirror neurons in monkeys, a number of transcranial magnetic stimulation, positron emission tomographic (PET), and functional magnetic resonance imaging (fMRI) studies have provided evidence that a similar "mirror neuron" system might also exist in humans (Buccino, Binkofski, Fink, Fadiga, & Fogassi, 2001; Grafton, Arbib, Fadiga, & Rizzolatti, 1996; Iacoboni et al., 1999). Mirror neuron findings have generated considerable excitement because they emphasize a number of important issues related to the embodied–embedded perspective. For instance, such findings demonstrate the functionally defined (rather than movement-oriented) nature of action and the commonality of perceiving another's actions and one's own action (self-action). Indeed, mirror neuron findings highlight how an action is not simply the enactment of the musculoskeletal system, but a process deeply connected with the flow of environment from the world involved with engaging in that action (or perceiving that action). Thus, the ripping of a paper, whether seen, felt, or heard, elicits a response, whereas meaningless movements of hands in an exact pattern, but serving no goal, does not elicit a response.

Perhaps most important for *all* perspectives within cognitive science is that the discovery of mirror neurons seems to provide direct neurological evidence of an inherent "resonance" between traditionally defined perceptual and motor systems. However, as highlighted by Brass and Heyes (2005), the argument that mirror neurons are the causal basis for such things as action understanding, language development, empathy, imitation, and social knowing (e.g., Gallese, 2003; Rizzolatti & Arbib, 1998; Rizzolatti & Craighero, 2004; Rizzolatti, Fogassi, &

Gallese, 2001) is far from convincing. Mirror neurons cannot cause the emergence of behavioral order alone, and any attempt to overemphasize their significance inevitably requires an implicit recourse to other causes. Most often, these "other causes" reflect a dependence on a centralized representational domain or neural simulation (e.g., Jacob & Jeannerod, 2005; Jeannerod, 2001; Wilson & Knoblich, 2005), both of which entail an a priori "code" or knowledge base. Interestingly, the existence of mirror neurons is also argued to provide evidence that such codes, knowledge, or representations exist. As such, many mirror neuron accounts of perceiving, acting, and knowing provide another good example of the pervasive and troublingly circular nature of the egocentric paradigm and, in this case, how it continues to draw many researchers to seek local and centrally defined neurophysiological explanations of behavioral order. Furthermore, by overemphasizing the role of neural activity in perception and action, the egocentric notion that mental cognition and the brain can account for systematicity of behavior is not only upheld, but, perhaps worse, also appears to be granted a tangible, physiological home.

CHALLENGING THE EGOCENTRIC VIEW OF BEHAVIOR

So what proves to challenge the egocentric understanding of behavioral order? What evidence is there to suggest that understanding human behavior might require adopting a more distributed, nonegocentric, mind–body–environment perspective? For what behaviors might it provide a better and more grounded understanding, and to what degree would it enable us to predict better the complex stabilities of that behavior? A number of theoretical developments and empirically well-understood phenomena allow us, we believe, to begin to address these questions. What follows is a discussion of just two, the ones most closely tied to our work, that challenge the egocentric notion of behavioral order by demonstrating how intra- and interpersonal coordinated action is a dynamic, self-organized consequence of the physical laws and informational constraints that are mutually structured across mind, body, and environment.[5] What is more, both of the phenomena we describe below demonstrate how coordinated perceiving–acting can transcend biological or anatomically defined notions of agency. Thus, the behavioral organization they entail cannot be attributed to any one internally defined set of cognitive or mental processes, but can only be understood, explained, and predicted as emergent properties of an animal–environment system.

Environmental and Interpersonal Rhythmic Coordination

A question that continues to drive the majority of research on perceptual–motor control focuses on how the exceedingly large number of degrees of freedom (*df*) present at the micro-levels of the perceptual–motor system (e.g., muscles, neurons, skeletal components, metabolic subsystems) are so effortlessly regulated to only a few collective *df* at the observed macro-level of behavior. With respect to everyday movements such as walking, reaching, grasping, and clapping, many contemporary researchers and theorists have moved away from the traditional neural or symbolic computational approach, turning instead to the laws that govern natural systems, namely, dynamical processes of self-organization (Kelso, 1995; Turvey, 1990). Accordingly, neural wiring conceptions, such as the afference and efference distinction, have been replaced by dynamically constrained synergistic linkages between muscles and limbs. Cognitive motor programs or representations have been replaced by equations of constraint that channel and guide a dynamic unfolding of behavior, whereby ordered behavior is not reduced to internal mechanisms or unconscious "mindful" control but is always understood to be the result of animal–environment couplings.

Key to understanding the self-organizing dynamics—namely, the free interplay of forces and mutual influences among components and properties of a system that tend toward equilibrium or steady states (Kugler, Kelso, & Turvey, 1980)—of ordered behavior is being able to conceive, model, and measure the equilibrium or attractor states that lawfully constrain the collective order and patterning of coordinated movements. This has been achieved most notably with respect to the behavioral patterns associated with coordinated rhythmical limb movements. These behavioral patterns are obvious to anyone who attempts to synchronize the oscillatory movements of two limbs, such as when one smoothly and continuously swings his or her two index fingers, wrists, or arms back and forth (readers are encouraged to try to synchronize their left and right hands as follows). To begin with, individuals can only coordinate their limbs in two possible ways: inphase or antiphase. *Inphase* refers to two limbs oscillating in the same parts of the cycle at the same time (e.g., both hands are in the same part of their backward or forward swings at the same point in time). *Antiphase* refers to the two limbs oscillating opposite parts of the cycle at the same time (e.g., while one hand is moving forward, the other hand mirrors the movement, but is moving backward). Further exploration has revealed that inphase is more stable than antiphase. This can be observed by instructing an individual who starts swinging his or her limbs in opposite directions (antiphase) slowly to increase the frequency (speed) of oscillation. At some point, namely, the critical frequency of oscillation, the individual will no longer be able to maintain antiphase and will spontaneously switch to inphase. The opposite does not occur, however. Individuals do not spontaneously switch from inphase to antiphase as the frequency of oscillation is increased, or back to antiphase as the frequency of oscillation is decreased. Thus, inphase reflects a more stable state (attractor) than antiphase because inphase can be produced across a wider range of frequencies. Still further exploration has revealed another defining quality of bimanual interlimb coordination. Specifically, for coordinating limbs that have different natural frequencies of oscillation (e.g., moving only the right index finger while moving one's entire left arm as a unit), the observed coordination pattern moves slightly away from perfect inphase or antiphase, with the faster limb segment (i.e., right index finger) leading the slower one (i.e., left arm). Such lead–lag behavior is also characterized by an increase in the variability of coordination, which, given the difference in stability of inphase and antiphase, is more pronounced for antiphase than for inphase.

These exact observations, as empirically studied by Kelso and others during the mid-1980s to the early 1990s (see Haken, Kelso, & Bunz, 1985; Kelso, 1995; Kugler & Turvey, 1987; Turvey, 1990), eventually led to the dynamic stabilities of within-person interlimb coordination being conceived and formally modeled as a system of coupled oscillators (see Figure 15.2). In this view, the stabilities and patterning of movement, as well as the frequency and amplitude at which such movements are naturally produced, are all understood to be a result of the physical and biomechanical constraints that naturally couple the different limbs or parts of the body together (Kelso, 1995; Kugler & Turvey, 1987). The importance of this dynamical model, known as the Haken, Kelso, and Bunz, or HKB model, is that it provides researchers with an elegant way of understanding how the stable patterns of interlimb coordination emerge, are maintained, and, conversely, how they become unstable and vanish. More importantly, it provides researchers with a much deeper understanding of how the perceptual–motor system regulates and orders its many *df* better than more traditional motor program accounts, in that the rhythmical coordination of two limbs (and their many neurons, muscles, etc.), is conceived as a single synergetic system or *coordinative structure*[6] (Kelso, 1995; Kugler & Turvey, 1987). On its own, then, the research on within-person rhythmical interlimb coordination challenges the egocentric notion of behavioral order by highlighting how complex patterns of perceptual–motor coordination can arise without recourse to internal or centrally defined mental causes or controllers. Even more significant than this, however, is the fact that the very same dynamic

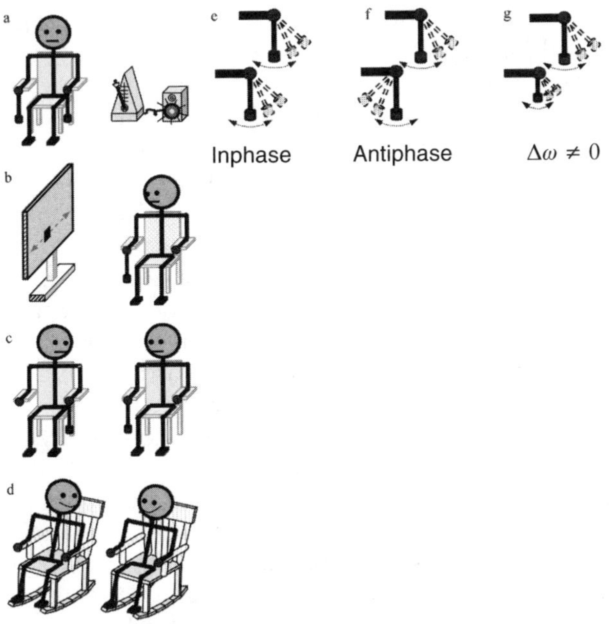

FIGURE 15.2. The HKB model captures the dynamic stabilities of rhythmic (a) intrapersonal, (b) environmental, and (c, d) interpersonal coordination using a motion equation for the collective variable of relative phase $\phi = (\theta_L - \theta_R)$—the difference in the phase angles of the left and right movements. This variable is referred to as "collective" because it quantifies in a single measure the spatial and temporal details of the two movements, irrespective of whether the movements are of fingers, arms, legs, wrist-pendulums, or rocking chairs. Typically, the motion equation takes the form

$$\phi = \Delta\omega - a \sin \phi - 2b \sin 2\phi$$

where ϕ is the rate of change of the relative phase angle and ϕ indexes where one movement is in its cycle relative to the other (Haken et al., 1985; Kelso et al., 1990). The sine functions of ϕ and 2ϕ, along with the coefficients a and b, govern the strength of the stable between-movement coordination patterns, (e) inphase ($\phi = 0°$) and (f) antiphase ($\phi = 180°$). $\Delta\omega$ is an index of frequency competition (the difference between the oscillators' natural frequencies; $\Delta\omega = \omega_L - \omega_R$). For movements that have the (e, f) same natural frequency, $\Delta\omega = 0$. For movements that have (g) different natural frequencies $\Delta\omega \neq 0$. Stable coordination only emerges when the coupling strength—captured by the ratio of b/a—is strong enough to overcome $\Delta\omega$. When the coupling strength is not strong enough to overcome $\Delta\omega$, no stable phase angle will emerge, but the movements will still be intermittently attracted toward 0° and 180° (Kelso & Ding, 1994). Such phase entrainment is known as relative coordination (von Holst, 1939/1973) and is a hallmark of unintentional coordination.

operates to constrain the rhythmical coordination that occurs between the rhythmical limb movements of an individual and a visual environmental rhythm (e.g., Bingham, 2004; Lopresti-Goodman, Richardson, Silva, & Schmidt, 2008; Schmidt, Richardson, Arsenault, & Galantucci, 2007) and, what is more, between the rhythmical limb movements of two or more visually interacting individuals (e.g., Schmidt, Bienvenu, Fitzpatrick, & Amazeen, 1998; Schmidt, Carello, & Turvey, 1990; Schmidt & Turvey, 1994); that is, even when there is no mechanical connection between the two oscillatory movements, individuals (without practice) are constrained by visual information to the same inphase and antiphase patterns of movement, with inphase being more stable than antiphase. Furthermore, any difference in the natural uncoupled frequencies of the visually coordinated movements results in a predictable lead–lag relationship, as well as an increase in the variability of coordination.

Perhaps even more profound are the research findings that demonstrate how the same coupled oscillator dynamic can constrain the coordination that occurs *unintentionally* between two interacting individuals or between an individual and an environmental rhythm (Lopresti-Goodman et al., 2008; Richardson, Marsh, Isenhower, Goodman, & Schmidt, 2007; Richardson, Marsh, & Schmidt, 2005; Schmidt & O'Brien, 1997; Schmidt & Richardson, 2008; Schmidt et al., 2007). In these studies, participants were asked to perform a rhythmical movement task, such as swinging a hand-held pendulum or rocking in a rocking chair, while visual information about movements of a coparticipant or an environmental rhythm was made available. Note that wrist pendulums and rocking chairs are used because they allow for the controlled manipulation of movement frequency (e.g., long wrist pendulums have a slower natural or comfort mode frequency than do short wrist pendulums). Despite the fact that participants were not instructed to coordinate their movements (participants were required to solve a puzzle or identification task and were unaware that movements were becoming coordinated), the results demonstrated that the participants' movements still became synchronized and, consistent with the patterns of intentional interpersonal and within-person coordination, were intermittently attracted toward an inphase or antiphase mode of coordination. Furthermore, the stability of the unintentional entrainment was influenced by frequency, detuning, and the strength of the information that couples the two movements (i.e., amount or availability of visual information).

In essence, these environmental and interpersonal rhythmical coordination phenomena affirm that the ordered behavior of rhythmical coordination has as much to do with the lawful relations and couplings that bind movements of the body to movements in the environment as it does with the particular anatomical and corporeal substrates of the human perceptual–motor system. Indeed, the organizational "system" in question is not the brain, centralized mental or cognition structures, or even the animal itself, but rather a functional perception–action synergy or coordinative structure defined and distributed across two individuals or across an individual and an environmental event. Therein lies the challenge to egocentric notions of behavioral order. This challenge is further endorsed by the fact that environmental and interpersonal coordination reveal that the coordinated patterning of rhythmical limb movements occurs independently of whether the coupling that links the oscillator components is biological (neuronal–muscular) or informational (i.e., visual, auditory, and haptic). Furthermore, the dynamics of within- and between-person and environmental coordination are not limited to human behavior but are actually a special instance of a more general coupled oscillator dynamic known to engender coordination phenomena across many scales of nature. First employed in the 17th century to explain how physical vibrations through a common support synchronize the motions of mechanical pendulum clocks (Huygens, 1673/1986), the lawful dynamics of a coupled oscillator system have more recently been used to explain phenomena ranging from the synchronous beating of pacemaker cells in the heart, the synchronous chirping of crickets (Walker, 1969) and flashing of fireflies (e.g., Hanson, 1978), the spontaneous asynchronous-to-synchronous-to-asynchronous applause transitions of an enamored audience (Néda, Ravasz, Brechet, Vicsek, & Barabási, 2000), and the different locomotive gaits and gait transitions that characterize all two-, four-, six-, and even eight-legged animals, insects, and perceiving–acting creatures (see Collins & Stewart, 1993; Kelso, 1995; Strogatz, 2003; Strogatz & Steward, 1993).

It is important to appreciate that centralized cognitive mechanisms, common codes, or neural simulations provide computationally untenable and far less parsimonious accounts of such coordination behavior. Moreover, while the neural connections and processes of the central nervous system play an important role in constraining the coordinated movements of humans and animals, without understanding the dynamical laws that underlie behavior, differentiating this activity adds little to the understanding of behavioral order beyond identifying an isomorphic set of patterns at the level of neuronal anatomy. In short, the centralized, microscopic, neural or cognitive processes that are involved in coordinated perceptual–motor behavior emerge as a consequence of the same natural laws that self-organize and constrain observed macroscopic behavior and thus also require adoption of a nonegocentric animal–environment approach.

The Perception and Actualization of Affordances

Although understanding the behavioral order of perceptual–motor coordination requires identifying the self-organizing dynamics that result from the mutual forces and couplings among mind, body, and environment, such phenomena indicate little with respect to the more abstract notions of knowing and meaning. Yet understanding what a behavioral agent, human or otherwise, is able to know, and what holds meaning for such agents, is what defines a perception–action synergy or coordinative structure as functional; such synergies or structures only exist with respect to some meaningful property or goal. A fitting question, then, is whether an understanding of knowing and meaning might also require adopting a nonegocentric stance?

Questioning whether knowing and meaning are the result of properties or processes distributed across mind, body, and environment is not new and underlies ecological psychology's conception of an affordance. Briefly stated, an *affordance* is an opportunity for action, and to perceive an affordance is to know what an environmental surface, object, or event means *relative* to the one's action capabilities. For example, a place or surface that supports human locomotion by being sufficiently hard and flat affords walking and/or running on and is perceived as such. Similarly, an object that is sufficiently small and can be grasped in an individual's hand is perceived to afford throwing, and when such an object is thrown with sufficient force and within sufficient range of another individual, it is perceived by that individual to afford catching.

As a psychological concept, the term *affordance* was first introduced by J. J. Gibson (1979) as a way of capturing both the complementarity of an animal and its environment, and the interdependence of perception and action. The term *affordance* emphasizes how knowing reflects an epistemic relation between an animal as a knowing agent and the environment that is to be known (Shaw, 2003; Turvey & Shaw, 1979). It thus challenges egocentric notions of behavioral order by recognizing that to understand what it is to know—perceive—one must identify the animal–environment relations that define what is knowable. Importantly, the use of an object or surface, and thus what it affords, cannot be said either to exist within the object in isolation from an animal or to be subjectively or socially imposed by an animal or social consensus. Rather, affordances are perceived by detecting lawfully structured information that invariantly specifies quantifiable features of a *particular* perception–action system in relation to quantifiable features of a *particular* surface, object, or event. In this sense, the perception of an affordance is direct and not mediated by mental computation or inference. Moreover, affordances are objective properties of a specific animal–environment system. What a surface, object, or event affords for one species or animal differs from what it affords another species. A water surface with adequate tension can afford locomotion for a bug but not a human. A Frisbee flying through the air is not a catchable object for an animal with no limbs or mouth with which to catch it; an adult, child, or dog may perceive a successfully thrown Frisbee as catchable, but an infant, snail, or beetle will not.

Starting with the foundational work of Warren (1984), who demonstrated that individuals perceive the climb-ability of stairs not by the height of the stair risers but by the height of the risers relative to the individual's own leg length, empirical support for the perception of affordances has been provided by identifying how individuals perceive environmental surfaces, objects, and events by means of intrinsic (dimensionless) action-scaled information (e.g., visual information specifying riser height taken with respect to one's leg length). The cross-ability of gaps (Burton, 1992; Jiang & Mark, 1994), the reach- and grasp-ability of objects (e.g., Cesari & Newell, 1999; van der Kamp, Savelsbergh, & Davis, 1998), the walk-through-ability of apertures (Warren & Whang, 1987), the walk-up-ability of slopes (Kinsella Shaw, Shaw, & Turvey, 1992) and the sit-ability of surfaces at different heights (e.g., Mark, 1987; Mark & Vogele, 1987) have all been shown to entail the detection of intrinsic, action-scaled information. In order to verify the direct (unmediated) specification of affordances, much of this research has also demonstrated that the information that specifies an affordance is invariant to differences in the absolute metrics of environmental properties or the properties of an individual's action system. For instance, the grasping patterns of 3- to 5-year-old children are determined by the same hand-to-object size ratio rather than the size of the object grasped or the size of the hand doing the grasping (e.g., Newell, Scully, Tenenbaum, & Hardiman, 1989). As a consequence, affordance research has demonstrated that the perception of an *affordance boundary*—the point at which an action such as reaching an object on a shelf is or is not possible—is also perceived by means of the same intrinsic, *action-scaled information* (e.g., information about how high the object is *relative* to one's reach). Moreover, detecting an affordance boundary dynamically self-organizes the mode of activity in which an individual engages in; that is, an individual's shift to a new mode of action (e.g., standing on tiptoe to reach an object, while steadying one's body with one hand and stretching hard with the other) is an emergent phenomena that occurs simultaneous with detecting the information (e.g., Mark, 1987; Warren & Whang, 1987). One example of this is derived from research on reaching behavior that has demonstrated how action-scaled information specifies what is reachable, and that perceiving the different means by which an object may be reached is dynamically constrained by a scaling of the distance and height of the objects to be reached (Carello, Grosofsky, Reichel, & Solomon, 1989; Mark et al., 1997).

Of most relevance is that the affordance concept, and the research that supports it, argues for meaning to be studied as a relative, yet objective, property of an animal–environment system rather than as a subjective property of a mind or brain. Thus, the concept of an affordance not only challenges egocentric notions of behavior by endorsing knowing and meaning as activities and properties of animal–environment systems but, more importantly, also seeks to dissolve the traditional boundaries historically set between animal and environment. To understand why this is, one must truly appreciate that affordances are not simply properties of an environment but are relational properties defined across mind, body, and environment. For a given animal–environment system, there is a set of affordances—an ecological niche—that is specific to the mutual relations between that animal and its environment (Reed, 1996; Turvey & Shaw, 1979). Moreover, for every affordance there is a corresponding *effectivity*. The term *effectivity*, coined by Shaw and Turvey (1981; Turvey & Shaw, 1979), refers to the functionally defined action systems used in the actualization of an affordance. For example, the human hand is the effectivity that makes a tennis ball graspable. Thus, affordances and effectivities are mutually defined concepts and, as such, the realization of an action possibility reflects the fit between animal and environment.

Consistent with the affordances to which they correspond, effectivities are defined not simply with respect to bodily encapsulated action capabilities, but more globally with respect to the action capabilities of the entire animal–environment system; that is, the effectivities that make the perception and actualization of an affordance possible can, and often do, involve action capabilities that have been extended by incorporating environmental objects or tools (Bongers, Michaels, & Smitsman, 2004; Smitsman, 1997; Wagman & Carello, 2003). For instance, 3 feet of fresh snow does not afford effective locomotion due to the small surface area of one's feet. However, once snow shoes are fitted, one's action system becomes more functionally refined, resulting in 3 feet of fresh snow affording effective locomotion. Similarly, that which an individual perceives as too high (un-sit-able) to sit upon will increase when blocks are attached to the feet (Mark & Vogele, 1987).

Environmental objects therefore have a dual function. Separated from a potential user's body, they afford certain actions, such as grasping and throwing. Once in use, however, they become functional parts of the user's action system, just as integral to the realization of affordances as bodily components (Gibson, 1979; Hirose, 2002; Richardson, Marsh,

& Baron, 2007; Shaw, Flasher, & Kadar, 1995; Smitsman & Bongers, 2003). Indeed, a cane is just as important for a blind person to perceive whether a surface or edge affords effective locomotion as the hand and arm the maneuvers it. That the cane *is* a part of the perception–action system, and not now something separate from it, is illustrated by the fact that one actually "feels" a surface or edge *at the end of the cane*, not at the juncture where the hand meets the cane! In many respects, other animals or individuals provide even more flexible and adaptive objects of an animal's environment than do inanimate ones. Thus, many affordances only exist and are only perceived with respect to interpersonal or social action systems. Recently, Richardson and colleagues (2007; Fowler, Richardson, Marsh, & Shockley, 2008; Isenhower, Marsh, Carello, Baron, & Richardson, 2005) have demonstrated how cooperating individuals spontaneously come together to actualize interpersonal grasping affordances. This research compared how a pair of participants shifted between the perception and actualization of solo and joint action possibilities in a task that required them to move short and long planks of wood, either alone or together. Understood from an affordance perspective, the emergence of cooperation (vs. autonomous action) was expected to be determined by a specific relation between an aspect of the actors' perception–action capabilities and an aspect of the environment. More specifically, the affordances of the situation—planks movable-alone or movable-with-two-people—were expected to be determined by information that specified the size of the two people's arm spans with respect to the length of the plank. Consistent with this prediction, the point of transition between solo and cooperative action was found to be dynamically constrained by the detection of action-scaled information, with short and tall arm span pairs transitioning from solo to joint and from joint to solo action in the same way and at the same invariant, arm span to plank length ratio. Consistent with research that indicates an individual can perceive the affordances of conspecifics (Ramenzoni, Riley, Shockley, Davis, & Snyder, 2005; Stoffregen, Gorday, Sheng, & Flynn, 1999), tall arm span participants who were paired with short arm span participants transitioned between solo and joint action at an action-scaled ratio that corresponded to the affordance boundary of their short arm span partners. The implicit commitment to act as a "plural subject" of action (Gilbert, 1996), that is, to choose to cooperate, was found to be something that emerged without prior planning or a priori expectations, in response to a meaningful relation defined across the individual–environment or, more specifically, the individual–individual system.

As illustrated in Figure 15.3, the similitude of mind and of perceiving and acting at multiple levels of an organism–environment system—the animal, the animal–tool, and the animal–animal systems—is being sug-

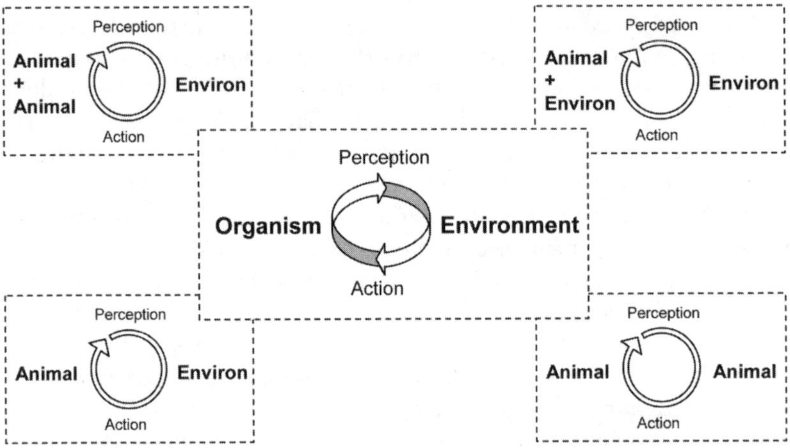

FIGURE 15.3. The similitude of perceiving and acting at multiple levels of the organism–environment system. Irrespective of whether a perception–action synergy entails an individual animal, an animal plus the environment, or two or more animals, the emergence of coordinated behavior for each system is a dynamic and self-organized result of the lawful process and informational constraints that bind and intimately couple mind, body, and environment.

gested here, where the emergence of coordinated behavior at each level (both intra- and interpersonal) is a dynamic and self-organized result of the lawful processes and informational constraints that bind and intimately couple mind, body, and environment. In addition, despite the intuition that cooperative action is totally different from solo action, an understanding of coordinated behavior in terms of affordances suggests that there is a similarity in how solo, joint, and even tool-based activity is constrained and organized (Marsh, Richardson, Baron, & Schmidt, 2006; Richardson, Marsh, & Baron, 2007). This is not to say the coordinated interpersonal or social activity is to be equated with simple tool use. On the contrary, cooperating with another individual can reflect the most substantial change to an individual's perception–action capabilities, producing a new social unit of perception–action that allows for the actualization of an extremely broad range of affordances, including many that can only be actualized by the unit acting as a whole. The action possibilities of a "we"—of a pair, or of a group—are emergent properties that differ in kind from the mere sum of the group members' capabilities considered at the individual level (Baron, 2007). However, tool and interpersonal affordances both challenge the classically defined separation between animal and environment that underscores egocentric notions of behavior by rejecting the idea that such separations should be viewed as fixed. What separates animal and environment is not always clear, with the boundary between what constitutes "animal" and what constitutes "environment" constantly shifting. To this extent, the action systems or effectivities that actualize affordances are perhaps best understood, like the perceptual–motor systems that characterize environmental and interpersonal coordination, as soft-molded perception–action synergies. Neither strictly "animal" nor strictly "environment," but both, these coordinative structures can be understood as being emergent properties of an animal–environment system, whereby that which is knowable, that which holds meaning and defines the functionality of these synergies, only does so in relation to an animal–environment (or animal–animal–environment) system and cannot be reduced to any individual part.

CONCLUSION

Our aim in this chapter was to challenge the traditional, egocentric approach to behavioral order, indicating how the explanations that stem from this approach focus more on the isolated and centralized mental, cognitive, and neural entities of minds, and, to their detriment, pay little attention to the embodied–embedded context of behavior. In challenging this approach, we briefly focused on two and socially situated (Smith & Semin, 2004) phenomena, environmental and interpersonal rhythmic coordination, as well as the perception and actualization of intra- and interpersonal affordances, which both demonstrate how the ordered regularity of behavior cannot be fully understood without identifying the nontrivial and lawful constraints that the body and environmental context impart on mind and brain. We further argued how the systematic and coordinated patterning of such activity is not determined and controlled by a context-free mind or brain, or an isolated and disembodied information-processing system, but is dynamically self-organized and results from the physical constraints and informational couplings that exist between animal and environment. Perhaps more profound is that by adopting a nonegocentric, animal–environment stance, these phenomena lead to the realization that the system or systems of interest are perception–action synergies, and that the organization of these synergies is not anatomically defined or hard-molded (restricted or fixed to biologically integrated or physically connected matter), but is soft-molded, with such synergies being assembled, disassembled, and reassembled in relation to the perception of mutually defined action possibilities and goals. Consequently, individuals perceiving and acting alone with environmental objects, or together with other conspecifics, can and should be understood as implausibly coherent organisms composed of diverse yet functionally related parts, and whose behavior cannot be understood by reducing the system to a disembodied set of centralized neural mechanisms or computational processes (Marsh et al., 2006, Rosen, 2000). Indeed, it is our view that to understand truly the systematic and coordinated patterns of human behavior will require nothing less than adopting this perception–action, animal–environment approach. We believe this to be true for the simple joint and interpersonal behaviors described earlier, as well as for more complex social behaviors, such as a cheerleading team doing a routine, a group of individuals clapping and yelling together, a work group cooperating to solve a problem, or a family preparing and sharing a meal together. We also believe that by studying social action systems as indivisible units or synergies, the attitudes, dispositional properties, and even self-conceptions of the individuals involved may ultimately be revealed as being emergent properties of embodied–embedded and socially entailed perception–action systems (see also Smith & Collins, Chapter 7, and Sinclair & Lun, Chapter 11, in this volume). Moreover, adopting this somewhat radical embodied–embedded approach will not only prove to completely dispel the ill-defined distinctions between perception and action, mind and body, animal and environment, and perhaps even individual and social, but will ultimately lead psychology and cognitive science to achieve a much deeper understanding of what it is to be a goal-directed, perceiving–acting agent.

NOTES

1. Observing that Jupiter had satellites (moons) was the first of many observations that led Galileo to adopt the "heliocentric" view of the universe/solar system previously proposed by Copernicus and Kepler. Others included the orbital phases of Venus and sunspots (see Langford, 1998, for more details).
2. In truth, the Copernican or heliocentric view of the universe that was championed by Galileo is only correct if we limit the discussion to our solar system. Moreover, the sun is not actually at the center of any planet's orbit, but rather is the focus of a planet's elliptical orbit.
3. Traditional approaches to connectionist modeling are largely a result of viewing cognition as a collection of disembodied, computational processes (Fodor & Pylyshyn, 1988; Hurley, 1998; von Eckardt, 1993).
4. Drawing from Haugeland (1998), we use the term *interactionist* to refer to the class of embodied and embedded approaches acknowledging that cognition cannot be understood without reference to the body and the environment, but still accept the premise that cognition is mental, centrally defined,

and by the nature of this mental centrality has some special feature that makes it essential for behavioral order, such as intentionality or normativity.

5. The arguments raised in this chapter are not drawn only from our own theorizing (see also Fowler, Richardson, Marsh, & Shockley, 2007; Marsh, Richardson, Baron, & Schmidt, 2006; Schmidt, 2007; Schmidt & Richardson, 2008) but from many others, particularly those working within the ecological and dynamical systems approaches. Arguments similar to the ones we present here were made over 20 years ago by Kelso, Holt, Kugler, and Turvey (1980), Kugler, Kelso, and Turvey (1980), Kugler and Turvey (1987), Gibson (1966, 1979), Michaels and Carello (1981), and Turvey and Shaw (1979)—among others. Most recently, Warren (2006) has also presented a similar set of arguments, drawing from his work on vehicle control and guided locomotion.
6. The term *coordinative structure* is borrowed from the field of thermodynamics and has been used in the human movement literature to refer to a set of relatively independent units (e.g., muscles, limbs, animals, or substances) that are temporarily constrained, both at short and long timescales, to act as a unitary functional unit (for more details, see Kugler et al., 1980; Kugler & Turvey, 1987; Tuller, Turvey, & Fitch, 1982).

REFERENCES

Bargh, J. A., & Chartrand, T. L. (1999). The unbearable automaticity of being. *American Psychologist*, *54*, 462–479.

Baron, R. M. (2007). Situating coordination and cooperation between ecological and social psychology. *Ecological Psychology*, *19*, 179–199.

Barsalou, L. W. (1999). Perceptual symbol systems. *Behavioral and Brain Sciences*, *22*, 577–660.

Beer, R. D. (1995). A dynamical systems perspective on agent–environment interaction. *Artificial Intelligence*, *72*, 173–215.

Beer, R. D. (1997). The dynamics of adaptive behavior: A research program. *Robotics and Autonomous Systems*, *20*, 257–289.

Bingham, G. P. (2004). A perceptually driven dynamical model of bimanual rhythmic movements (and phase entrainment). *Ecological Psychology*, *16*, 45–53.

Bongers, R. M., Smitsman, A. W., & Michaels, C. F. (2004). Variations of tool and task characteristics reveal that tool-use postures are anticipated. *Journal of Motor Behavior*, *36*(3), 305–315.

Brass, M., & Heyes, C. (2005). Imitation: is cognitive neuroscience solving the correspondence problem? *Trends in Cognitive Sciences*, *9*, 489–495.

Brooks, R. A. (1986). A robust layered control system for a mobile robot. *IEEE Journal of Robotics and Automation*, *2*, 12–23.

Brooks, R. A. (1991). New approaches to robotics. *Science*, *253*, 1227–1232.

Brooks, R. A. (1995). Intelligence without reason. In L. Steels & R. A. Brooks

(Eds.), *The artificial life route to artificial intelligence* (pp. 25–81). Hillsdale, NJ: Erlbaum.

Buccino, G., Binkofski, F., Fink, G. R., Fadiga, L., & Fogassi, L. (2001). Action observation activates premotor and parietal areas in a somatotopic manner: An fMRI study. *European Journal of Neuroscience, 13*, 400–404.

Burton, G. (1992). Nonvisual judgment of the crossability of path gaps. *Journal of Experimental Psychology: Human Perception and Performance, 18*, 698–713.

Carello, C., Grosofsky, A., Reichel, F. D., & Solomon, H. Y. (1989). Visually perceiving what is reachable. *Ecological Psychology, 1*(1), 27–54.

Cesari, P., & Newell, K. M. (1999). The scaling of human grip configurations. *Journal of Experimental Psychology: Human Perception and Performance, 25*(4), 927–935.

Chartrand, T. L., & Bargh, J. A. (1999). The chameleon effect: The perception–behavior link and social interaction. *Journal of Personality and Social Psychology, 76*(6), 893–910.

Clark, A. (1997). The dynamical challenge. *Cognitive Science, 21*, 461–481.

Collins, J. J., & Stewart, I. (1993). Coupled nonlinear oscillators and the symmetries of animal gaits. *Journal of Nonlinear Science, 3*, 349–392.

Dijkstra, K., Kaschak, M. P., & Zwaan, R. A. (2007). Body posture facilitates retrieval of autobiographical memories. *Cognition, 102*, 139–149.

Di Pellegrino, G., Fadiga, L., Fogassi, L., Gallese, V., & Rizzolatti, G. (1992). Understanding motor events: A neurophysiological study. *Experimental Brain Research, 91*, 176–180.

Fodor, J. (2000). *The mind doesn't work that way: The scope and limits of computational psychology*. Cambridge, MA: MIT Press.

Fodor, J. A., & Pylyshyn, Z. (1988). Connectionism and cognitive architecture: A critical analysis. *Cognition, 28*, 3–71.

Fowler, C. A., Richardson, M. J., Marsh, K. L., & Shockley, K. D. (2008). Language use, coordination, and the emergence of cooperative action. In A. Fuchs & V. Jirsa (Eds.), *Coordination: Neural, behavioral and social dynamics* (pp. 261–280). Berlin: Springer.

Gallese, V. (2003). The manifold nature of interpersonal relations: The quest for a common mechanism. In C. Frith & D. Wolpert (Eds.), *The neuroscience of social interaction* (pp. 159–182). New York: Oxford University Press.

Gallese, V., Fadiga, L., Fogassi, L., & Rizzolatti, G. (1996). Action recognition in the premotor cortex. *Brain, 119*, 593–609.

Gibbs, R. W. (2007). *Embodiment and cognitive science*. Cambridge, UK: Cambridge University Press.

Gibson, J. J. (1966). *The senses considered as perceptual systems*. Boston: Houghton Mifflin.

Gibson, J. J. (1979). *The ecological approach to visual perception*. Boston: Houghton Mifflin.

Gilbert, M. (1996). *Living together: Rationality, sociality, and obligation*. Lanham, MD: Rowman & Littlefield.

Grafton, S. T., Arbib, M. A., Fadiga, L., & Rizzolatti, G. (1996). Localization of grasp representations in humans by PET: 2. Observation compared with imagination. *Experimental Brain Research*, *112*, 103–111.

Haken, H., Kelso, J. A. S., & Bunz, H. (1985). A theoretical model of phase transitions in human hand movements. *Biological Cybernetics*, *51*, 347–356.

Hanson, F. E. (1978). Comparative studies of firefly pacemakers. *Federation Proceedings*, *37*(8), 2158–2164.

Haugeland, J. (1998). *Having thought.* Cambridge, MA: Harvard University Press.

Hirose, N. (2002). An ecological approach to embodiment and cognition. *Cognitive Systems Research*, *3*, 289–299.

Hommel, B., Müsseler, J., Aschersleben, G., & Prinz, W. (2001). The theory of event coding (TEC): A framework for perception and action planning. *Behavioral and Brain Sciences*, *24*, 849–937.

Humphrey, G. (1933). *The nature of learning.* New York: Harcourt Brace.

Hurley, S. L. (1998). *Consciousness in action.* Cambridge, MA: Harvard University Press.

Hutchins, E. (1995). *Cognition in the wild.* Cambridge, MA: MIT Press.

Huygens, C. (1986). *The pendulum clock or geometrical demonstrations concerning the motion of pendula as applied to clocks* (R. J. Blackwell, Trans.). Ames: Iowa State University Press. (Original work published 1673)

Iacoboni, M., Woods, R. P., Brass, M., Bekkering, H., Mazziotta, J. C., & Rizzolatti, G. (1999). Cortical mechanisms of human imitation. *Science*, *286*, 2526–2528.

Isenhower, R. W., Marsh, K. L., Carello, C., Baron, R. M., & Richardson, M. J. (2005). The specificity of intrapersonal and interpersonal affordance boundaries: Intrinsic versus absolute metrics. In H. Heft & K. L. Marsh (Eds.), *Studies in perception and action VIII* (pp. 54–58). Mahwah, NJ: Erlbaum.

Jacob, P., & Jeannerod, M. (2005). The motor theory of social cognition: A critique. *Trends in Cognitive Sciences*, *9*(1), 21–25.

James, W. (1890). *Psychology: The briefer course.* New York: Holt.

Jeannerod, M. (2001). Neural simulation of action: A unifying mechanism for motor cognition. *NeuroImage*, *14*, S103–S109.

Jiang, Y., & Mark, L. S. (1994). The effect of gap depth on the perception of whether a gap is crossable. *Perception and Psychophysics*, *56*(6), 691–700.

Kelso, J. A. S. (1995). *Dynamic patterns: The self-organization of brain and behavior.* Cambridge, MA: MIT Press.

Kelso, J. A. S., DelColle, J. D., & Schöner, G. (1990). Action–perception as a pattern formation process. In M. Jeannerod (Ed.), *Attention and performance XIII* (Vol. 5, pp. 139–169). Hillsdale, NJ: Erlbaum.

Kelso, J. A. S., & Ding, M. (1994). Fluctuations, intermittency, and controllable chaos in biological coordination. In K. M. Newell & D. M. Corcos (Eds.), *Variability in motor control* (pp. 291–316). Champaign, IL: Human Kinetics.

Kelso, J. A. S., Holt, K. G., Kugler, P. N., & Turvey, M. T. (1980). On the concept of coordinative structures as dissipative structures: II. Empirical lines of convergence. In G. E. Stelmach & J. Requin (Eds.), *Tutorials in motor behavior* (pp. 49–70). New York: North Holland.

Kinsella Shaw, J. M., Shaw, B., & Turvey, M. T. (1992). Perceiving "walk-on-able" slopes. *Ecological Psychology*, *4*(4), 223–239.

Knoblich, G., & Flach, R. (2003). Action identity: Evidence from self-recognition, prediction, and coordination. *Consciousness and Cognition: An International Journal. Special Issue: Self and Action*, *12*(4), 620–632.

Kugler, P. N., Kelso, J. A. S., & Turvey, M. T. (1980). On the concept of coordinative structures as dissipative structures: I. Theoretical lines of convergence. In G. E. Stelmach & J. Requin (Eds.), *Tutorials in motor behavior* (pp. 3–47). Amsterdam: North Holland.

Kugler, P. N., & Turvey, M. T. (1987). *Information, natural law, and the self-assembly of rhythmic movement*. Hillsdale, NJ: Erlbaum.

Lakoff, G., & Johnson, M. (1999). *Philosophy in the flesh: The embodied mind and its challenge to western thought*. New York: Basic Books.

Langford, J. J. (1998). *Galileo, science and the church* (3rd ed.). Sound Bend, IN: St. Augustine's Press.

Liberman, A. M., Cooper, F. S., Shankweiler, D. P., & Studdert-Kennedy, M. (1967). Perception of speech code. *Psychological Review*, *74*, 431–461.

Lopresti-Goodman, S., Richardson, M. J., Silva, P. L., & Schmidt, R. C. (2008). Period basin of entrainment for unintentional visual coordination. *Journal of Motor Behavior*, *40*, 3–10.

Mark, L. S. (1987). Eyeheight-scaled information about affordances: A study of sitting and stair climbing. *Journal of Experimental Psychology: Human Perception and Performance*, *13*(3), 361–370.

Mark, L. S., Nemeth, K., Gardner, D., Dainoff, M. J., Paasche, J., Duffy, M., et al. (1997). Postural dynamics and the preferred critical boundary for visually guided reaching. *Journal of Experimental Psychology: Human Perception and Performance*, *23*(5), 1365–1379.

Mark, L. S., & Vogele, D. (1987). A biodynamic basis for perceived categories of action: A study of sitting and stair climbing. *Journal of Motor Behavior*, *19*(3), 367–384.

Marsh, K. L., Richardson, M. J., Baron, R. M., & Schmidt, R. C. (2006). Contrasting approaches to perceiving and acting with others. *Ecological Psychology*, *18*, 1–37.

Michaels, C. F., & Carello, C. (1981). *Direct perception*. Englewood Cliffs, NJ: Prentice-Hall.

Néda, Z., Ravasz, E., Brechet, Y., Vicsek, T., & Barabási, A. L. (2000). The sound of many hands clapping, *Nature*, *403*, 849–850.

Newell, K. M., Scully, D. M., Tenenbaum, F., & Hardiman, S. (1989). Body scale and the development of prehension. *Developmental Psychobiology*, *22*(1), 1–13.

Pfeifer, R., & Lida, F. (2005). New robotics: Design principles for intelligent systems. *Artificial Life*, *11*, 99–120.

Prinz, W. (1997). Perception and action planning. *European Journal of Cognitive Psychology, 9*, 129–154.

Proffitt, D. R. (2006). Embodied perception and the economy of action. *Perspectives on Psychological Science, 1*, 110–122.

Ramenzoni, V. C., Riley, M. T., Davis, T., & Snyder, J. (2005). Perceiving whether or not another person can use a step to reach an object. In H. Heft & K. L. Marsh (Eds.), *Studies in perception and action VIII* (pp. 41–44). Mahwah, NJ: Erlbaum.

Reed, E. S. (1996). *Encountering the world: Toward an ecological psychology.* New York: Oxford University Press.

Richardson, M. J., Marsh, K. L., & Baron, R. M. (2007). Judging and actualizing intrapersonal and interpersonal affordances. *Journal of Experimental Psychology: Human Perception and Performance, 33*, 845–859.

Richardson, M. J., Marsh, K. L., Isenhower, R., Goodman, J., & Schmidt, R. C. (2007). Rocking together: Dynamics of intentional and unintentional interpersonal coordination. *Human Movement Science, 26*, 867–891.

Richardson, M. J., Marsh, K. L., & Schmidt, R. C. (2005). Effects of visual and verbal information on unintentional interpersonal coordination. *Journal of Experimental Psychology: Human Perception and Performance, 31*, 62–79.

Rizzolatti, G., & Arbib, M. A. (1998). Language within our grasp. *Trends in Neurosciences, 21*(5), 188–194.

Rizzolatti, G., & Craighero, L. (2004). The mirror-neuron system. *Annual Review of Neuroscience, 27*, 169–192.

Rizzolatti, G., Fogassi, L., & Gallese, V. (2001). Neurophysiological mechanisms underlying the understanding and imitation of action. *Natural Review of Neuroscience, 2*, 661–670.

Rosen, R. (2000). *Essays on life itself.* New York: Columbia University Press.

Schmidt, R. C. (2007). Scaffolds for social meaning. *Ecological Psychology, 19*, 137–151.

Schmidt, R. C., & O'Brien, B. (1997). Evaluating the dynamics of unintended interpersonal coordination. *Ecological Psychology, 9*(3), 189–206.

Schmidt, R. C., & Richardson, M. J. (2008). Dynamics of interpersonal coordination. In A. Fuchs & V. Jirsa (Eds.), *Coordination: Neural, behavioral and social dynamics* (pp. 281–308). Berlin: Springer.

Schmidt, R. C., Richardson, M. J., Arsenault, C., & Galantucci, B. (2007). Unintentional entrainment to an environmental rhythm: Effect of eye tracking. *Journal of Experimental Psychology: Human Perception and Performance, 33*(4), 860–870.

Schmidt, R. C., & Turvey, M. T. (1994). Phase-entrainment dynamics of visually coupled rhythmic movements. *Biological Cybernetics, 70*(4), 369–376.

Searle, J. R. (1980). Minds, brains, and programs. *Behavioral and Brain Sciences, 3*, 417–457.

Shaw, R. E. (2003). The agent–environment interface: Simon's indirect or Gibson's direct coupling? *Ecological Psychology, 15*, 37–106.

Shaw, R. E., Flasher, O. M., & Kadar, E. E. (1995). Dimensionless invariants for intentional systems: Measuring the fit of vehicular activities to environmental layout. In J. M. Flach, P. A. Hancock, J. Carid, & K. J. Vicente (Eds.), *Global perspective on the ecology of human–machine systems* (pp. 293–357). Hillsdale, NJ: Erlbaum.

Shaw, R. E., & Turvey, M. T. (1981). Coalitions as models of ecosystems: A realist perspective on perceptual organization. In M. Kubovy & J. Pomeranz (Eds.), *Perceptual organization* (pp. 343–415). Hillsdale, NJ: Erlbaum.

Smith, E. R., & Semin, G. R. (2004). Socially situated cognition: Cognition in its social context. *Advances in Experimental Social Psychology, 36,* 53–117.

Smitsman, A. W. (1997). The development of tool use: Changing boundaries between organism and environment. In C. Dent-Read & P. Zukow-Goldring (Eds.), *Evolving explanations of development* (pp. 301–329). Washington, DC: American Psychological Association.

Smitsman, A. W., & Bongers, R. M. (2003). Tool use and tool making: A dynamical developmental perspective. In J. Valsiner & K. J. Connolly (Eds.), *Handbook of developmental psychology* (pp. 172–193). London: Sage.

Stoffregen, T. A., Gorday, K. M., Sheng, Y. Y., & Flynn, S. B. (1999). Perceiving affordances for another person's actions. *Journal of Experimental Psychology: Human Perception and Performance, 25*(1), 120–136.

Strogatz, S. H. (2003). *Sync: The emerging science of spontaneous order.* New York: Hyperion Books.

Strogatz, S. H., & Stewart, I. (1993). Coupled oscillators and biological synchronization. *Scientific American, 269,* 102–109.

Thelen, E., & Smith, L. B. (1994). *A dynamic systems approach to the development of cognition and action.* Cambridge, MA: MIT Press.

Tuller, B., Turvey, M. T., & Fitch, H. L. (1982). The Bernstein perspective: II. The concept of muscle linkage or coordinative structure. In J. A. S. Kelso (Ed.), *Human motor behavior: An introduction* (pp. 253–270). Hillsdale, NJ: Erlbaum.

Turvey, M. T. (1990). Coordination. *American Psychologist, 45*(8), 938–953.

Turvey, M. T., & Shaw, R. E. (1979). The primacy of perceiving: An ecological reformulation of perception for understanding memory. In L. G. Nilsson (Ed.), *Perspectives on memory research: Essays in honor of Uppsala University's 500th anniversary* (pp. 167–222). Hillsdale, NJ: Erlbaum.

Turvey, M. T., & Shaw, R. E. (1999). Ecological foundations of cognition: I. Symmetry and specificity of animal-environment systems. *Journal of Consciousness Studies, 6,* 95–110.

Turvey, M. T., Shaw, R. E., Reed, E. S., & Mace, W. M. (1981). Ecological laws of perceiving and acting: In reply to Fodor and Pylyshyn (1981). *Cognition, 9*(3), 237–304.

van der Kamp, J., Savelsbergh, G. J. P., & Davis, W. E. (1998). Body-scaled ratio as a control parameter for prehension in 5- to 9-year-old children. *Developmental Psychobiology, 33*(4), 351–361.

Varela, F., Thompson, E., & Rosch, E. (1991). *The embodied mind.* Cambridge, MA: MIT Press.

Viviani, P., & Stucchi, N. (1992). Motor–perceptual interactions. *Tutorials in Motor Behavior: 2. Advances in Psychology*, *87*, 229–248.

von Eckardt, B. (1993). *What is cognitive science?* Cambridge, MA: MIT Press.

von Holst, E. (1973). The collected papers of Eric von Holst: Vol. 1. The behavioral physiology of animal and man. In R. Martin (Ed.), *The collected papers of Eric von Holst.* Coral Gables, FL: University of Miami Press. (Original work published 1939)

Wagman, J. B., & Carello, C. (2003). Haptically creating affordances: The user–tool interface. *Journal of Experimental Psychology: Applied*, *9*(3), 175–186.

Walker, T. J. (1969). Acoustic synchrony: Two mechanisms in the snow tree cricket. *Science*, *166*, 891–894.

Warren, W. (2006). The dynamics of perception and action. *Psychological Review*, *113*, 358–389.

Warren, W. H. (1984). Perceiving affordances: Visual guidance of stair climbing. *Journal of Experimental Psychology: Human Perception and Performance*, *10*(5), 683–703.

Warren, W. H., & Whang, S. (1987). Visual guidance of walking through apertures: Body-scaled information for affordances. *Journal of Experimental Psychology: Human Perception and Performance*, *13*(3), 371–383.

Wilson, M. (2001). The case for sensorimotor coding in working memory. *Psychonomic Bulletin and Review*, *8*, 44–57.

Wilson, M. (2002). Six views of embodied cognition. *Psychonomic Bulletin and Review*, *9*, 625–636.

Wilson, M., & Knoblich, G. (2005). The case for motor involvement in perceiving conspecifics. *Psychological Bulletin*, *131*, 460–473.

16

On the Vices of Nominalization and the Virtues of Contextualizing

LAWRENCE W. BARSALOU
CHRISTINE D. WILSON
WENDY HASENKAMP

The chapters in this volume document the importance of context across diverse literatures, including genetics, neuroscience, perception, action, cognition, emotion, social interaction, and culture.[1] Specifically, three dominant themes emerge from this interdisciplinary collection.

- **Theme 1.** *Extensive evidence exists for context effects.* Regardless of one's theoretical orientation, there can be no doubt that context effects are ubiquitous. When a phenomenon is studied carefully, it typically does not behave the same way across contexts. Regardless of whether the phenomenon is genetic, neural, cognitive, behavioral, social, or cultural, it is likely to exhibit extensive sensitivity to context, as the diverse chapters of this volume illustrate.
- **Theme 2.** *Taking context into account is more effective than ignoring it.* When a mechanism is specified independently of context, it may capture some variance of the phenomena it explains. Nevertheless, taking context into account usually explains significantly more variance. When a mechanism contributes to a phenomenon, context shapes the expression of its contribution.
- **Theme 3.** *Mechanisms as dynamic, context-sensitive processes.* As Barrett, Mesquita, and Smith (Chapter 1) document, lay individuals

and scientists alike gravitate toward decontextualized ways of thinking that simplify and objectify mechanisms. From this perspective, modular mechanisms exist that operate exactly the same way across contexts, using additional processes to adapt a mechanism's behavior to each context in which it operates (e.g., Fodor, 1983). A classic example is Chomsky's (1965) decontextualized rules of syntax that remain constant across contexts, while performance rules map them to specific utterances. Fodor's (1975) decontextualized representations of concepts operate similarly. Barrett and colleagues provide many additional examples of decontextualized mechanisms in science.

Some mechanisms may indeed operate across contexts in a relatively invariant manner. For example, DNA remains constant across different contexts whereas RNA expresses it dynamically (Harper, Chapter 2), and occasionally, a classically conditioned stimulus–response relation does not change across contexts (e.g., Bouton, Chapter 12). Nevertheless, the form of many mechanisms depends inherently on context. Following Barrett and colleagues' *context principle*, such mechanisms emerge from context, with context contributing to the expression of the mechanism on each occasion (see also Bechtel, 2007; Bechtel & Richardson, 1993). Rather than being constant in each context, the mechanism itself changes, reflecting contextual contributions to its emergent form. Many authors in the current volume construe their mechanisms of interest this way, namely, as dynamic context-sensitive processes, not as objectified context-free mechanisms.

Ultimately, distinguishing between these two possibilities must be addressed for any mechanism. Given the strong epigenetic character of virtually everything at systems-level neuroscience and higher in complex organisms, it seems likely that many of the relevant mechanisms will turn out to be inherently context-sensitive. Furthermore, the exquisite sensitivity of cognitive processes to repetition priming, statistical structure, and expertise, together with the widespread belief that context-sensitive patterns in memory underlie such phenomena, suggest that modular context-free mechanisms in the brain may be relatively unusual.

THE VICES (AND VIRTUES) OF NOMINALIZATION

If the evidence for context effects is so overwhelming, why do people continue to exhibit *Platonic blindness*, namely, the failure to see the importance of context (Dunham & Banaji, Chapter 10)? One possibility is that Platonic blindness reflects a more general and basic phenomenon associated with coercing processes into noun concepts. For example, coercing cognitive processing into the noun "cognition" causes us to view cognition as a more discrete, isolable, and context-free system than it really is.[2] Perhaps nominalizing cognitive processing in this manner, along with other intelligent processes, invites the false belief that cognition, affect, perception, and action constitute modular systems in the brain that can be studied independently of each other. Conversely, the verb "cognizing" does not seem to invite such inferences, suggesting instead that cognition is a process that varies dynamically over time as a function of contextual influences.

Origins of Process Simplification

This section speculates on the origins of nominalizing processes and the associated effects of simplifying and objectifying them. According to this proposal, an intuitive theory about nouns develops during childhood, which specifies that prototypical noun concepts exhibit the properties of countable physical objects. Once this intuitive theory is in place, it coerces nominalized processes into conceptualizations that are relatively modular and context-free.[3]

Before proceeding further, two important points must be made. First, it is often argued that nouns essentialize their referents, simplifying their representations by endowing them with inherent invisible properties that constitute their true nature (e.g., Gelman, 2003; Medin & Ortony, 1989; see also Barrett et al., Chapter 1). The account to follow extends this view, proposing that manipulable object categories motivate an intuitive theory of nouns, which, in turn, shapes thought by making things appear simpler than they really are.[4]

Second, this account focuses on Western cultures where count nouns and object categories are salient. In non-Western cultures, where verb categories and/or mass nouns are important, this account is less applicable. Indeed, much evidence suggests that verbs and contextual relations become increasingly important in these other cultures, relative to nouns and object categories (e.g., Nisbett, 2003). Notably, however, the account to follow predicts such cultural modulation: To the extent that nouns and manipulable object categories are not central in a culture, the intuitive theory that prototypical nouns exhibit the properties of physical objects should have less impact on thought.

Ease of Learning Manipulable Object Categories

Dunham and Banaji (Chapter 10) suggest that people's proclivity for decontextualizing processes originates in knowledge about manipulable object categories. Much research suggests that these categories are indeed privileged in human cognition.

Consider evidence from developmental psycholinguistics. In general, manipulable object categories associated with nouns are acquired earlier than process categories associated with verbs for actions and events. A common explanation is that the members of manipulable object categories are individuated more easily in perception than the members of process categories (e.g., Gentner & Boroditsky, 2001; Piccin & Waxman, 2007).

To see this, consider the ease of individuating an object such as a *chair* relative to the ease of discriminating a process such as *convince.* Objects typically have clear physical and perceptual boundaries such that they pop out in the visual field; objects remain relatively constant over time and across contexts (in shape, components, behavior, etc.); objects are readily manipulated and acted upon; and objects enter into relatively simple contact causality. Conversely, processes are relatively amorphous in perception, often not being clearly bounded physically or perceptually; processes typically change significantly over time and vary significantly with context; acting upon processes is often more complex than manipulating objects; and processes typically enter into complex, often intentional (psychological) causal relations. For these reasons, manipulable object categories such as *chair* are easier to individuate in perception than process categories such as *convince.*

Because manipulable object categories are easier to individuate than process categories, object categories are easier for children to learn. Identifying their instances in complex perceptual fields is easier, as is establishing their shared properties. Additionally, storing category information in memory is easier, as is retrieving and using it. Because of these advantages, manipulable object categories tend to be acquired earlier in development than process categories.

Not only do manipulable object categories have physical properties that make them easy to individuate, but they also benefit from biological predispositions that anticipate these properties. At an early age, infants expect objects to have clear boundaries, to remain relatively constant across time and context, to be easily manipulable, and to exhibit contact causality. Some theorists propose that these predispositions reflect innate determinants (e.g., Baillargeon, 2008; Spelke, 2000), whereas others propose that they reflect weaker biological determinants coupled with epigenesis (e.g., Elman et al., 1996). Regardless, the evidence for such predispositions is overwhelming. Most importantly for our purposes here, these predispositions establish strong expectations about the salient properties that make manipulable object categories easy to individuate.

Cross-cultural research further illustrates the salient nature of manipulable object categories (e.g., Malt, 1995). Across diverse cultures, including ones not exposed to Western science, highly similar categories for plants and animals develop at the generic (basic) level of taxonomies. Furthermore, these categories are generally consistent with scientific categories grounded originally in morphological structure and later in genetics. According to Malt (1995), this strong consistency across cultures reflects the salience of these categories, both physically and perceptually. Physically, the members of a genus-level category share a common morphological structure, namely, a common configuration of parts. Butterflies, for example, exhibit one shared morphology, whereas crickets and bees exhibit others. Perceptually, a powerful shape-processing system has evolved in the ventral stream of the brain that extracts shared morphological structure and establishes categories around it (e.g., Biederman, 1987; Milner & Goodale, 1996; Rosch, Mervis, Gray, Johnson, & Boyes-Braem, 1976; Ungerleider & Haxby, 1994). Because these morphological structures are well bounded, relatively constant across time and contexts, and readily manipulable, they yield highly similar categories across cultures, regardless of cultural beliefs and practices. As we saw for category learning in development, object categories are associated with properties that make them salient and easy to learn.

Nouns and an Intuitive Theory about Their Associated Concepts

Most languages (perhaps not all) distinguish grammatically among nouns, verbs, and other grammatical classes. One common way of viewing these distinctions in linguistics is that nouns represent individuals, whereas verbs and modifiers predicate processes and properties of these individuals (for recent reviews and theories, see Bisang, in press; Croft, 2007).

Notably, linguistic theories often associate the general semantic properties of nouns with the salient properties of manipulable object categories (e.g., Frawley, 1992; Langacker, 1987). Nouns are prototypically associated with referents that are well-bounded and relatively constant across time and contexts. Clearly, nouns can refer to many other kinds of referents as well, such as mass nouns that are not well bounded (e.g., "sand") and processes that change across time and contexts (e.g., a "jump" varies over time, and also across entities that jump, such as children, horses, and crickets). Nevertheless, prototypical noun concepts are generally characterized as manipulable objects. Frawley (1992), for example, characterizes nouns as exhibiting informational, temporal, and cognitive stability at the levels of discourse, ontology, and concepts.

How might manipulable object categories come to define the prototypical noun concept? From a developmental perspective, many nouns are learned early for manipulable object categories, as we just saw (e.g., Gentner & Boroditsky, 2001; Piccin & Waxman, 2007). As a result, these early categories come to dominate children's intuitive theories about what a noun is.[5] Prototypically, a noun comes to mean categories whose members have clear boundaries, remain relatively constant across time and contexts, are manipulable, and exhibit simple contact causality. Even though children ultimately learn that nouns can refer to many other kinds of things, including events and mental states, these latter categories remain relatively atypical and peripheral to the prototypical conception. When people first think of noun categories, manipulable object categories come to mind.

Much evidence supports this claim. The first exemplars learned for a category tend to be typical (Mervis & Pani, 1980), with these typical exemplars continuing to dominate the category's representation into adulthood (Rosch & Mervis, 1975). Generalizing this pattern to noun concepts, the early association of manipulable object categories with nouns results in these categories becoming prototypical conceptions of nouns more generally.

The shape bias in early conceptual development further supports this proposal (e.g., Pereira & Smith, 2009). During early noun learning, children believe that shape is the central property for defining the category associated with a noun for a manipulable object category. When learning the noun's meaning, children assume that the object's shape is common across objects associated with the word. The shape bias illustrates that an expectancy about shape comes to bias children's beliefs about manipulable object categories in general. Analogously, the proposal here is that manipulable object categories come to bias people's expectations about noun meanings more generally.

Finally, the overemphasis on manipulable object categories in the adult categorization literature further supports their central role in the conceptualization of nouns. In this literature, a common complaint is that too much research focuses on manipulable object categories because they are relatively simple, well defined, and context independent (e.g., Medin, Lynch, & Solomon, 2000). Much less research addresses more amorphous noun categories for events and abstract entities. Thus, manipulable object concepts appear unusually prototypical of nouns, not only to lay individuals but also to scientists.

All this evidence supports the proposal that manipulable object categories become central to people's intuitive theory of nouns. As a result, when someone uses a noun or nominalizes a process, the properties of manipulable object categories become active implicitly and automatically, structuring cognition.

Coercing Processes into Object Concepts via Nouns

Once this intuitive theory about nouns exists, to what mischief might it be put to use? Coercing processes into object-like concepts seems like a particularly relevant example.

Coercion is a basic linguistic phenomenon whereby a lexical concept is restructured conceptually by a syntactic structure that contains it. Consider the intransitive English verb "sneeze." An agent can sneeze (Melanie sneezes), but the act of sneezing does not take an object in the way that a transitive verb like "push" does (e.g., "Melanie pushes the pillow" vs. "Melanie sneezes the pillow"). Structurally speaking, "push" takes a syntactic and semantic object, but "sneeze" does not.

Consider, however, the sentence, "Lisa sneezed the foam off her beer." Interestingly, this sentence seems perfectly grammatical. According to construction grammar (Goldberg, 1995), this grammatical use results from embedding "sneeze" in the *caused motion construction*, a syntactic and semantic pattern that English speakers use to describe agent-caused motion. Most importantly, when an intransitive verb such as "sneeze" is inserted in the verb argument of the caused motion construction, the transitive properties of the verb argument are coerced onto the verb. Even though the verb is normally intransitive, it develops transitive properties.

Coercion is a general phenomenon that goes beyond verbs, for example, operating on nouns as well (Michaelis, 2004, 2005; see also Lupyan, 2008). Consider the sentence, "After hogging the only pillow on the bed, Emily moved over and gave her younger sister some pillow." As illustrated by the first usage of "pillow" in this sentence, "pillow" is normally a count noun, referring to a kind of well-bounded object that can be counted, such as chairs or birds. As illustrated by the second usage, however, "pillow" can be coerced into a mass noun, namely, a physical object with amorphous boundaries, such as air or sand. The evidence for coercion is that "pillow" now enters into the type of noun phrase associated with mass nouns ("*some* pillow" comparable to "*some* air"), rather than entering into the type of noun phrase associated with count nouns ("*the* pillow" comparable to "*the* chair"). Once the concept of *pillow* has been coerced into the conceptualization of a mass noun, reasoning about it changes, such that an agent can share some of it.

More generally, coercion can be viewed as a form of perspective taking, an ability that appears unique to humans (e.g., Tomasello, Kruger, & Ratner, 1993). Because of this ability, humans can radically change how they experience something of interest. A specific situation, for example, can be viewed from different spatial perspectives (e.g., a theatrical play from before vs. behind the stage). Similarly, a situation can be viewed from different conceptual perspectives (e.g., a house from the perspective of a home buyer vs. a thief), or from different emotional perspectives (e.g., the outcome of a basketball game from the perspectives of winning vs. losing). Coercion appears to reflect similar changes in perspective, as when viewing *sneezing* in intransitive versus transitive manners. Thus, the nominalization of processes may reflect a more general perspective-taking ability that has evolved in humans.

Consequences of Nominalizing Processes

Conceptual Simplification

Taken together, the preceding sections suggest that nominalizing a process should coerce its conceptualization toward a manipulable object category. Nominalizing cognitive processing as "cognition," for example, should increase the conception of cognition as a modular, stable, and simple entity. Once the intuitive theory associated with nouns is applied to the process, its conceptualization is simplified and objectified. Rather than being viewed as something that exhibits diffuse boundaries, varies across time and context, is complex to control, and enters into complex causal relationships, the process is viewed as something that exists discretely, remains relatively constant across time and context, is easy to manipulate, and enters into simple causal relationships. Platonic blindness follows, viewing the process as a context-free mechanism, analogous to a simple manipulable object.

Vices and Virtues of Platonic Blindness in Everyday Cognition

Nominalizing a process may license a variety of (mistaken) assumptions about it: (1) A simple, well-defined representation suffices to capture the process's content (analogous to object well-boundedness); (2) the process is relatively stable across time and contexts (analogous to object constancy); (3) the process is easy to manipulate and influence (analogous to manipulating an object); and (4) the process enters into relatively simple causal relationships (analogous to contact causality).

Although nominalizing a process distorts it, advantages may result as well, warranting the simplification. Indeed, nominalizing may have virtues as well as vices! Nominalized processes, for example, may be relatively easy to learn, store, and retrieve; they may be relatively easy to communicate; they may be well suited to various types of reasoning, including class inclusion, induction, and causal analysis. Because nominalized representations are relatively simple, compact, and stable, they are efficient cognitive units.

Consider thinking about oneself. Nominalizing behavior as traits may simplify the process of establishing one's self-concept and conveying it to others, especially when doing so is important, as in Western cultures (Kitayama & Imada, Chapter 9). Rather than having to list a series of trait–situation interactions, people simply summarize their identities as traits, even if doing so oversimplifies their actual personality and behavior (Mischel & Shoda, Chapter 8). Simplified trait descriptions similarly make it easier for others to remember an individual's identity, and to communicate and reason about it.

In general, nominalizing processes may streamline cognition in a variety of ways that include learning, representation, storage, communication, and inference. Indeed, these compact streamlined units of representation may be essential—or at least highly useful—for many basic cognitive functions that humans perform regularly. In many processing contexts, more complex and cumbersome representations might make efficient processing difficult, if not impossible, especially when survival and other issues of fitness are at stake. Notably, however, these benefits come at the cost of oversimplifying the associated processes.

Vices and Virtues of Platonic Blindness in Science

The contributions to this volume suggest that, in science, nouns are often associated with process simplification (e.g., Barrett et al., Chapter 1). Nouns typically capture these simplifications, as we saw for the concepts of *emotion*, *trait*, *self-concept*, *prejudice*, and *stimulus–response behavior.* No level of analysis is immune to process simplification, from *gene* and *neuron*, to *perception* and *cognition*, to *self* and *culture*. Again, when these same concepts are verbified (e.g., *emoting*, *perceiving*, *cognizing*), they acquire a more dynamic, context-sensitive feel, perhaps because an intuitive theory associated with verbs makes these properties salient.

Science is well known for valuing elegance, parsimony, and power in theoretical and empirical research. When possible, scientists like to avoid messy complexity, imprecision, and weak effects. In general, scientists prefer tractable domains that are amenable to formal analysis, in particular, domains that allow linear, compositional, and closed-form analysis. As domains become increasingly dynamical, nonlinear, and multiply determined by many weak causes interacting in complex ways, scientists become increasingly reluctant to wallow in them. Thus, it should not be surprising if a rigorous examination of scientific practice found that the act of nominalizing a process promotes increased elegance in theory and empirical assessment. Idealization in science is pervasive and clearly highly productive in many cases.

Nominalizing processes may further reflect an emphasis on understanding the internal structure of mechanisms, analogous to understanding the internal structure of objects. Often scientific interest focuses on identifying the components of a mechanism and establishing the relations between them. Of less interest is understanding the mechanism's external relations to other mechanisms in relevant contexts. As a result, the number of external relations is minimized, with those addressed supporting an elegant analysis of the mechanism's internal structure. The overall effect is a simplification of the mechanism as being relatively context-free. If the full set of external relations were considered, then the complexity of the mechanism's internal structure might increase as well, making it appear as more of a context-sensitive process than as a context-free object.

In reaction to the oversimplification of scientific problems, scientists often call for less emphasis on idealized elegance and more emphasis on natural complexity. In categorization research, for example, category learning is often studied in extremely simplified contexts, such that only a few well-controlled variables affect learning, thereby enabling powerful mathematical models to explain it. Other categorization researchers, however, argue that this oversimplified approach distorts the true nature of the process (e.g., Murphy, 2002, 2005). In a similar spirit, the contributors to this volume argue that complexity is not a nuisance factor, but it is central for understanding everything, from genes to the self. Lewontin (2000) makes a similar argument for research in genetics.

Interestingly, even context-appreciative scientists often find it necessary to simplify processes at lower levels of analysis. Mischel and Shoda (Chapter 8), for example, focus on the importance of context at the level of person–situation interactions. At the lower levels of their cognitive–affective processing system (CAPS) model, however, the units for cognition, affect, and behavior are presented in relatively context-free ways. If pressed, Mischel and Shoda would almost certainly agree that these units are context sensitive as well. Nevertheless, thinking about context sensitivity at these lower levels overcomplicates the analysis of context effects at the level of person–situation interactions. Simplification (idealization) is useful—and probably necessary—in most scientific contexts, with the caveat that dynamic, context-sensitive processes may actually constitute processes all the way down.

THE VIRTUES OF CONTEXTUALIZING

As we have just seen, both the lay public and scientists exhibit strong predispositions to view the world through the lens of simple, objectified noun concepts. Contrary to this view, extensive evidence exists that the world does not work this way. Instead, the fundamental building blocks of everything, from genetics to culture, appear to be dynamic, context-sensitive processes.

Context Effects are Universal

Examples from the Current Volume

In genetics, it has become overwhelmingly clear that context plays central roles via epigenesis, with an organism's body and environment contributing to gene regulation (Harper, Chapter 2). In the brain, a neural circuit is modulated by other circuits that contain it, rather than operating independently (Sporns, Chapter 3; also Barrett et al., Chapter 1). In social endocrinology, the body's current hormonal context modulates the perception of social stimuli (van Anders, Chapter 4).

In general, the body and the environment serve as contexts for cognition, with environmental and bodily states not only modulating cognitive processes but being essential for them (Richardson, Marsh, & Schmidt, Chapter 15; see also Sporns, Chapter 3; Smith & Collins, Chapter 7). The body and environment similarly modulate learning (Bouton, Chapter 12). In perception, processing objects and events is modulated by background knowledge and theories (Schwarz, Chapter 6), and also by various other contextual factors, including the current motivational state and the potential for action (Barrett et al., Chapter 1; Richardson et al., Chapter 15).

In personality, a person's social behavior does not result from situation-independent traits but instead from situational patterns of meaning-making, affect, and action (Mischel & Shoda, Chapter 8). Similarly, a person's self-concept reflects the cultural context (Kitayama & Imada, Chapter 9; see also Smith & Collins, Chapter 7), and emotion is not just a discrete response to a stimulus, but reflects the larger social situation, in turn regulating it (Mesquita, Chapter 5).

In social cognition, various aspects of processing people, including categorization, attribution, and attitude, are modulated by the race of the perceiver and the perceived (Dunham & Banaji, Chapter 10). Similarly, a person's prejudice toward a particular group is not rigid but is instead adapted to different individuals and groups, reflecting evolutionary pressure to interact effectively with the people present (Sinclair & Lun, Chapter 11).

In the larger social context, the perception of a person's behavior is interpreted relative to the background norms of social groups (Prentice & Trail, Chapter 13; see also Smith & Collins, Chapter 7). More generally, a person's behavior is interpreted relative to the history of behaviors, situations, and cultural practices that accumulate in social settings, what Adams, Salter, Pickett, Kurtiş, and Phillips (Chapter 14) call "social sediment." Extensive amounts of previous behavior serve as the context for interpreting current behavior. Unless past behavior is taken into account, explaining current behavior is difficult.

Calling All Context Effects

Several authors here note the significance of bringing research on context together in one volume. Doing so demonstrates the ubiquity of context effects and their importance, suggesting that dynamic context-sensitive processes constitute central mechanisms in natural organisms.

It is worth noting that the evidence for such processes goes significantly beyond these chapters. Consider some prominent examples that document how situations contextualize diverse processes.[6] In language comprehension, texts can be incomprehensible when the relevant situation is not known (e.g., Bransford & McCarrell, 1974). During conversations, situations are central to establishing common ground between speakers (e.g., Clark, 1992) and also in nonhuman communication (e.g., Smith, 1977). Widespread evidence indicates that people use situation models to represent the meanings of texts (e.g., Zwaan & Radvansky, 1998). Across levels of analysis, language comprehension is a heavily situated process (Barsalou, 1999; Sanford & Garrod, 1981). In problem solving and reasoning, it is often difficult to draw valid conclusions without the support of concrete situations (e.g., Cheng & Holyoak, 1985; Gick & Holyoak, 1980; Johnson-Laird, 1983). In developmental psychology, the Vygotskian tradition stresses the importance of situations in acquiring cognitive and social skills (e.g., Vygotsky, 1991). In linguistics, the importance of situations motivated the theory of construction grammar, where grammatical structures evolve from familiar situations (e.g., Goldberg, 1995). In philosophy, the importance of situations motivated the theory of situation semantics, where logical inference is optimized when performed in the context of specific situations (e.g., Barwise & Perry, 1983). In artificial intelligence, situating action in physical environments enhances robotic intelligence (e.g., Brooks, 1991; Kirsh, 1991).

General arguments about the central role of situations in cognition can be found in Clark (1997), Dunbar (1991), Glenberg (1997), Greeno (1998), Spivey (2007), Barsalou (2003), and Barsalou, Breazeal, and Smith (2007). Robbins and Aydede's *Handbook of Situated Cognition* (2008) documents situation effects extensively across diverse domains and provides theoretical accounts. Even at the level of galaxies, context effects exist, with a galaxy's internal operation depending on neighboring galaxies (Cho, 2009). Much other work not cited here further documents diverse context effects.

Context Sensitivity Even in Nouns

Based on the earlier analysis of nouns, one might assume that nouns for manipulable object categories are relatively context-free, referring to entities that are well bounded, stable across time and contexts, easily manipulated, and causally simple. Nevertheless, much evidence shows that nouns for manipulable object categories are highly context sensitive, just like everything else.

As we have already seen, the adult categorization literature focuses on the study of nouns for manipulable object categories. In this literature, context effects are extensive, exhibiting two general themes (Yeh & Barsalou, 2006). First, strong associations exist between manipulable objects and the situations in which they occur. On processing *chairs*, for example, relevant settings and events come immediately to mind, such as *office* and *sitting* (Wu & Barsalou, 2009). Second, the conceptual content activated for a noun varies with the situation in which it is processed. Thus, the content activated for *basketballs* depends on whether basketballs are processed in a gym (they bounce) or on a lake (they float) (Barsalou, 1982). As Yeh and Barsalou (2006) document, overwhelming evidence exists that the nouns for manipulable object concepts exhibit these two forms of context sensitivity. Even though the intuitive theory for nouns suggests that their content is context-free, it is not.

If the conceptual content for nouns is not context-free, then it seems certain that the conceptual content for word classes associated with processes is not context-free either. Much evidence supports this conclusion as well. Many authors have noted the strong dependence of verbs on context (e.g., Gentner & Boroditsky, 2001; Langacker, 1987). For example, the verb "run" depends on the entity or process that is running (e.g., toddler, sprinter, grandparent, dog, sparrow, spider, engine, meeting). As the entity or process changes, the conceptual content for "run" changes as well. Many authors have similarly noted the strong dependence of abstract concepts on context (e.g., Barsalou & Wiemer-Hastings, 2005; Wiemer-Hastings & Graesser, 1998; Wiemer-Hastings,

Krug, & Xu, 2001). The meaning of "truth," for example, depends on whether it is processed in a principle's office, a courtroom, a church, or a course on logic.

Contexts Optimize and Simplify Processing

Why do context effects exhibit such ubiquity? As we saw earlier, nouns are associated with optimizing and simplifying processes. Interestingly, so are contexts! Taking context into account both optimizes and simplifies the implementation of a process. Each benefit is addressed in turn.

Optimizing Processing

Applying a single constant form of a mechanism typically does not produce optimal performance across different contexts. To see this, imagine that a single constant concept for *chairs* existed, such as a definition or rigid prototype. Essentially, such a concept would have to be the lowest common denominator across *chairs*, capturing information true of most instances at a relatively abstract level (e.g., seat, back, legs, used for sitting). Problematically, this constant form would falsely describe some instances, such as bean bag chairs. Most significantly, even when this constant form is correct, it fails to provide much relevant information essential for successful goal-directed action. On a jet, for example, this constant form fails to provide the following relevant information: Chairs on jets have a unique shape and structure adapted for air travel; chairs on jets are reclinable, but at the risk of cramping the person behind you; chairs on jets contain controls for audio and video systems; chairs on jets have seat belts that should remain fastened. Furthermore, optimal knowledge about chairs on jets is context sensitive to time, persons, and a host of other factors. Seat belts, for example, need not be fastened once a comfortable cruising altitude is reached, although it is recommended that they remain fastened. When holding a child in one's lap, the seat belt should not be placed around the child but only around the adult. Clearly, a single stable representation of *chairs* does not support everything one needs to know about chairs on jets. Instead, context-sensitive representations retrieved at the correct points in time optimize successful interactions with these objects. The contributions to this volume document many analogous ways in which context optimizes processing.

Context-Specific Knowledge Simplifies Processing

Extensive evidence indicates that processing becomes easier with practice (e.g., Chase & Ericsson, 1981). When an organism has experience with a particular situation, the subsequent learning produces expertise that simplifies later processing and performance. Conversely, when an organism does not have such experience, more effortful processing is necessary to produce a novel response, often associated with trial and error. As practice on the task increases, accompanied by feedback, effortful responding becomes relatively unnecessary, with performance becoming increasingly automatic.

According to many theories, expertise results from storing situation-specific chunks or exemplars in long-term memory that represent how to perform a task in a specific situation (e.g., Anderson, 1983; Chase & Simon, 1973; Logan, 1988; Medin & Schaffer, 1978; Newell, 1990; Nosofsky, Palmeri, & McKinley, 1994; Palmeri, Wong, & Gauthier, 2004). Rather than having to use executive processes to figure out an appropriate response, a situation-specific pattern in memory becomes active that specifies what to do. Simple pattern matching replaces reasoning to produce expert performance, with effort decreasing and automaticity increasing.

Thus, optimal processing is often associated with simple processing. Most importantly, both optimal processing and simple processing reflect context specificity. Optimal processing results from taking context into account. Simple processing results from retrieving situation-specific patterns stored in memory from previous experience. Most processing, most of the time, probably proceeds as optimally as it does because relevant context-specific patterns reside in memory. When such patterns are absent, processing tends to become more difficult and less optimal.

Nouns in Context

As we saw earlier, nominalizing processes has virtues, producing compact cognitive units that are easy to represent and process. These compact units have further virtues as described next, playing important roles in contextual processing. Although this section focuses on nouns, the principles presented apply to all word classes, including verbs, adjectives, and adverbs. The focus on nouns reflects our general emphasis on understanding the process of nominalization and its relations to contextualization.

Roles of Nouns in Context-Sensitive Systems

A noun serves the important goal of integrating diverse situational information for its associated concept. Consider nouns for physical object categories. Even though the relevant knowledge for *cars* varies widely across situations, it may be useful to integrate all this knowledge using a single index, namely, the noun "car." Integrating all this knowledge serves multiple purposes. A common index can cue many different instances of the same category, such as various cars one has experienced. A common index can cue the diverse situations in which cars occur, such as on the highway, in the gas station, at the mechanic, in the parking lot, in an accident, in transporting purchases, and so forth. A common index can motivate searches for common information across instances and situations, should such information become important (e.g., for certain types of relatively abstract induction that attempt to generalize across situations). A mechanism that strengthens shared information and weakens unique information across situations may underlie the emergence of common decontextualized information for nouns (e.g., Watkins & Kerkar, 1985).

Nouns may serve similar functions in other domains besides physical objects. Trait and emotion nouns, for example, may serve to integrate similar types of behavior across individuals and situations, again for the purposes of later being able to retrieve it, abstract over it, generate broad inductions, and so on. Similarly, decontextualizing a mechanism in science may serve as an index that integrates diverse context-specific knowledge about the mechanism and later supports broad inductions about it (e.g., the constructs of fluency, prejudice, gait).

Modern theories of grammar suggest that nouns perform another important role. In sentences, nouns typically represent individuals, whereas verbs (with their associated constructions) typically elaborate on these individuals (e.g., Bisang, in press; Croft, 2007; Langacker, 1987). In "The car crawled along the narrow unpaved road," the nouns "car" and "road" serve as individuals elaborated by the remainder of the sentence. Essentially this elaboration can be viewed as contextualizing the individuals, especially the subject noun ("car"). The car of interest is driving (not being fueled) along a road that is unpaved and narrow (not a freeway). Because nouns are always being contextualized in this manner by sentences, decontextualizing the nouns (at least to some extent) may facilitate this process. If a noun's meaning can be represented as a compact decontextualized cognitive unit, then contextualizing it in a new way is easier. If a noun were always retrieved with detailed context, then retrieved context could interfere with elaborating it the new context. Thus, decontextualization serves contextualization across situations.[7]

Such decontextualization may similarly serve contextualization in other domains, such as traits, emotions, and scientific mechanisms. Again, decontextualizing a construct may make it easier to process in new contexts.

In summary, decontextualized nouns play central roles in context-sensitive systems. Problems arise, however, when we reify decontextualized noun concepts as stable independent entities and forget that they belong to contextual systems in which they constantly develop emergent forms.

Context-Sensitive Processing of Noun Concepts

Under normal circumstances, noun concepts typically appear in contexts, not in isolation. In language processing, noun concepts for manipulable objects often occur in familiar situations (e.g., a *car* on the highway, a *car* in the gas station, a *car* in a parking deck). Many theories propose that the conjunction of an object noun and a familiar situation activates entrenched knowledge about that object in the situation. A car on a highway, for example, activates knowledge about the car's engine running and a driver controlling it, whereas a car in a gas station activates knowledge about the engine being off, with the driver outside pumping fuel. Even though one might be tempted to believe that a decontextualized representation of *car* exists, the moment that the *car* concept is placed in context, a relevant situated representation is retrieved and an emergent form of *car* is constructed. Much evidence supports this claim (for reviews, see Barsalou, 2003, 2008; Barsalou et al., 1993; Yeh & Barsalou, 2006).

Mechanisms in other domains operate similarly. Although the cognitive system may be capable of constructing decontextualized representations of traits and emotions, once these representations are processed in familiar contexts, they become contextualized and emergent forms appear (Mischel & Shoda, Chapter 8; Mesquita, Chapter 5). Similarly, scientists may be able to articulate decontextualized mechanisms in nature, but placing them in context illustrates their context-sensitivity (e.g., genes: Harper, Chapter 2; neural circuits: Sporns, Chapter 3; fluency: Schwarz, Chapter 6; stimulus–response relations: Bouton, Chapter 12; gait: Richardson et al., Chapter 15).

In summary, it is possible to conceptualize nouns in decontextualized ways, and these decontextualizations play important roles. We err, however, when we mistakenly believe that these decontextualized mechanisms refer to meaningful entities in isolation, and forget that they operate intrinsically in contexts and depend on contexts for their realization. The mechanism indexed by a noun integrates a large system of situated patterns, with this system usually producing an emergent form well-suited to the current situation.

LEARNING TO CONTEXTUALIZE

Is it possible to alter human cognition so that it is less inclined to coerce processes into objectified noun concepts when doing so is counterproductive? Is it possible to more readily appreciate the contextual nature of things? The final section explores these issues.

Developing Awareness of Contextual Impact

Dunham and Banaji (Chapter 10) suggest that developing awareness of contextual influences can decrease people's tendency to simplify dynamic, context-sensitive processes. As a domain is studied increasingly, it may often become clear that its central mechanisms are not as simple and context-free as believed initially. As it becomes clear that these mechanisms are context sensitive, people may come to view them as complex dynamic processes rather than as simple rigid mechanisms.

To the extent that the media, educational institutions, political systems, and occupational environments adopt these contextualized accounts, they may be transmitted broadly to lay individuals. In turn, the cognition and behavior practiced widely in the culture may change. Such change may also be transmitted individual to individual, via the relationships into which individuals enter.

It is not clear how best to make this happen. What seems most likely is that these ideas will take hold to the extent that they increase quality of life. Concrete benefits of contextualized thinking will get people's attention, change their cognition, and redirect their behavior (cf. Cohen, 2001).

Cultural Enhancement of Contextualizing

Some cultures appear to exhibit the context principle more than others. Kitayama and Imada (Chapter 9) review evidence that an interdependent orientation to self can result from individuals living in close proximity across many generations (e.g., in Asian cultures). More specific factors that result from living this way—high levels of pathogens, farming, low social mobility, and no frontiers—cause people to become interdependent. Most importantly, interdependency creates an appreciation of context. Individuals perceive themselves as an intrinsic part of a larger culture, realize that who they are reflects their culture, and see that their behavior contributes to it. Because thinking this way is important to optimal living in close proximity across generations, it makes cognition relational and context sensitive (see also Nisbett, 2003).

Under these conditions, thinking contextually produces rewards in everyday life and increases fitness. Again this may be what it takes to foster contextual thinking. Only when the conditions of living reach a point where contextual thinking is advantageous will people adopt it. Otherwise, more independent forms of thought, as in Western cultures, may offer different advantages well suited for other living conditions (e.g., living on a rapidly changing frontier with relatively few people). Even under these latter conditions, one could argue that seeing oneself as part of nature, or as part of a local ecosystem, would produce concrete rewards (Atran & Medin, 2008). Nevertheless, the data suggest that independent orientations to self are adaptive under some conditions (Kitayama & Imada, Chapter 9).

Western cultures may be rapidly approaching the point where contextual thinking is increasingly essential. As population density continues to grow, along with pressure on social, political, and environmental systems, interdependency may become increasingly fit. Cultures may increasingly enforce interdependent thinking, and people's cognitive systems may become increasingly sensitive to context (cf. Cohen, 2001).

Formal Practices for Contextualizing

Because Eastern cultures have exhibited an appreciation for interdependency and the importance of context over millennia, it is perhaps not surprising that sophisticated methods for developing these modes of thought have evolved in these cultures. Not only are these practices relevant to the lay public, they are relevant for scientific thought.

Buddhism offers a well-known example of such practices, containing various techniques across many traditions for transforming objectified cognition into contextual cognition. Although Buddhist meditation is often known for focusing attention to create calmness, these attention-based practices are primarily a tool for achieving deeper conceptual changes in cognition (e.g., Dalai Lama & Berzin, 1997; Thrangu Rinpoche, 2004).[8] Once it becomes possible to focus attention with minimal distraction, attention is focused on all mental activity, from perception to thought. As mental activity is observed, attempts to understand its nature follow. A conceptual apparatus typical of many Buddhist approaches supports this introspective examination, focusing on the objectivization versus contextualization of conscious experience. On the one hand, constructs such as *essence*, *object*, and *concept* refer to undesirable mental states that are experienced subjectively as being true, real, and of an independent objectified nature. On the other hand, constructs such as *emptiness* (*voidness*), *dependent origination*, and *impermanence* refer to the dynamic context-sensitive process of experience. From this latter perspective, all conscious experience is *empty* (*void*), namely, it is not inherently real, as it may seem to be, but is simply mental activity constructed by the mind. Even when a mental state corresponds to a perceived entity, the mental state is not the real entity, but a mental state constructed to represent it (e.g., the experience of color constructed from physical wavelength). In general, the qualia of experience are mental constructions, not to be confused with perceived counterparts that may contribute to them. Furthermore, all experience results from *dependent origination*; that is, no experience exists as an independent object, but instead emerges from a wide variety of contextual factors acting together, including the current situation, other knowledge, the brain, the environment, culture, and so forth. Finally, all experience is *impermanent*; that is, it is never a permanent object but ever changing.[9]

Of particular interest is the self. Although the self appears to exist as an independent objectified entity, this is an illusion, according to Buddhism. Instead, there is no real self, with thoughts of oneself being empty (mental constructions), dependent on numerous contextual factors, and impermanent.

During conceptual analysis of experience in Buddhist practice, various logical approaches are adopted to deconstruct the essentialist objectified nature of experience. A particular experience, such as a thought, a perception, or one's self concept, is examined with formal questions designed, first, to undermine its appearance as a real object and, second, to reveal its true nature as a temporary, interdependent, highly contextualized construction of the mind. Rather than simply focusing attention to produce calmness, attention focuses on experience, while this conceptual apparatus operates. Even when a mental state corresponds to a perceived entity, the mental state is viewed as distinctly different from the entity, being a dynamic inter-dependent construction that in itself is not real.

This approach to meditation—*Mahamudra*—is considered relatively difficult and advanced. Nevertheless, it is widely viewed as powerful and effective when performed correctly at the appropriate time in a meditation practice. It is a reliable technique for contextualizing cognition profoundly.

Mindfulness-based stress reduction (MBSR), practiced increasingly in Western cultures, can be viewed as a Westernized form of Buddhist meditation, drawing techniques from many traditions, including *Mahamudra* (Kabat-Zinn, 1994, 2005; Kabat-Zinn & Chapman-Waldrop, 1988). In MBSR, attention is distributed across experience—from the body, to thought, to the environment—as the mind produces experience from one moment to the next. Experience flows uninterrupted, unless some aspect of experience is grasped, thereby causing the practitioner to leave the moment and become engrossed in thought. As the ability to follow successive experiential states without distraction develops, these states increasingly come to be viewed as transient thoughts rather than as objectified events that appear real. The less real thoughts seem, the less self-interest and affect they produce, thereby reducing stress and negative affect. Although standard MBSR does not explicitly engage a Buddhist conceptual apparatus (e.g., *emptiness*, *dependent origination*, *impermanence*), some of the benefits nevertheless result, perhaps because the presence of such an apparatus is implicit. By viewing experience as a continual flow of temporary mental states that pass quickly rather than as real objects that exist indefinitely with continuing implications, experience acquires a sense of impermanence and dependence on the mind rather than as objectified reality in the world. Increasing research documents the benefits of this simple practice in psychotherapy, medical treatment, and education (e.g., Baer, 2003).

MBSR is becoming increasingly widespread in Western cultures, not only to treat physical and mental health problems, but also to improve the quality of life and relationships. Following Kitayama and Imada (Chapter 9), the nature of Western culture may be changing such that contextualized practices like MBSR are increasingly fit. As it becomes clear that we are all one global community, and that each individual's actions have implications for others, practices such as MBSR may produce contextual awareness that optimizes living under these conditions.

ACKNOWLEDGMENTS

Work on this chapter was supported by Grant No. DPI OD003312 from the National Institutes of Health to Lisa Feldman Barrett at Boston College, subcontract to Lawrence Barsalou at Emory University. We are grateful to the editors for the opportunity to write this chapter. We are also grateful to Brooke Dodson-Lavelle, John Dunne, Lisa Feldman Barrett, David Kemmerer, Anne Klein, Batja Mesquita, Brendan Ozawa-de Silva, and Phil Wolff for helpful suggestions.

NOTES

1. Throughout this chapter, "context" refers to the background in which something of focal interest occurs in the attentional foreground. As the chapters in this volume illustrate, such backgrounds are highly diverse, including genetic material, neural circuits, hormonal contexts, physical settings, social interactions, cultures, and so forth.
2. Quotes are used to indicate linguistic forms, and italics are used to indicate categories and their associated concepts. Thus, "cognition" is a linguistic form (a word in this case), whereas *cognition* indicates the associated category and concept.
3. Nominalization typically refers to the use of a verb or an adjective as a noun, with or without morphological transformation, so that the word can act as the head of a noun phrase. In this chapter, however, "nominalization" is generalized to include creating a noun as the name for a process.

4. For the sake of simplicity, "manipulable object categories" from this sentence on will refer to *countable* physical objects (e.g., *chairs*, *birds*). Whenever categories for mass objects are relevant (e.g., *air*, *sand*), this will be indicted explicitly.
5. An intuitive theory is a coherent system of background beliefs that helps lay individuals explain a focal entity of interest, often specifying properties and relations relevant to understanding and predicting the entity (e.g., Murphy, 2002; Murphy & Medin, 1985).
6. "Situation" is used in this section and elsewhere as the subset of contexts that typically contain agents and objects performing meaningful goal-directed events in a setting (e.g., Barsalou, 2003, 2005, 2008; Barsalou, Niedenthal, Barbey, & Ruppert, 2003).
7. This account does *not* assume that there is a single, stable decontextualized representation that exists for a noun. Instead, it is highly likely that these decontextualized representations vary dynamically across occasions as a function of numerous factors, including the frequency and recency of information associated with the noun's referents. As a result, numerous decontextualized forms of a noun occur over time.
8. Many religions, not just Buddhism, attempt to increase awareness of the extensive interdependence that exists among people and in the world. In particular, practices for fostering compassion across religions often appear to have the effect of reducing isolation and connecting individuals with their social and environmental contexts.
9. Buddhist approaches vary considerably in their assumptions about the physical world (e.g., Dunne, 2005). Some approaches are dualistic, adopting a strict distinction between mind and physical matter. Others amount to philosophical idealism, assuming that only mind exists. Still others are nondualistic, viewing the physical world as an energy field, not unlike modern physics. In all cases, it is agreed that sensory experience *at least appears* to involve an external, physical world, and that from a *conventional* perspective, an extramental world cannot be denied. Regardless of the stance taken, the focus is typically on the mental experience of reality—whatever form it takes—and on seeing that this experience is inherently empty, interdependent, and impermanent.

REFERENCES

Anderson, J. R. (1983). *The architecture of cognition.* Cambridge, MA: Harvard University Press.

Atran, S., & Medin, D. L. (2008). *The native mind and the cultural construction of nature.* Cambridge, MA: MIT Press.

Baer, R. A. (2003). Mindfulness training as a clinical intervention: A conceptual and empirical review. *Clinical Psychology: Science and Practice, 10,* 125–143.

Baillargeon, R. (2008). Innate ideas revisited: For a principle of persistence in infants' physical reasoning. *Perspectives on Psychological Science*, *3*, 2–13.

Barsalou, L. W. (1982). Context-independent and context-dependent information in concepts. *Memory and Cognition*, *10*, 82–93.

Barsalou, L. W. (1999). Language comprehension: Archival memory or preparation for situated action. *Discourse Processes*, *28*, 61–80.

Barsalou, L. W. (2003). Situated simulation in the human conceptual system. *Language and Cognitive Processes*, *18*, 513–562.

Barsalou, L. W. (2005). Continuity of the conceptual system across species. *Trends in Cognitive Sciences*, *9*, 309–311.

Barsalou, L. W. (2008). Situating concepts. In P. Robbins & M. Aydede (Eds.), *Cambridge handbook of situated cognition* (pp. 236–263). New York: Cambridge University Press.

Barsalou, L. W., Breazeal, C., & Smith, L. B. (2007). Cognition as coordinated non-cognition. *Cognitive Processing*, *8*, 79–91.

Barsalou, L. W., Niedenthal, P. M., Barbey, A., & Ruppert, J. (2003). Social embodiment. In B. Ross (Ed.), *The psychology of learning and motivation* (Vol. 43, pp. 43–92). San Diego, CA: Academic Press.

Barsalou, L. W., & Wiemer-Hastings, K. (2005). Situating abstract concepts. In D. Pecher & R. Zwaan (Eds.), *Grounding cognition: The role of perception and action in memory, language, and thought* (pp. 129–163). New York: Cambridge University Press.

Barsalou, L. W., Yeh, W., Luka, B. J., Olseth, K. L., Mix, K. S., & Wu, L. (1993). Concepts and meaning. In K. Beals, G. Cooke, D. Kathman, K. E. McCullough, S. Kita, & D. Testen (Eds.), *Chicago Linguistics Society 29: Papers from the parasession on conceptual representations* (pp. 23–61). Chicago: University of Chicago, Chicago Linguistics Society.

Barwise, J., & Perry, J. (1983). *Situations and attitudes*. Cambridge, MA: MIT Press.

Bechtel, W. (2007). *Mental mechanisms: Philosophical perspectives on cognitive neuroscience*. Mahwah, NJ: Erlbaum.

Bechtel, W., & Richardson, R. C. (1993). *Discovering complexity: Decomposition and localization as strategies in scientific research*. Princeton, NJ: Princeton University Press.

Biederman, I. (1987). Recognition-by-components: A theory of human image understanding. *Psychological Review*, *94*, 115–147.

Bisang, W. (in press). Word classes. In J. J. Song (Ed.), *The Oxford handbook of language typology*. Oxford, UK: Oxford University Press.

Bransford, J. D., & McCarrell, N. S. (1974). A sketch of a cognitive approach to comprehension: Some thoughts about understanding what it means to comprehend. In W. B. Weimer & D. S. Palermo (Eds.), *Cognition and the symbolic processes* (pp. 377–399). Hillsdale, NJ: Erlbaum.

Brooks, R. A. (1991). Intelligence without representation. *Artificial Intelligence*, *47*, 139–159.

Chase, W. G., & Ericsson, K. A. (1981). Skilled memory. In J. R. Anderson

(Ed.), *Cognitive skills and their acquisition* (pp. 141–189). Hillsdale, NJ: Erlbaum.
Chase, W. G., & Simon, H. A. (1973). The mind's eye in chess. In W. G. Chase (Ed.), *Visual information processing* (pp. 215–281). New York: Academic Press.
Cheng, P. W., & Holyoak, K. J. (1985). Pragmatic reasoning schemas. *Cognitive Psychology, 17,* 391–416.
Cho, A. (2009). The tales told by lonely galaxies. *Science, 324,* 1262–1263.
Chomsky, N. (1965). *Aspects of a theory of syntax.* Cambridge, MA: MIT Press.
Clark, A. (1997). *Being there: Putting brain, body, and world together again.* Cambridge, MA: MIT Press.
Clark, H. H. (1992). *Arenas of language use.* Chicago: University of Chicago Press.
Cohen, D. (2001). Cultural variation: Considerations and implications. *Psychological Bulletin, 127,* 451–571.
Croft, W. (2007). The origins of grammar in the verbalization of experience. *Cognitive Linguistics, 18,* 339–382.
Dalai Lama, XIV, & Berzin, A. (1997). *The Gelug/*Kagyü *tradition of Mahamudra.* Ithaca, NY: Snow Lion Publications.
Dunbar, G. (1991). *The cognitive lexicon.* Tübingen, Germany: Gunter Narr Verlag.
Dunne, J. D. (2005) "Mahāyāna philosophical schools of Buddhism." In L. Jones (Ed.), *Encyclopedia of religion* (2nd ed., pp. 1203–1213). New York: Macmillan.
Elman, J. L., Bates, E. A., Johnson, M. H., Karmiloff-Smith, A., Parisi, D., & Plunkett, K. (1996). *Rethinking innateness: A connectionist perspective on development.* Cambridge, MA: MIT Press.
Fodor, J. A. (1975). *The language of thought.* New York: T.Y. Crowell.
Fodor, J. A. (1983). *The modularity of mind: An essay on faculty psychology.* Cambridge, MA: Bradford Books, MIT Press.
Frawley, W. (1992). *Linguistic semantics.* Hillsdale, NJ: Erlbaum.
Gelman, S. A. (2003). *The essential child: Origins of essentialism in everyday thought.* Oxford, UK: Oxford University Press.
Gentner, D., & Boroditsky, L. (2001). Individuation, relativity, and early word learning. In M. Bowerman & S. Levinson (Eds.), *Language acquisition and conceptual development* (pp. 215–256). Cambridge, UK: Cambridge University Press.
Gick, M. L., & Holyoak, K. J. (1980). Analogical problem solving. *Cognitive Psychology, 12,* 306–355.
Glenberg, A. M. (1997). What memory is for. *Behavioral and Brain Sciences, 20,* 1–55.
Goldberg, A. (1995). *Constructions: A construction grammar approach to argument structure.* Chicago: University of Chicago Press.
Greeno, J. G. (1998). The situativity of knowing, learning, and research. *American Psychologist, 53,* 5–26.

Johnson-Laird, P. N. (1983). *Mental models.* Cambridge, MA: Harvard University Press.

Kabat-Zinn, J. (1994). *Wherever you go there you are.* New York: Hyperion.

Kabat-Zinn, J. (2005). *Guided mindfulness meditation.* Louisville, CO: Sounds True.

Kabat-Zinn, J., & Chapman-Waldrop, A. (1988). Compliance with an outpatient stress reduction program: Rates and predictors of program completion. *Journal of Behavioral Medicine, 11,* 333–352.

Kirsh, D. (1991). Today the earwig, tomorrow man. *Artificial Intelligence, 47,* 161–184.

Langacker, R. W. (1987). *Foundations of cognitive grammar: Vol. I. Theoretical prerequisites.* Stanford, CA: Stanford University Press.

Lewontin, R. (2000). *The triple helix.* Cambridge, MA: Harvard University Press.

Logan, G. D. (1988). Toward an instance theory of automatization. *Psychological Review, 95,* 492–527.

Lupyan, G. (2008). From chair to "chair": A representational shift account of object labeling effects on memory. *Journal of Experimental Psychology: General, 137,* 348–369.

Malt, B. C. (1995). Category coherence in cross-cultural perspective. *Cognitive Psychology, 29,* 85–148.

Medin, D. L., Lynch, E. B., & Solomon, K. O. (2000). Are there kinds of concepts? *Annual Review of Psychology, 51,* 121–147.

Medin, D. L., & Ortony A. (1989). Psychological essentialism. In S. Vosniadou & A. Ortony (Eds.), *Similarity and analogical learning* (pp. 179–195). New York: Cambridge University Press.

Medin, D. L., & Schaffer, M. (1978). A context theory of classification learning. *Psychological Review, 85,* 207–238.

Mervis, C. B., & Pani, J. R. (1980). Acquisition of basic object categories. *Cognitive Psychology, 12,* 496–522.

Michaelis, L. A. (2004). Type shifting in construction grammar: An integrated approach to aspectual coercion. *Cognitive Linguistics, 15,* 1–67.

Michaelis, L. A. (2005). Entity and event coercion in a symbolic theory of syntax. In J. O. Oestman & M. Fried (Eds.), *Construction grammar(s): Cognitive grounding and theoretical extensions. Constructional approaches to language* (Vol. 3, pp. 45–87). Amsterdam: Benjamins.

Milner, A. D., & Goodale, M. A. (1996). *The visual brain in action.* Oxford, UK: Oxford University Press.

Murphy, G. L. (2002). *The big book of concepts.* Cambridge, MA: MIT Press.

Murphy, G. L. (2005). The study of concepts inside and outside the laboratory: Medin versus Medin. In W. Ahn, R. Goldstone, B. Love, A. Markman, & P. Wolff (Eds.), *Categorization inside and outside the lab: Essays in honor of Douglas L. Medin* (pp. 179–195). Washington, DC: American Psychological Association.

Murphy, G. L., & Medin, D. L. (1985). The role of theories in conceptual coherence. *Psychological Review, 92,* 289–316.

Newell, A. (1990). *Unified theories of cognition.* Cambridge, UK: Cambridge University Press.
Nisbett, R. A. (2003). *The geography of thought: How Easterners and Westerners think differently ... and why.* New York: Free Press.
Nosofsky, R. M., Palmeri, T. J., & McKinley, S. C. (1994). Rule-plus-exception model of classification learning. *Psychological Review, 101*, 53–79.
Palmeri, T. J., Wong, A. C. N., & Gauthier, I. (2004). Computational approaches to the development of perceptual expertise. *Trends in Cognitive Science, 8*, 378–386.
Pereira, A., & Smith, L. B. (2009). Developmental changes in visual object recognition between 18 and 24 months of age. *Developmental Science, 12*, 67–80.
Piccin, T. B., & Waxman, S. R. (2007). Why nouns trump verbs in word learning: New evidence from children and adults in the Human Simulation Paradigm. *Language Learning and Development, 3*, 295–323.
Robbins, P., & Aydede, M. (Eds.). (2008). *Cambridge handbook of situated cognition.* New York: Cambridge University Press.
Rosch, E., & Mervis, C. B. (1975). Family resemblances: Studies in the internal structure of categories. *Cognitive Psychology, 7*, 573–605.
Rosch, E., Mervis, C. B., Gray, W. D., Johnson, D. M., & Boyes-Braem, P. (1976). Basic objects in natural categories. *Cognitive Psychology, 8*, 382–439.
Sanford, A. J., & Garrod, S. C. (1981). *Understanding written language: Explanations of comprehension beyond the sentence.* Chichester, UK: Wiley.
Smith, W. J. (1977). *The behavior of communicating: An ethological approach.* Cambridge, MA: Harvard University Press.
Spelke, E. S. (2000). Core knowledge. *American Psychologist, 55*, 1233–1243.
Spivey, M. (2007). *The continuity of mind.* New York: Oxford University Press.
Thrangu Rinpoche, K. (2004). *Essentials of Mahamudra: Looking directly at the mind.* Somerville, MA: Wisdom Publications.
Tomasello, M., Kruger, A., & Ratner, H. (1993). Cultural learning. *Behavioral and Brain Sciences, 16*, 495–552.
Ungerleider, L. G., & Haxby, J. V. (1994). "What" and "where" in the human brain. *Current Opinion in Neurobiology, 4*, 157–165.
Vygotsky, L. S. (1991). Genesis of the higher mental functions. In P. Light, S. Sheldon, & M. Woodhead (Eds.), *Learning to think: Child development in social context* (Vol. 2, pp. 32–41). London: Routledge.
Watkins, M. J., & Kerkar, S. P. (1985). Recall of a twice-presented item without recall of either presentation: Generic memory for events. *Journal of Memory and Language, 24*, 666–678.
Wiemer-Hastings, K., & Graesser, A. C. (1998). Contextual representation of abstract nouns: A neural network approach. In *Proceedings of the 20th Annual Conference of the Cognitive Science Society* (pp. 1036–1042). Mahwah, NJ: Erlbaum.

Wiemer-Hastings, K., Krug, J., & Xu, X. (2001). Imagery, context availability, contextual constraint, and abstractness. In *Proceedings of the 23rd Annual Conference of the Cognitive Science Society* (pp. 1134–1139). Mahwah, NJ: Erlbaum.

Wu, L. L., & Barsalou, L. W. (2009). Perceptual simulation in conceptual combination: Evidence from property generation. *Acta Psychologica, 132*, 173–189.

Yeh, W., & Barsalou, L. W. (2006). The situated nature of concepts. *American Journal of Psychology, 119*, 349–384.

Zwaan, R. A., & Radvansky, G. A. (1998). Situation models in language comprehension and memory. *Psychological Bulletin, 123*, 162–185.

Index

Page numbers followed by *f* indicate figure; *n*, note; *t*, table

D

T

V

W